T0191486

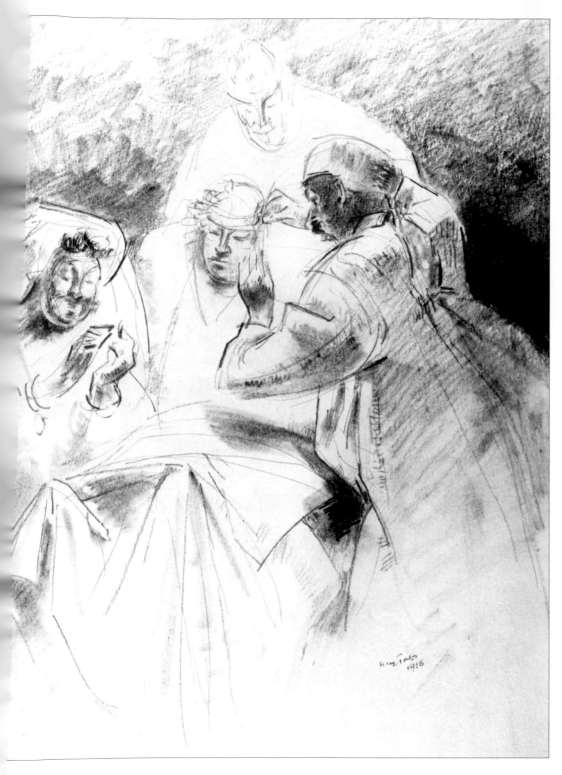

...ing by Henry Tonks of Gillies operating at the Cambridge Military Hospital, Aldershot, in 1916. (Reproduced

...of the Gillies Archives, Queen Mary's Hospital, Sidcup)

Reconstructing Faces

Dra

courte

Reconstructing Faces

THE ART AND WARTIME SURGERY *of*

Gillies, Pickerill, McIndoe & Mowlem

MURRAY C. MEIKLE

This book is dedicated to the men and women who sacrificed life and limb in two world wars to preserve our freedom, and members of the armed forces who continue to do so.

First published 2013
Reprinted 2015

Text copyright © Murray C. Meikle
Volume copyright © Otago University Press
The moral rights of the author have been asserted.

ISBN 978-1-877578-39-7

A catalogue record for this book is available from the National Library of New Zealand.

This book and DVD are copyright. Except for the purpose of fair review, no part may be stored or transmitted in any form or by any means, electronic or mechanical, including recording or storage in any information retrieval system,without permission in writing from the publishers. No reproduction may be made, whether by photocopying or by any other means, unless a licence has been obtained from the publisher.

Editor: Gillan Tewsley
Design/layout: Fiona Moffat
Printed in China through Asia Pacific Offset Ltd

Front cover: *An Advanced Dressing Station in France* by Henry Tonks. (IWM: ART 1922. Reproduced with the kind permission of the Imperial War Museum, London)

The DVD

Inside the back cover of this book is a DVD containing a series of four 16-mm cinematographic instructional films, *Techniques in Plastic Surgery*, produced in 1945 by the J Arthur Rank Organisation Ltd for the British Council, showing Mowlem performing a variety of plastic operations at Hill End. Originally made for trainee surgeons to show how various plastic operations are performed, the films are accompanied by a commentary describing in some detail the sequence of steps involved in each procedure. When the Plastic Unit moved from Mount Vernon Hospital, they were saved from the skip by Brian Morgan, and are reproduced here courtesy of the Antony Wallace Archive. See p. 172 of the book for more information on the films.

CONTENTS

Contributors

Andrew N Bamji MB, FRCP. Consultant Rheumatologist, Queen Mary's Hospital, Sidcup (Retired). Honorary Curator, Gillies Archive, Queen Mary's Hospital, Sidcup, Kent.

Robert (Bob) R Marchant. Honorary Curator, Queen Victoria Hospital Museum, East Grinstead. Honorary Secretary to the Guinea Pig Club. Former operating department assistant to Sir Archibald McIndoe.

Brian Morgan MB FRCS. Consultant Plastic Surgeon, Mount Vernon and University College Hospitals, London (Retired). Honorary Archivist, Antony Wallace Collection, British Association of Plastic, Reconstructive and Aesthetic Surgeons, Royal College of Surgeons of England.

Preface

When I retired as Professor of Orthodontics at Guy's, King's and St Thomas' Dental Institute (as it was then called) in 2003, I was fortunate enough to be offered an appointment by my *alma mater* – the University of Otago in Dunedin, where I had been a dental student 40 years earlier. At the time the local newspaper, the *Otago Daily Times*, ran a short quiz of five questions on the front page each day, and one morning (25 April 2005) the following question was included … 'Name the famous plastic surgeon born in Dunedin – and the answer they gave was Sir Archibald McIndoe.' I was moved to point out to the editor that although technically correct, *the* famous plastic surgeon born in Dunedin was actually Sir Harold Gillies, McIndoe's older cousin, who was pioneering the subject during the First World War while McIndoe was still a schoolboy at Otago Boys' High School. I was familiar with the story of Gillies at Queen Mary's Hospital, Sidcup, and McIndoe at the Queen Victoria Hospital, East Grinstead – both hospitals were on our senior registrar and registrar training rotations. I also had a number of personal points of contact because my mother-in-law, Sadie Barbara Nixon, had been taught by Henry Tonks at the Slade, and Sir William Kelsey Fry's great grand-daughter Victoria had been a patient of mine at Guy's Hospital; both Tonks and Kelsey Fry had worked closely with Gillies at Aldershot and Sidcup. Quite by chance, we also happened to be living in a house built on land which originally formed part of the McIndoe farm that had been bought for Elizabeth McIndoe by her father John Gillies, *paterfamilias* of the Gillies and McIndoe families.

It soon became clear on making further enquiries that McIndoe was the name associated with plastic surgery in the mind of most New Zealanders, as it is in the United Kingdom with the ongoing publicity surrounding the Guinea Pig Club. In an attempt to put the part played by both men into some sort of perspective, I wrote a short commentary for *The Surgeon* (the journal of the Royal Colleges of Surgeons of Edinburgh and Ireland) published in 2006, later expanded into the present volume while a visiting professor at the National University of Singapore. But Gillies and McIndoe are only half the story – less well known but also important are the contributions of two other surgeons. Henry Pickerill, foundation Dean of the Dental School who came to Dunedin from England in 1907, and Rainsford Mowlem, a contemporary of McIndoe at the University of Otago Medical School in the 1920s.

Gillies, McIndoe (two) and more recently Pickerill have all been the subject of biographies. However, the Gillies and McIndoe books were written 50 years ago shortly after their deaths, and while valuable sources of information from their immediate contemporaries covers their whole lives. The aim of the present volume is to focus instead on how the lives of these men were fashioned by a small mid-19th-century Scottish settlement at the bottom of the South Island of New Zealand, and more importantly, what they actually did to revolutionise the surgical treatment of facial injuries – in other words, what were the reconstructive problems faced by maxillofacial surgeons in the First and Second World Wars and how were they solved? Furthermore, Gillies *et al.* did not work alone. They were the most visible representatives of a vast surgical enterprise with a supporting cast of thousands that included surgeons, dentists, anaesthetists, artists and photographers, not to mention the nursing and orderly staff, many of whom went on to distinguished careers in their own right. Who were these people and what was their background? For that reason I have included short biographical notes on some of the key players; these will not be to everyone's taste except for those who enjoy reading obituaries, but some interesting patterns emerge. For example, most of the surgical staff of the British Section at Sidcup in 1917–18 had specialized in ENT surgery before the war. They were drawn almost exclusively from the English Public School system, followed by either (1) the Natural Sciences Tripos at Cambridge and clinical training at a London teaching hospital, or (2) the full medical course at one of the London medical schools. The dental surgeons on the staff at Sidcup had a similar public school background and more than half had studied both medicine and dentistry, again at a London medical and/or dental school. For the dental surgeons, time spent at a maxillofacial unit turned out to be a good career move, particularly during the Second World War: five future Deans of the Dental Faculty of the Royal College of Surgeons of England worked with Gillies, McIndoe or Mowlem.

In many ways, I was sorry to come to the end this project because numerous people made it such an enjoyable and satisfying project. First, on behalf of all those who have benefited from their generosity and time, I should like to pay tribute to Andrew Bamji, Bob Marchant and Brian Morgan for their untiring commitment over many years to preserving the priceless clinical and historical records of Sidcup, Rooksdown House, East Grinstead and Hill End Hospitals, and above all, making them available to myself and numerous other individuals. This volume and many other books, newspaper articles and academic papers would not have been possible without their help. Second, I am indebted to Philip Kidd and Richard McIntyre of Octagon Books, 32 Moray Place, Dunedin (incidentally, judged by the freelance Irish writer Derbhile Dromey of the Irish *Independent News* in 2009 to be the seventh best second-hand bookshop in the world in a field of 10), who from the beginning patiently guided my reading through New Zealand's colonial history – and much else besides. Members of the Hocken Library of the University of Otago were also unfailingly helpful with advice, access to records and the provision of photographs from their collections.

The late David Billing of Otago Boys' High School went to considerable trouble searching the dusty OBHS archives and school magazines for photographs and information about McIndoe, as did Richard Bourne for Gillies at Wanganui Collegiate School. Many thanks go to Dorothy Mowlem for information regarding Rainsford Mowlem's family background; Paul Paton, archivist at Auckland Grammar School, who kindly provided the information about his school career; and Donald Cochrane, curator of photographs at Knox College, who came up trumps when he discovered a rare image of a youthful Rainsford Mowlem in the 1922 College photograph. John 'Jock' McIndoe of Dunedin (McIndoe's nephew) kindly provided the origins and history of the McIndoe name and the Gillies–McIndoe family tree, and several descendants of Sir Harold Gillies living in Cambridge (Joanna, daughter; Nigel Harrison, grandson) and New Zealand (Jane Waller (née Gillies), grand-daughter and Gavin Harrison, grandson) were kind enough to meet and relate their personal reminiscences. I am also grateful to Harvey Brown, author of the recent biography of

Henry Pickerill and Daryl Tong, for discussions concerning Pickerill's surgical career.

For the biographical notes and information about the NZ Section at Sidcup, I am particularly indebted to the following: Dr Brian Adams (Christchurch) for his interest and persistent research into the life of William S Seed; the University of Otago Alumni Office and the University of Pennsylvania for information about James McD Turner; Waitaki Boys' High School, Oamaru, for Angus McP Marshall's outstanding sporting and academic record; Dr Basil Hutchinson (Auckland) for his personal memoir of Marshall and a copy of the coroner's report into his suicide; Sydney 'Tommy' Rhind's daughter, Mrs Gillian Martin (Adelaide), for information regarding her father's early family life in NZ and Belgium, and who was kind enough to provide a copy and permission to reproduce photographs from her father's album of cases treated at Sidcup; the NZ Dental Association and Nelson College for information about the early career of John N Rishworth; Ross Parkes (Timaru) for the photograph of the visit of his grandfather, Colonel WH Parkes CMG (Director of Medical Services, NZEF) and other dignitaries to Sidcup, and for comments on Chapter 6; Donald Gordon, Ross Grimmett, Ralph Body, Lyndal Kilgour and Hugh Tohill, who all responded to a letter in the *Otago Daily Times* (27 March 2007) requesting information about Herbert R Cole, artist to the NZ Section, which cleared up my confusion – there were in fact two Herbert Coles, both artists and both born in England. Many thanks also to the NZ Defence Force Archives for providing copies of the military records for each of the above.

The priceless help of Sue Light and her formidable knowledge of the history of the Army Nursing Service (accessible on her website www.scarletfinders.co.uk) provided valuable information regarding the wartime career of Sir Auguste Charles Valadier, and by taking the trouble to visit the National Archives, helped solve the mystery of the name change of No 13 Stationary Hospital to No 83 (Dublin) General. In addition, she kindly provided copies of the relevant pages from Catherine Black's autobiography recalling her experiences at Aldershot, and put me in touch with Sheila Brownlee whose grandmother had worked as a British Red Cross nurse at No 13 Stationary, and supplied rare cuttings and photographs of the hospital. Derek Marrison, Curator of the Army Medical Services Museum at Aldershot, provided helpful advice and access to Valadier's Service and Career File, and Dr Ian Kelsey Fry kindly supplied excerpts from the diary of Colonel Stockwell, Commanding Officer, 1st Battalion, Royal Welch (spelt with a 'c') Fusiliers, and directed me to comments about his father, 'the little doctor', in *Memoirs of an Infantry Officer* by Siegfried Sassoon. Thanks also to: (1) The Hunterian Museum and the Photographic Unit of the Royal College of Surgeons of England for generously providing images of the Tonk's pastels and Orpen drawings; (2) The British Council for having the foresight to commission the 16 mm films of Mowlem operating at Hill End Hospital in 1945, and (3) The Imperial War Museum and National Portrait Gallery for providing images from their art and photographic collections.

Alexandra Le Maître, Queen Victoria Hospital, East Grinstead, kindly provided access to the Guinea Pig records and arranged for scanned copies of relevant case notes and clinical photographs to be made available, including those used in Chapter 8. My thanks also to Mrs Angela Lodge, Tom Gleave's daughter; the family of Geoffrey Page; the late Jack Allaway and Mrs Brian Kingcome for permission to reproduce these and other photographs; Ray Reed, fellow orthodontist from student days, and Simon Millar kindly provided photographs, documents and information about Rooksdown House and the Rooksdown Club. I am also grateful to my former colleague at Guy's and St Thomas', Mark McGurk, for his encouragement and kind comments during the preparation of the manuscript.

Dirk Bister, also of Guy's and St Thomas', once again provided translations of German texts without complaint, and Barry Cardno (Wanaka) was of considerable help in compiling Appendix III: Members of the Guinea Pig Club - a task that involved trawling through all *The Guinea Pig* magazines in an attempt to establish their first names and nationality. Together with the efforts of Sergeant Chris Turner from RAF Shawbury and Bob Marchant who added the decorations and squadrons, several names not included amongst the 642 listed on the honours board in the Canadian Wing at QVH have been uncovered; these have been included as an *ad addendum* to Appendix II. Many thanks also to my son Alastair for his computer skills in the restoration and preparation of many of the illustrations, and to my wife Harriet for her forbearance over the long gestation period of this book.

Finally, I wish to acknowledge with gratitude the work of the team at Otago University Press, who, with great patience and attention to detail, skilfully managed the manuscript and brought the project to fruition: Wendy Harrex and Rachel Scott, publishers; Fiona Moffat, production and design; Gillian Tewsley, editor; Diane Lowther, indexer; and Imogen Coxhead, editorial assistant.

MURRAY C. MEIKLE
Singapore, May 2013

Abbreviations

AB, AM	Bachelor, Master of Arts	FFARCS	Fellow of the Faculty of Anaesthetists, Royal College of Surgeons
ADC	Aide-de-Camp		
AEF	American Expeditionary Force		
AFC	Air Force Cross	FLS	Fellow of the Linnean Society
AIF	Australian Imperial Force	FRACP	Fellow of the Royal Australasian College of Physicians
ANZAC	Australia and New Zealand Army Corps		
		FRACS	Fellow of the Royal Australasian College of Surgeons
BA	Bachelor of Arts		
BAO	Bachelor of the Art of Obstetrics	FRCS	Fellow of the Royal College of Surgeons
Bart, Bt	Baronet		
BChir	Bachelor of Surgery, Cambridge	GC	George Cross
BDS	Bachelor of Dental Surgery	GMC	General Medical Council
BEF	British Expeditionary Force	GCMG	Knight Grand Cross of the Order of St Michael and St George
BRCS	British Red Cross Society		
BS	Bachelor of Surgery	GCVO	Knight Grand Cross of the Royal Victorian Order
CAMC	Canadian Army Medical Corps		
CB	Companion of the Order of the Bath	IWM	Imperial War Museum
CBE	Commander of the British Empire	KBE	Knight of the British Empire
CCS	Casualty Clearing Station	KCVO	Knight Commander of the Royal Victorian Order
ChB	Bachelor of Surgery		
CM	Master of Surgery, Edinburgh	KStJ	Knight of St John of Jerusalem
CMG	Commander of the Order of St Michael and St George	LDSRCS (LDS)	Licentiate in Dental Surgery of the Royal College of Surgeons
DA	Diploma in Anaesthetics		
DCM	Distinguished Conduct Medal	LLB	Bachelor of Laws
DFC	Distinguished Flying Cross	LCC	London County Council
DFM	Distinguished Flying Medal	LLD	Doctor of Laws
DMD	Doctor of Dental Medicine	LMSSA	Licentiate in Medicine and Surgery of the Society of Apothecaries
DD	Doctor of Divinity		
DDS	Doctor of Dental Surgery	LRCP	Licentiate of the Royal College of Physicians
DSc	Doctor of Science		
DSO	Distinguished Service Order	OBE	Order of the British Empire
ED	Efficiency Decoration	MA	Master of Arts
EMS	Emergency Medical Service	MB	Bachelor of Medicine
ENT	Ear, Nose and Throat	MBE	Member of the British Empire
FACS	Fellow of the American College of Surgeons	MC	Master of Surgery, Cambridge (changed to MChir after WWI)
FDSRCS	Fellow in Dental Surgery of the Royal College of Surgeons	MC	Military Cross
		MD	Doctor of Medicine

MDS	Master of Dental Surgery	QAIMNS	Queen Alexandra's Imperial Military Nursing Service
MHR	Member of the House of Representatives, NZ's Parliament	RA	Royal Academy
MM	Military Medal	RADC	Royal Army Dental Corps
MP	Member of Parliament	RAF	Royal Air Force
MRC	Medical Research Council	RAMC	Royal Army Medical Corps
MRCS	Member of the Royal College of Surgeons	RMO	Regimental Medical Officer
MS	Master of Surgery	RNZAF	Royal New Zealand Air Force
MSc	Master of Science	RSO	Resident Surgical Officer
NCO	Non-commissioned Officer	SLdr	Squadron Leader
NZDC	New Zealand Dental Corps	UK	United Kingdom
NZEF	New Zealand Expeditionary Force	VAD	Voluntary Aid Detachment
NZMC	New Zealand Medical Corps	VC	Victoria Cross
POW	Prisoner of War	W/C	Wing Commander
		YMCA	Young Men's Christian Organisation

CHAPTER 1

Edinburgh in the South Pacific

TWO WORLD WARS PLAYED an important role in the evolution of plastic and maxillofacial surgery during the first half of the twentieth century. At the outbreak of the Second World War there were four full-time plastic surgeons in the United Kingdom: Gillies, Kilner, McIndoe and Mowlem, known to all British and American plastic surgeons as the 'Big Four'. Three were from New Zealand; two were born in Dunedin (Harold Gillies and Archibald McIndoe) and two (McIndoe and Rainsford Mowlem) had studied medicine in Dunedin at the University of Otago. By any measure this is an impressive record for one of the more remote outposts of the British Empire.

The story of Gillies and McIndoe is familiar to many. Less well known are the contributions of Mowlem and of Henry Pickerill, foundation Dean of the University of Otago Dental School, and how the lives of these men were shaped by a small nineteenth-century Scottish settlement at the bottom of the South Island of New Zealand.[1] The following is a brief account of the origins of the settlement and how it came to have New Zealand's first university, with the only medical and dental schools in the country.

Origins of the Otago scheme

The systematic colonisation of New Zealand did not begin until the late 1830s, so there were few Scots who settled in the country as a result of the Highland Clearances. The reason many left to start a new life abroad can be traced to the Industrial Revolution, which changed Scotland from a thinly populated agricultural society into an urban industrialised one, producing a vast amount of wealth of benefit to a relatively small section of the community.[2,3] The migration of farm workers from the countryside seeking work, rapid population growth, and an influx of Irish after the potato famine all combined to depress wages to an artificially low level and impoverish the working class. Between 1801 and 1840, around 350,000 people – nearly four times the 1801 population of Glasgow – crowded into the factories that sprang up on the coalfields along the Clyde valley. The new centres of Scottish industry, Glasgow and Paisley, were subjected to a bitter cycle of unemployment, starvation, misery and disease. Against this background of Dickensian squalor, it is hardly surprising that many of the more energetic among the economically depressed took advantage of any opportunity to leave their homeland.[2]

The Otago scheme ('Otago' was the transliteration of the Ngai Tahu pronunciation of Otakou, 'the place where the red earth abounds') had its genesis in 1842 when George Rennie, the multi-talented Scottish-born Liberal MP for Ipswich, proposed to the New Zealand Company that a Scottish Presbyterian colony be founded on the Wakefield system in the South Island: 'We shall found a New Edinburgh in the Antipodes, that shall one day rival the old.'[4] The scheme had an early supporter in Captain William Cargill, memorably described as 'a man in his late fifties, who apart from his fine army record and the fact that he had brought into the world seventeen children, had done little to distinguish himself in any way'.[5] Cargill was willing to emigrate provided he could secure some occupation suitable to his position.[2] The New Zealand Company gave a cautious blessing to the scheme, but the Disruption that occurred within the Presbyterian Church the following year was to profoundly affect the character of the proposed settlement.

The central issue of the Disruption was feudal patronage. The Disruptors believed that each congregation should have the freedom to appoint the minister of their choice, rather than have one imposed on them by the state or by local gentry. Led by the Reverend Dr Thomas Chalmers (1780–1847), in 1833 the Disruptors won control of the General Assembly of the Church of Scotland, and in 1834 they asserted the right to shape the constitution by passing the *Veto Act*. This empowered congregations to reject a patron's nomination without giving reasons.[3] The effect of the Act was to polarise positions within the Church and inevitably bring it into conflict with the state. In 1843, after the 'Ten Years' Conflict', one third of the Church of Scotland's ministers were no longer willing to submit to state control and patronage. They followed Chalmers out of the established church and founded the Free Church of Scotland.

For Rennie and Cargill, the Disruption identified a body of prospective colonists. They approached the Free Church leaders, who endorsed the proposal, appointing the Reverend Thomas Burns, a nephew of the poet Robbie Burns, as spiritual leader of the planned settlement. Cargill and Burns, two dour and inflexible men, worked loyally with Rennie for a time, but a conflict of ideas was inevitable and Rennie's liberal views of a comprehensive Scottish scheme soon gave way to the exclusive Free Church settlement wanted by Burns. As a consequence, Rennie became marginalised, leaving him little

choice but to withdraw. He departed for the South Atlantic not long afterwards to become Governor of the Falkland Islands. By 1845 Cargill was the undisputed leader of the scheme – a man who drew inspiration from the *Mayflower* Pilgrims of New England, whose 'wise and holy example' would guide the Otago pioneers.[4]

Dunedin: Edinburgh of the South

As in all the colonies planned under the inspiration of that erratic genius Edward Gibbon Wakefield (1796–1862) – a man who developed his ideas on penal and social reform while an inmate of Newgate prison, having abducted a 15-year-old heiress – the main aim was to establish a community of two classes which, in its social structure, would represent a cross-section of English life:[6] investors with capital, who would purchase land to farm, start businesses and provide employment; and wage-earning labourers whose passage would be paid for or assisted out of funds arising from land sales.[7] Wakefield argued that to promote a civilised society, land should be charged at what he called 'a sufficient price' – this would ensure that few immigrants would be able to afford to buy land and, as a result, the landowning class would have labourers to work for them. (Most New Zealanders regard themselves as being members of an egalitarian society, but the seeds of a class structure based on education and wealth were sown from the very beginning of the colony.)

In 1844, 400,000 acres of land was purchased for £2400 from the Maori at Otakou by Frederick Tuckett, the New Zealand Company surveyor charged with choosing a suitable site for the proposed settlement.[7] One hundred and twenty members of the Ngai Tahu tribe were present, and the chiefs and twenty-two members of the tribe signed the agreement.[8] A block of 144,600 acres was selected and surveyed into 2400 properties; 2000 were available for purchase by immigrants and were allocated by ballot. Each property consisted of three allotments: a rural section of 50 acres, a suburban section of 10 acres, and a quarter-acre town section.[9] The 'sufficient price' was set at £2 per acre.

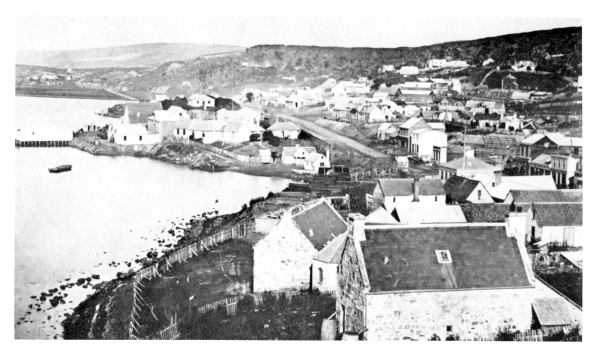

FIGURE 1.1. *The settlement of Dunedin in the 1850s looking south from Bell Hill (present site of the First Church of Otago). The bay in the foreground is where the first settlers landed from a boat off the* John Wickliffe *on 23 March 1848; the dirt track behind is present-day Princes Street. The event is commemorated by a memorial plaque inserted into the pavement at the corner of Princes and Water Streets.* (From McDonald (1965), City of Dunedin: A Century of Civic Enterprise. *Photograph by FA Coxhead, reproduced by permission of Dunedin City Council)*

Originally the name of the new town was to be New Edinburgh, but there were objections to the naming of places 'new this and new that', and besides, a New Edinburgh already existed in the bogs of Darien (the result of a failed attempt to colonise the isthmus of Panama in 1698). It was decided that the name should be Dunedin – the ancient Gaelic name of Edinburgh – suggested earlier by William Chambers.[9] There was an instruction from the New Zealand Company to Charles Kettle, who completed Tuckett's survey in 1846, that the town plan should reproduce the features of the Scottish capital as far as possible; but as any visitor to Dunedin will quickly observe, although the surrounding hills have a certain familiarity, the town plan bears little resemblance to that of Edinburgh, apart from the names of the streets – and even these do not follow a recognisable pattern.

The Free Church appealed to Scotland's aspiring middle class – people who were often of humble background, but ambitious, resourceful and energetic (confirming JM Barrie's observation about his fellow countrymen – that there was no more impressive sight than a Scotsman on the make). Those with status and wealth tended to remain loyal to the established church.[3] At first the New Zealand Company, which had been sponsoring the project through the Lay Association of the Free Church, had difficulty in attracting sufficient investors to make the project financially viable. With plenty of choice closer to home, particularly in North America, the Scots were reluctant to emigrate to such a distant and unknown land. In addition the Colonial Office, as was its custom, tried to obstruct the scheme; in its view Britain already had enough colonies. In 1846 the New Zealand Company's fortunes improved, however, when the British government agreed to underwrite its current liabilities, in addition to all expenses incurred over the next three years.[6] Cargill was appointed Company Agent at a salary of £500 per annum, and he sailed with 97 settlers from Gravesend on 22 November 1847 and Portsmouth on 14 December 1847, in the *John Wickliffe* (662 tons), reaching Otago Harbour on 23 March 1848. Three weeks later the *Philip Laing* (459 tons) arrived, having sailed from Greenock on the Clyde on 23 November 1847 and Milford Haven on 20 December 1847, with 247 passengers including the Reverend Burns.

For the first 10–12 years, the progress of Dunedin was slow, hampered to a large extent by the efforts of Cargill and Burns to maintain the exclusive Free Church character of the settlement, and by their quarrel with the Anglican minority known as the 'Little Enemy', some of whom were much-needed capitalists.[3] The rigid military and clerical upbringing of Cargill and Burns had not equipped either of them with the social skills and liberality of thought to deal with an independent-thinking colonial society. By 1860 the population had only reached 2262. The situation was changed dramatically, however, by two events. The first was the discovery of gold in May 1861 by Australian prospector Gabriel Read, in a creekbed (now called Gabriels Gully) close to the banks of the Tuapeka River near present-day Lawrence. By the end of the year 14,000 miners had arrived in Otago, many of them veterans of the California and Victorian goldfields. The second event was the intermittent warfare between the colonial government and Maori tribes from 1860 to 1870 in Taranaki and the Waikato, which deterred many prospective immigrants from settling in the North Island.

By 1863 the population of Otago Province had reached 79,000. Dunedin was the first city in New Zealand to become industrialised, and it became the major financial, business and cultural centre in the country – a position it held into the twentieth century.[7] The largest population centre today is Auckland with 1.5 million, while Dunedin remains a small university town of about 120,000, including 20,000 tertiary students.

The University of Otago

Under the contract drawn up between the New Zealand Company and the Otago Association, one of the conditions was that one-eighth of the money raised from the sale of land should be set aside for religious and educational purposes. In keeping with the Scottish tradition of higher education for all classes, the idea of creating a university was included in the original prospectus: 'the scheme embraces provision for religious ordinances, schools and *a College* [my emphasis].'[9] The Scots were justifiably proud of their national system of parish schools, set up by Reformers in the sixteenth century. The system was crowned by five universities – St Andrews (1413), Glasgow (1451), Aberdeen (1495), Edinburgh (1582) and Marischal College, Aberdeen (1593) – attended by a higher proportion of the population than in any other European country; England by this time had four. The money acquired from this one-eighth was to be paid over by the company to trustees representing the Church. The trustees appointed under the Trust Deed of 1847 were the Reverend Thomas Burns, Captain Cargill, John McGlashan and Edward Lee.[9]

In 1852 the governance of New Zealand underwent a dramatic change when the British government passed the New Zealand Constitution Act, which provided the colony with two distinct forms of government:[6]

1. A General Assembly: Composed of the Governor; a nominated Legislative Council (which fulfilled the role of an Upper House), made up of no fewer than ten members who held their seats for life; and an elected House of Representatives or parliament, which was to consist of 'not more than forty-two nor less than twenty-four' members who were elected for a term of five years.

2. Provincial Councils: New Zealand was divided into six provinces: Auckland, New Plymouth (renamed Taranaki), Wellington, Nelson, Canterbury and Otago, each with a Superintendent and a provincial council of no fewer than nine members elected by popular vote for a four-year term of office. This gave the provinces unparalleled powers of self-government and control over local affairs, until they were abolished on 31 December 1876.[2]

In the early days of the Otago settlement little money was raised from Church endowments. After seven years, barely 450 properties had been sold and only 3600 acres of land was under cultivation. Otago was suffering from the same problem as the settlements further north – insufficient men with capital to buy land; and a preponderance of labourers, for whom there was consequently little work.[10]

However, with the increase in population following the goldrush, demand for sections increased and Church income rose rapidly. The provincial government had by this time taken over provision for primary and secondary education, so in 1866 the Church proposed that a proportion of the trust funds should be used to support higher education, including the endowment of chairs in connection with a college in Dunedin. As pointed out by Thompson in his *History of the University of Otago*, the distinction in terminology between a university and a college observed in England did not apply in Scotland or in the United States.[9] As we will see later, the difference between the Scottish and English university systems was to prove a difficulty for the proposed institution in Dunedin. There was a great deal of debate about the wisdom of founding a university. Many thought it premature, including a Joint Committee of the House of Representatives and Legislative Council, who advised against the foundation of a colonial university, proposing instead the creation of eight scholarships to enable young men to study in Britain.[9] However, the wealth created by the goldrush, sheep farming (by 1861 there were 694,000 sheep in the province) and the proceeds of the educational fund, not to mention the determination of James Macandrew, Superintendent of the province, to have his way, enabled the Otago Provincial Council to ignore the recommendations of the Joint Committee. On 3 June 1869 they realised their ambition by passing the University of Otago Ordinance 'with the intent to promote sound learning in the province of Otago', thereby establishing the first university in New Zealand (and the third in Australasia, after Sydney

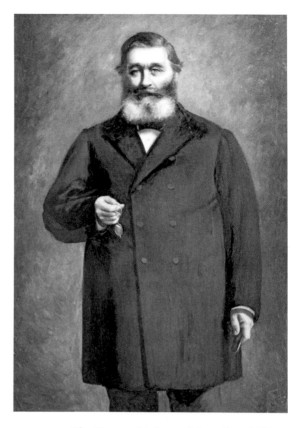

FIGURE 1.2. *The Honourable James Macandrew MHR, Superintendent of the Province of Otago (1867–76). The portrait, painted in 1885 by Eleanor Kate Sperry (1862–1893), hangs on the stairs of the Clocktower building.* (Courtesy of the Hocken Collections, Uare Taoka o Hakena, University of Otago)

and Melbourne), with an endowment of 100,000 acres of pastoral land, and with the Reverend Burns as Chancellor. The Cross of St Andrew features prominently in the university coat of arms and the motto *Sapere aude* (Dare to be wise), a popular Enlightenment quotation, was borrowed from Horace and Immanuel Kant. At the time the other provinces had neither the money nor, apart from Canterbury, the inclination to establish a university of their own.

On 30 September 1870 the University Council made its first two appointments to chairs; there were 62 candidates for each. This may seem a large number for an appointment in one of the more remote colonies of the Empire, but given the small number of universities in the United Kingdom, few academic opportunities in higher education were then available. This enabled the university to appoint men of outstanding ability. George Samuel Sale, MA (Cantab), a former Fellow of Trinity College, Cambridge, was appointed to the chair of Classics, and John Shand MA (Aberdeen), Head of Mathematics at the Edinburgh Academy, to the chair of Mathematics and Natural Philosophy. The selection of the Professor of Mental and Moral Philosophy was left to a Scottish committee, who appointed Duncan MacGregor, MA (Aberdeen), MB, CM (Edinburgh), a young man of twenty-seven and a former Ferguson Scholar in Philosophy (a scholarship open to graduates of all the Scottish universities). And with the appointment on 22 February 1871 of James Gow Black, MA, DSc (Edinburgh) as Professor of Natural Science, the staff of the University of Otago was for the time being complete. Each was on an annual salary of £600 plus class fees.[11]

The university officially opened its doors on 5 July 1871 with an enrolment of 81 students. Student numbers never fell below 50, which proved to be a much greater attendance during its early years than at either the University of Sydney (39 students in 1861, 10 years after its foundation) or Melbourne (which opened in 1864 with twenty-seven students).[9] Women were admitted from the beginning: New Zealand was the first university in the British Empire to admit women to degrees.[9] At first the university occupied a building in Princes Street that had been intended as the Post Office and later became the Stock Exchange (since demolished in the 1960s in an act of corporate vandalism), but in 1877 land was purchased beside the Water of Leith, and work on the Clocktower Building was begun the same year.

University of Otago or University of New Zealand?

The independent action of the Otago Provincial Council forced the hand of the colonial government, which had to decide on the status of the new university – was it to be a provincial or a colonial institution, with the power to award degrees? In 1870 a parliamentary committee representing each province was duly appointed. It recommended by a large majority that a University of New Zealand should immediately be established and, after amalgamation with the University of Otago, should have its seat in Dunedin.[9,11] Nevertheless, opposition to the decision of the committee came from a small but powerful group in the government, which included Henry Tancred and William Rolleston, both Englishmen from Canterbury. Tancred, the younger son of a baronet, had been educated at Rugby School under Dr Thomas Arnold, and Rolleston had attended Rossall School and Emmanuel College, Cambridge. Both men were convinced of the superiority of the English university system – to them a university was purely an examining and degree-awarding body under which were ranked affiliated teaching colleges.[9] Their opposition denied the University of Otago the right to its title.

The model they suggested was that of the federal University of London that had been established in 1836, but Oxford and Cambridge had operated such a system for hundreds of years. The charter of the University of London had been the solution of the government to the application of University College – a secular institution founded in 1825 ('that Godless institution in Gower Street', according to Dr Arnold) – for a charter of incorporation as a university. The response of the Duke of Wellington (then Prime Minister), the Archbishop of Canterbury and the Anglican Church had been King's College, founded in 1829 by Royal Charter for 'instruction in the various branches of literature and science and the doctrines and duties of Christianity'. This charter, however, conferred no power to award degrees. The charter of 1836, on the other hand, empowered the newly constituted University of London 'to grant degrees … after examination to candidates holding certificates of having completed a course of instruction at University College, King's College and such other institutions as might hereafter be

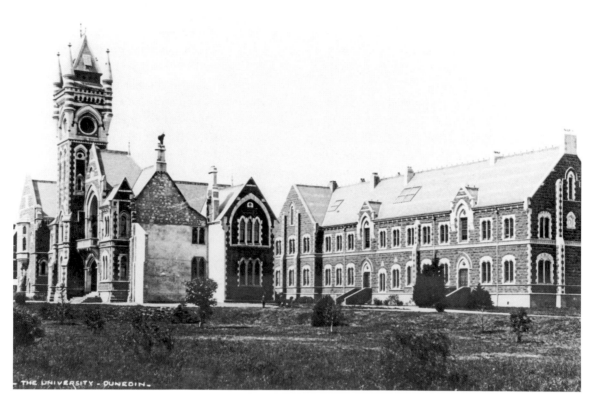

FIGURE 1.3. *University of Otago, 1879. The Clocktower complex designed in the Gothic Revival style by the engineer and architect Maxwell Bury (1825–1912). The winning entry in a design competition, it shows the influence of Sir George Gilbert Scott's design for the University of Glasgow – the clock, a gift of Sir Thomas Sidey, was not added until 1931. The building to the right was occupied by the Medical School until 1917, when it was relocated to the new Scott Building in Great King Street.* (Courtesy of the Hocken Collections, Uare Taoka o Hakena, University of Otago: accession number E4909/4)

approved for the purpose'.[9] This ordinance remains in place to the present day, although it is potentially under threat from some of the larger and more ambitious constituent colleges.

Eventually, after much acrimonious debate, protracted negotiation and two New Zealand University Acts (1870 and 1874), Otago reluctantly agreed to become an affiliated college of the University of New Zealand (which would be purely an examining body), provided it could retain its endowments and the title University of Otago. The University of New Zealand came into being in 1874, with the University of Otago and Canterbury College (1873) as its constituent colleges (and Henry Tancred as Chancellor); these two were later joined by Auckland University College (1883) and Victoria University College in Wellington (1897). Canterbury College remained true to the principles of its founders until 1933, when its name was changed to Canterbury University College. The University of New Zealand existed in name only and never occupied more than one floor in a smallish building in Wellington, until the federal system of tertiary education in New Zealand was dissolved in 1961 and the constituent colleges given full university status with degree-granting powers.

The Medical School

The University of Otago Ordinance of 1869 intended that degrees would be granted in Arts, Medicine, Law and Music, and in 1871 steps were taken to establish classes in law and medicine. The provincial council reserved 10,000 acres in Southland and 100,000 acres in the Waitaki District in North Otago for the University, and it is clear the Superintendent had in mind a medical school when he made the grant.[9,11] Given the need to obtain course recognition for licensing and examination purposes by the General Medical Council and Royal Medical Colleges in Britain, this was seen by many as a very rash undertaking.

Nevertheless, fortune favours the brave and after a number of false starts, in 1875 four students began a course of instruction under Dr Millen Coughtrey, the inaugural Professor of Anatomy and Physiology. This enabled students to take the first two preclinical years at Otago, and then complete their clinical training at Edinburgh, Glasgow or Trinity College Dublin. Within a few days, however, the class was reduced by two – one decided to transfer to law and the other left to train in Edinburgh. Furthermore, to supplement his income, Coughtrey had been seeing private patients in contravention of the terms of his contract, and was forced to resign. The Medical School was thus reduced to one room, two students and no staff. The *Otago Daily Times* recommended closure.

James Macandrew was not about to see his pet project fail, however. He persuaded the University Council to persevere and in 1877, on the recommendations of William Turner, Professor of Anatomy at Edinburgh, and John McKendrick, Professor of Physiology at Glasgow, John Halliday Scott was chosen from a field of twenty-five and appointed Professor of Anatomy and Physiology. Scott, who was twenty-six, had recently been awarded an MD and gold medal at Edinburgh. For many years the only full-time member of staff, he almost single-handedly brought the Otago Medical School into being: under his leadership it slowly began to find its feet and become firmly established. Part-time appointments to the faculty continued to be made and in 1878, the year in which the two-year course could be said to be fully operational, the Medical School moved into the bluestone buildings by the Leith. There were five students in the first class (including Macandrew's son Herbert), four of whom completed their degrees in Edinburgh.[12] The right to award the MB ChB (NZ) degrees had been approved by the Senate of the University of New Zealand in 1877; from 1883 the full medical course of four years could be completed in Dunedin. By 1900, 56 students had gone through the whole of their course in Otago, 46 of whom then went into practice in New Zealand. In addition, 90 students had taken part of their course in Dunedin and completed their training in the United Kingdom.[9]

The Dental School

During the nineteenth century the practice of medicine in the United Kingdom was under attack by reformers. It became increasingly organised and regulated by Parliament: first with the Apothecaries' Act of 1815, which required apothecaries (who had evolved into the general medical practitioners of the day) in England and Wales to have served an apprenticeship of five years and to be examined for a licence by the Society of Apothecaries;[13] and second, with the Medical Act of 1858 – 'An Act to regulate the Qualifications of Practitioners in Medicine and Surgery' – which led to the formation of the General Medical Council (GMC) and a Medical Register.

It was during this period of profound institutional change that the dental profession gradually emerged from obscurity with the introduction of the LDSRCS (Eng) in 1860, followed by the passing of the Dentists Act in 1878, the first legislation aimed to restrict dental practice to qualified dentists by creating a Dentists' Register.[13] Up until the passing of the Act, the practice of dentistry in the United Kingdom had been unregulated – practitioners ranged from surgeon-dentists and surgeon-apothecaries to numerous others, including chemists and druggists (who had taken over the pharmaceutical function of the apothecary), blacksmiths, and out-and-out quacks and charlatans who offered to extract teeth or provide patent medicines for curing toothache and other ailments. The 1878 Act enabled dentistry to transform itself from a trade into a profession with, eventually, near-equal status to medicine, and full equality in terms of income.[14]

By the end of the nineteenth century, the training of dentists by apprenticeship was being phased out in many countries and replaced by formalised training programmes – a movement that began in the United States with the foundation of the Baltimore College of Dental Surgery in 1840. The founders of the Baltimore College – all doctors of medicine – had hoped to develop dentistry in association with medicine at the University of Maryland, but their proposal was rejected by the Medical Faculty, with the result that dentistry outside Continental Europe evolved largely as a separate profession. The Baltimore College was also the birthplace of the Doctor of Dental Surgery (DDS), although the requirements for the degree were not particularly onerous. The first academic year at Baltimore College opened on 3 November 1840 with five students; instruction continued until the latter part of February, and the first class of two graduated on 9 March 1841. The status of dentistry was considerably enhanced, however, when in 1867 the first school of dentistry affiliated with a medical school was established at Harvard University. By 1884 nine other universities in the United States had followed Harvard's example and founded dental schools.[15] In contrast, it was not until the foundation of the University of Birmingham in 1900 that dentistry was elevated to university status in the United Kingdom.

An important political figure in this transformation in New Zealand was Sir Thomas Kay Sidey, the Liberal member of the House of Representatives for Caversham (1901–08) and South Dunedin (1908–28), and a member of the University of Otago Council. In 1904 Sidey introduced the Dentists' Act as a private member's bill – legislation which was to lead to the establishment of the Dental School in Dunedin. The Act established matriculation as a prerequisite for entry, followed by at least two years' study at the University of Otago. It also raised the status of the profession by bringing the training, examination and registration

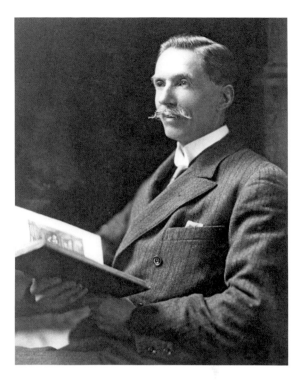

FIGURE 1.4. *Sir Thomas Kay Sidey KBE, Liberal member of the House of Representatives (1901–28) who introduced the 1904 Dentists' Act as a private member's bill. Photograph by SP Andrew Ltd, Dunedin.*

(Courtesy of the Hocken Collections, Uare Taoka o Hakena, University of Otago: accession number 84.3007)

of dentists within the control of the University of New Zealand.[9] Under the existing Dental Act of 1880, there were no entry requirements to judge the fitness of students for training – a three-year apprenticeship with a practising dentist, followed by an examination, was all that was required. Moreover, the training was not recognised outside New Zealand. In the United Kingdom, not only were courses in the theory and practice of dentistry available in institutions affiliated to universities, but in every case the course was four years in length – as was the case in the colonies of Victoria and New South Wales.

The change in the law made it necessary to establish a Dental School plus a Dental Hospital, to provide patients for instruction, without delay. In view of the location of the Medical School, and despite heavy lobbying from Auckland, the balance was tipped in favour of siting the school in Dunedin. The rapid advances taking place in the medical sciences and the expansionist mood of the university were important factors in the final decision; and Professor Scott as Dean of the Medical School was a major supporter. Dentistry benefited from being seen as a branch of medicine, and a dental school was viewed as increasing the importance of the Medical Faculty.

The estimated cost of a suitable building was £2500. The newly reconstituted New Zealand Dental Association raised £1000 towards the cost, and the government paid the balance of £1500. In 1907 the University of Otago Dental School was completed on the corner of Castle and Union Streets, to the design of J Louis Salmond (1868–1950). It opened that same year, with Dr HP Pickerill as Dean and Director of Dental Studies. The Otago Dental School was the third dental school to be founded in Australasia, after the University of Melbourne (1902) and the University of Sydney (1906).

The early years of the school were difficult. There were few students, and the regulations governing the new four-year degree of Bachelor of Dental Surgery (BDS) were framed to satisfy the demands of the General Medical Council of Great Britain (which kept the Dentists' Register), so that the qualification could be recognised abroad. In keeping with the entrance requirements of the Medical School, the matriculation examination had been replaced by a special Medical Preliminary Examination. Candidates had to be at least 16 years of age, and were required to pass in six compulsory subjects – English, Latin, Arithmetic, Algebra, Geometry, Mechanics and Hydrostatics – plus two optional subjects chosen from Greek, French, German, Logic, Moral Philosophy, Higher Mathematics, Higher Natural Philosophy, Inorganic Chemistry, Botany and Geology,[8] by modern-day academic standards a rather impressive and formidable list.

Few who passed the medical preliminary chose to study dentistry in preference to medicine with its higher status, and the first class to graduate BDS (NZ) in 1911 consisted of just three students. One was Charles Hercus, who went on to study medicine, eventually becoming Sir Charles Hercus, Dean of the Medical School. Another, William Seed, went on to play an important role in the rehabilitation of soldiers with facial injuries at the Queen's Hospital, Sidcup, during the First World War, and later in Dunedin following the Armistice (see Chapter 6).

A more serious impediment to the success of university-based training in dentistry was a concession in the law which allowed those already working as bona fide apprentices at the time of the 1904 Act to continue to do so until 1910. This was the result of considerable lobbying of local MPs as well as special pleading by those affected by the new legislation.[14] Prominent among these was a man who was about to make his name at Gallipoli and France during the First World War and become New Zealand's most famous soldier: Lieutenant-General Sir Bernard Freyberg VC, DSO and three bars. (Freyberg commanded the New Zealand 2nd Division in the Second World War and as Lord Freyberg became Governor-General of New Zealand (1946–52), and subsequently, Lieutenant-Governor of Windsor Castle.) Freyberg had been apprenticed to a Morrinsville dentist and admitted to the Dentists' Register in 1911, later practising in Hamilton and Levin. Like many of his contemporaries, he was rescued from obscurity by the outbreak of war.

The shortage of applicants to study dentistry was not resolved until bursaries for dental students were established. Once again TK Sidey came to the rescue with an offer of £100 per annum for three years – a sum that would carry a government subsidy of a like amount. This had the desired effect: by the end of 1917, bursaries had been granted to 16 applicants, all of whom resided outside Dunedin; in 1919 the number of dental students in training had risen to 33. By 1923 the school was quite inadequate for the numbers, and in 1926 a new Dental School building to accommodate 60 students was opened in Great King Street adjacent to the Medical School and Dunedin Hospital.

CHAPTER 2

Gillies and Pickerill: The first generation

Two of the important figures in the development of plastic and maxillofacial surgery during the First World War were Harold Gillies and Henry Pickerill. Gillies, a New Zealander, was head of the British Section at the Queen's Hospital at Sidcup in Kent, and Pickerill, an Englishman, was head of the New Zealand Section. Both had completely different personalities and came from very different family, educational and social backgrounds. Gillies was also much better company.

The Gillies family

Harold Delf Gillies came from a prosperous and influential Dunedin family. His grandfather, John Gillies (1802–1871), was born in the Royal Burgh of Rothesay on the Isle of Bute, the son of crofters. He was educated at the local parish school and, at the age of 17, was articled to Alexander Irvine, the local Town Clerk, Sheriff and Comptroller of Customs. In 1832 he himself was appointed Town Clerk, Clerk to the Harbour Trustees, and was admitted to practise as a Notary Public (since notaries in Scotland are solicitors, he must have sat the qualifying examinations set by the Law Society of Scotland). Ten years later he drafted the local bill to provide a police force, water supply and lighting for Rothesay, and supervised its passage through Parliament in London.[1] Active in church affairs, in 1830 Gillies was ordained an elder in the Church of Scotland, and after the Ten Years' Conflict he supported the withdrawal of his local minister from the established church. He subsequently became a prominent Free Churchman, representing his parish in Free Church assemblies after the Disruption.[1,2] At the age of 49, he decided to emigrate to the settlement of Otago for health reasons and arrived in 1852 with his wife Isabella, four sons, two daughters and a daughter-in-law on the *Slains Castle*, a ship which brought to the province a large number of emigrants and a cargo consisting almost exclusively of alcohol.[3]

John Gillies had clearly been raised in the Scots tradition of thrift. Despite having sufficient capital to purchase a town section, a 10-acre suburban section at Halfway Bush near Dunedin and a 100-acre (40 ha) farm for £1000 on the Tokomairiro Plains, about 30 miles south of Dunedin, the family travelled in steerage on the *Slains Castle*,[4] a particularly unpleasant way to spend three months at sea. As if that was not bad enough, they had to endure putrid drinking water from the River Thames, and a mutiny by 16 members of the crew who, unbeknown to the captain and the ship's officers, had been helping themselves liberally to the contents of the cargo.[3]

On arrival in Dunedin, John Gillies quickly made his mark in the colony. He was admitted as a barrister and solicitor (unlike in the United Kingdom, in New Zealand the legal profession was 'fused', allowing lawyers to practise at both), and entered into a legal partnership with John Hyde Harris, a son-in-law of William Cargill. In 1853 he was elected to the first Otago Provincial Council, and in 1857 was appointed Resident Magistrate in Dunedin, being noted for the tolerance and integrity of his judgments.[1,2] Resident magistrates seem to have been chosen for their administrative rather than their legal qualifications, so Gillies was unusually well qualified for the position. Their duties included decisions regarding the construction of roads, other public works and buildings; land purchases; and the investigation and adjustment of land claims. No local official could incur any unauthorised expenditure without the sanction of the Resident Magistrate.[5] From 1861 Gillies was also Registrar for Births, Deaths and Marriages for Otago. In a family of high-achievers, three sons – Thomas, John and Robert – all became members of the House of Representatives. From 1869 to 1873 his eldest son, Thomas Bannatyne Gillies, was also Superintendent of the Auckland Provincial Council and a Cabinet minister who held the positions of Attorney-General (1861–62), Minister of Finance (1872) and, in 1875, was appointed a Supreme Court judge.[6] Gillies Avenue in Epsom, Auckland, is named after Thomas.

Harold Delf Gillies

Harold Delf Gillies (1882–1960) was born at 44 Park Street, Dunedin, on 17 June 1882, the youngest of eight children of Robert Craig Gillies and his English wife Emily Street. For a long time it was thought that Harold had been born at Transit House (Colour plate 3); however, a time capsule dated 24 June 1882 that was discovered in the foundations adjacent to the front entrance to the house suggests he was born in an adjacent property, previously occupied by the family.[7]

Harold's father Robert had spent a year at the University of Glasgow before the family emigrated to Otago, and after working on the Tokomairiro farm for five years entered the provincial surveying service, where he remained until 1861.[8] He then moved to Dunedin, which proved to be the right place at the right time – Dunedin during the goldrush – and formed a partnership with Charles Street from Birtley near Guildford in Surrey. They speculated successfully in real estate, and Robert married Charles Street's daughter Emily, a great niece of Edward Lear, the celebrated author of *A Book of Nonsense* (1843). Robert Gillies himself became a leading figure in Dunedin's public, commercial and scientific life and was the first chairman of the *Otago Witness* and the *Otago Daily Times*. He was elected to the House of Representatives in 1884, but sat for only one session before retiring because of ill health. He died in 1886 at the age of only 51, leaving his widow and children well provided for, and the family subsequently moved to Auckland.

When Harold was eight he was sent to Lindley Lodge, a preparatory school near Rugby in England. As he wrote more than 50 years later in *The Wanganui Collegian*, 'the prefects took every opportunity to beat me up'[9] – no doubt for being from the colonies.

Gillies at Wanganui Collegiate School

Gillies returned to New Zealand for his secondary education at Wanganui Collegiate School, an institution with an interesting, if somewhat complex and irregular beginning. It had been founded in 1852 by a land grant of 250 acres from the Governor, Sir George Grey, to the Anglican Bishop of New Zealand, George Augustus Selwyn, for the purpose of establishing a school. Intended to educate the Maori and local immigrant community, it was originally called the Native and Industrial School and opened in January 1854 with one Pakeha (European) and 24 Maori pupils. The local Maori, however, proved reluctant students and within 12 months had all absconded. After struggling on for a further six years, the Native and Industrial school eventually closed.

Following a good deal of debate about what kind of school it should be, it re-opened in 1867 as the Wanganui Collegiate School, a fee-paying school for boys, including boarders.[10] (The New Zealand Education Act of 1877 provided free, secular, compulsory primary education, but did

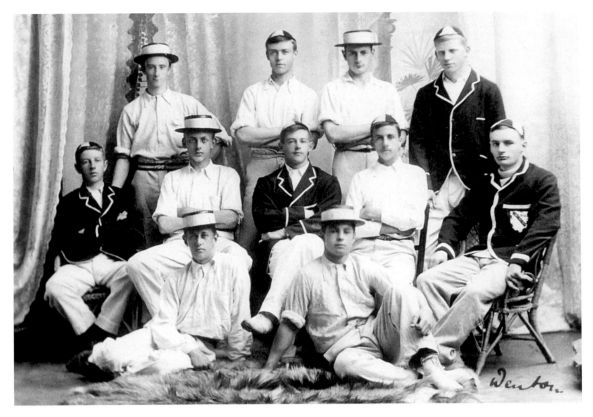

FIGURE 2.1. *Wanganui Collegiate School First Cricket XI 1899. Back Row: DB Maunsell, WT Ritchie, JFD Hewitt, RStC Stewart. Middle Row: ET Wilder, FH Moore, FS Simcox (Captain), HD Gillies, RF-R Beetham. In Front: EP Simcox, DHS Riddiford. Gillies was captain in 1900 and left at the end of the summer term; consequently, he does not appear in the photograph of the First XI taken later in the year.* (Photograph courtesy of Richard Bourne, WCS Museum Trust)

not provide for secondary education, which at the time was still fee-paying. It was not until the passing of the Secondary Schools Act of 1903 by the Seddon government that qualified pupils were eligible for free education at a secondary or district high school.) The choice of the name 'Collegiate School' implied an English grammar or 'public' school, providing a course of instruction leading to university.

One is bound to ask why Gillies was sent to a school with such an erratic history. The answer was the appointment as headmaster in 1882 of the Reverend Dr BW Harvey, the man who, in the space of five years, managed to turn the school around. Bache Wright Harvey (1834–1888) had been educated at the Royal Free Grammar School, Mansfield, and St John's College, Cambridge, where he was a wrangler – gaining a First in the Mathematical Tripos. (At the head of the list stood the Senior Wrangler, while the candidate with the lowest score in the third-class honours list received the wooden spoon – a term that has now passed into common usage.) Harvey's instructions were to transform the school into an institution run on English public school lines, and he set about the task with enthusiasm, recruiting pupils (in 1881 there were barely 40 boys on the roll; by 1886 there were 154, with 84 boarders from all parts of New Zealand), raising money and embarking on an extensive building programme.[10] After Harvey's premature death, his successor as headmaster, Walter Empson (Charterhouse and

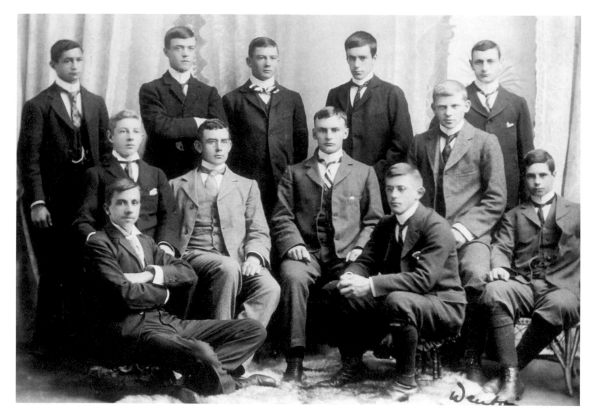

FIGURE 2.2. *Wanganui Collegiate School prefects, 1899. Back Row: J Holden, WT Ritchie (later represented Scotland at rugby while at Cambridge), IF Johnston, GH Dive, JFD Hewitt. Middle Row: ET Wilder, JEP Allen, R Beetham, RStC Stewart. In Front: HD Gillies, FS Simcox, DHS Riddiford.* (Photograph courtesy of Richard Bourne, WCS Museum Trust)

Trinity College, Oxford, where he had read law) built on this tradition. Two of Gillies' older brothers had been pupils at the school, and by the time he arrived in 1895 as a boarder, Wanganui Collegiate School was one of the most highly regarded schools in the country.

Throughout his life Gillies excelled as a sportsman. At school he was in the First Cricket XI for three years and captain in 1900, the year he played for a combined Wanganui–Taranaki XI against the touring Melbourne Cricket Club, captained by the legendary Hugh Trumble. Trumble, described by CB Fry as 'one of the greatest cricketers of all time', bowled medium paced off-spin,[11] and Gillies was justifiably proud of the 20 he scored with late cuts off Trumble that day (Trumble's bowling average in 32 tests for Australia was 19.79). According to Trumble, the best players in the combined XI were 'a broken down parson' (the Reverend JM Marshall, a teacher at the school) and a schoolboy (Gillies).[10] In the last match of the season he distinguished himself by making the first century (105) ever made for the school. His greatest delight as a golfer at the time seems to have been hitting balls over the local 5 o'clock train as it passed by – a sign, as it happens, of things to come. Accomplished academically, Gillies was awarded the Gold Medal for Science and runner-up (*proxime accessit*) in Mathematics, Latin and French during his final year. He was also a prefect, and rose to the rank of lieutenant in the Cadet Corps – the Boer War was in full swing and unlike today, military training was an important part of school life – although later photographs of

Gillies, taken during the First World War, suggest that during this period he did not acquire a military bearing. He played the violin, took part in school debates and performed in school plays, where he gained valuable acting experience – later put to good use in the impersonations and disguises he was to assume on various occasions throughout his life.[12,13]

Gillies at Cambridge

At the turn of the century the prosperous middle classes in New Zealand sent their sons to university in the United Kingdom (commonly referred to as 'Home'). In 1901 Gillies matriculated at Gonville and Caius College, Cambridge, as an exhibitioner. The college was originally founded in 1348 as

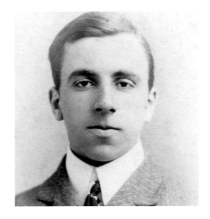

FIGURE 2.3. *Harold Delf Gillies as an undergraduate at Gonville and Caius College, Cambridge, reading Natural Sciences.* (Photograph taken in 1902 by Messrs Stearn, Cambridge. Courtesy of the Gillies Archives, Frognal Centre, Queen Mary's Hospital, Sidcup)

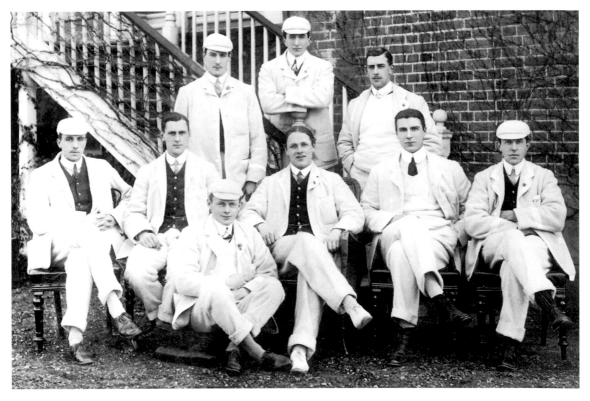

FIGURE 2.4. *Cambridge University Boat Race Crew, 1904. Back Row: RV Powell, No 5 (Eton and 3rd Trinity); SM Bruce, No 2 (Melbourne and Trinity Hall); BC Johnstone, No 3 (Eton and 3rd Trinity). Middle Row: HD Gillies, No 7 (Wanganui and Caius); H Sanger, Bow (Dunstable and Lady Margaret); PH Thomas, No 6 (Eton and 3rd Trinity); AL Lawrence, No 4 (Rugby and 1st Trinity); MV Smith, Stroke (Eton and Trinity Hall). In Front: BGA Scott, Cox (St Paul's and Trinity Hall). Coaches: FJ Escombe; CWH Taylor.* (Photograph courtesy of Cambridge University Boat Club and the Syndics of Cambridge University Library)

Gonville Hall by Edmund Gonville, and refounded in the sixteenth century by John Keys. It is usually referred to simply as Caius (pronounced 'keys'), since John Keys latinised his name after studying in Italy. While at Caius, Gillies acquired the nickname 'Giles', which remained for the rest of his life.

Gillies was the embodiment of *mens sana in corpore sano* (a healthy mind in a healthy body). He gained Second Class Honours in the Natural Sciences Tripos (BA Cantab, 1904) and, in the same year, a rowing blue at No 7 in the Cambridge boat – despite weighing in at just 10 stone 5 pounds. Oxford were beaten by four and a half lengths. He also represented Cambridge at golf for three consecutive years, gaining three half-blues, and in 1903 reached the semi-finals of the Amateur Championship at St Andrew's. In 1913 at Sandwich he won the St George's Grand Challenge Cup, one of the premier amateur prizes in the United Kingdom, and during 1925–27 was awarded six caps by the English Golf Union for matches against Scotland.[14] His party piece was to tee off by placing a golfball on the top of an empty beer bottle – something not widely appreciated by the more staid members of the golfing establishment, including the Royal and Ancient at St Andrew's. Gillies also happened to be a gifted amateur artist, enthusiastic fly fisherman, and a practical joker with a wicked sense of humour, presumably inherited from his great-uncle. He was one of those individuals who seemed to be infuriatingly good at everything.

Clinical training at St Bartholomew's Hospital

After three years at Cambridge, Gillies moved for his clinical training to St Bartholomew's Hospital at Smithfield in the City of London (otherwise known as Bart's, London's oldest surviving hospital founded by Rahere in 1123 on land granted by Henry I). By all accounts an excellent student, he did not take the Cambridge MB, BChir examinations, but chose instead to sit the conjoint MRCS (Eng), LRCP (Lond), which he passed in 1908. After holding house appointments at Bart's, including ear, nose and throat (ENT), in 1910 he won the Luther Holden Research Scholarship and passed the FRCS examination of the English College. He

then specialised in otolaryngology as assistant to Sir Milsom Rees, the reigning ENT consultant at St Bartholomew's Hospital and consultant laryngologist to the royal family and the Royal Opera House, Covent Garden. Apparently the interview, which was conducted at 18 Upper Wimpole Street, consisted largely of a discussion about golf and a demonstration of his stance for various shots, using Sir Milsom's golf clubs.[13] One wonders what Rees and Gillies would make of the current cult of managerialism, reverse discrimination and political correctness and its obsession with job descriptions, person specifications and appointment committees, which while increasing the bureaucratic process and producing identikit candidates, appears not to have measurably improved candidate selection. One thing is certain, however: Gillies retained an eccentric approach to interviews for the rest of his life, if the experience of Denis Sugrue in a letter published in the *British Medical Journal* is anything to go by. It also gives an interesting insight into Gillies' character:

> At the outbreak of the Second World War a plastic and jaw unit was established by Sir Harold Gillies at Rooksdown House, Basingstoke. In 1954 I applied for a post in plastic surgery. The subsequent interview was held at the hospital, a strange looking building which had been the private block of Park Prewett Hospital.
>
> On inquiry at the porter's office, I was directed by an elderly gentleman to wait in the main hall along with the other candidates. Being last in line for interview I was left in glorious isolation until joined by the porter who proceeded to make conversation. His opening gambit was to inquire how much fishing I had done in Ireland, to which I replied in the negative. As to other sporting activities, I admitted there were none at that particular time. There followed a few desultory questions about my surgical activities, which I thought were none of his business. Returning to the question of sport, he expressed further curiosity regarding my sporting interests in the past. Feeling slightly irritated and intimidated by the old man's persistence I announced that I

had been a member of the Irish Olympic rowing team which competed at Henley in 1948. He was most interested in this information and casually mentioned that he had rowed for Cambridge in the Boat Race. It emerged that he had also played golf for England and that painting and fishing were his main interests apart, of course, from plastic surgery.

Shortly afterwards I was called in to see the medical superintendent who, after a few perfunctory remarks, told me that Sir Harold Gillies had interviewed me in the hall and that my application was satisfactory. During the ensuing three years at Rooksdown House, Sir Harold made no reference to our unconventional interview.[15]

As assistant to Sir Milsom Rees, Gillies was paid £500 per annum, plus any private patients he could pick up for himself – a considerable improvement on his salary of about £50 as a registrar. In the period leading up to the First World War, in addition to his West End practice, Gillies also worked as a surgeon at the ENT Department of the Prince of Wales General Hospital, Tottenham, and as a pathologist at the Royal Ear Nose and Throat Hospital in Golden Square, London.

The University of Birmingham

In common with many of the universities founded in England during the nineteenth century, the University of Birmingham had its origins in the movement to provide higher education for all social classes irrespective of religion, social class, gender or race that began with the founding of University College London (UCL) in 1825. Up until the abolition of religious tests by act of Parliament in 1871, entry to and employment at the universities of Oxford, Cambridge and Durham were restricted to practising members of the Church of England. The University Tests Act abolished subscriptions to the Thirty-Nine Articles of the Church of England, all declarations and oaths respecting religious belief, and all compulsory attendance at public worship.

It was also clear that if Britain was to compete with an industrialised and increasingly self-confident Germany, there was a need for university-level training in practical subjects such as science, engineering, commerce and medicine. During the first half of the nineteenth century the ancient universities had been forced into reforming their curricula and examinations, but the administration of Oxford and Cambridge as working institutions were still in the control of the colleges and their heads – Anglican clergymen to a man.[16] After the second royal commission's enquiry into the Universities of Oxford and Cambridge in 1872, it was apparent that there were contrasting views of the role and function of the modern university: those who upheld the primacy of the colleges and the tutors; and those who thought the university should serve as a centre of scholarship and research. Despite these conflicting views, the subsequent executive commissions completed the process by which Oxford and Cambridge ceased to be clerical corporations attached to the Church of England and became modern universities.[16]

It was during this period of enormous social and political upheaval that the institutions that eventually formed the nucleus of the University of Birmingham had their origins. Although the university was formally established by a Royal Charter granted by Queen Victoria on 24 March 1900 as the successor to Mason University College, its origins can be traced back to the Birmingham Medical School founded in 1825 by William Sands Cox, a surgeon who began teaching medical students in his father's house. In 1843 the Birmingham Medical School became known as Queen's College, but after internal quarrelling, the medical and scientific departments with their staff and 250 students split from Queen's and joined nearby Mason Science College, founded in 1875 by Sir Josiah Mason, a local industrialist and philanthropist.

This greatly increased the importance of Mason Science College, and in 1898 the merged institution became known as Mason University College.[17] Birmingham was the first so-called redbrick university to receive a Royal Charter, and came into being in large part due to the ambition of the Right

Honorable Joseph Chamberlain MP (an alumnus of Mason Science College and father of Neville Chamberlain of 'Peace in Our Time'), who was Colonial Secretary, a former Mayor of Birmingham and the university's first chancellor. Appropriately for a university founded by industrialists in a city with enormous business wealth, Birmingham was the first in Britain to have a Faculty of Commerce.[17]

The city already had a tradition of dental education by the time the university was established. Birmingham Dental Hospital had been in existence since 1858, making it arguably the oldest in the country, and included a Dental School with three professorships – Dental Surgery and Pathology, Dental Anatomy and Physiology, and Dental Mechanics. These had been part of Queen's College since 1880, and had moved with the Medical Faculty to Mason Science College.[18,19] However, the only examination available to dental students in the United Kingdom at the time was the Licentiate in Dental Surgery (LDSRCS) of one of the Royal Surgical Colleges. University status enabled the university to award degrees and diplomas in dentistry, and Birmingham was the first university in the United Kingdom to introduce the degree of Bachelor of Dental Surgery (BDS).

Henry Percy Pickerill

Henry Percy Pickerill (1879–1956), known in the family as Percy, was born in Hereford, England, on 3 August 1879, the oldest child and only surviving son of Thomas Pickerill and his wife Mary Ann Gurney. His father was a commercial clerk and later managing director of the Lugwardine Tile Works of WH Godwin, a company that made ornate porcelain tiles.[20] At the time of his birth the family lived at 34 Harold Street, Hereford. When Pickerill was nine, the family moved to 1 Montrose Villas at 13 Harold Street, a substantial semi-detached house that suggests the family was comfortably off. Pickerill was educated at the Chandos School, the Collegiate School of Hereford, one of several private schools in the area, and then at Hereford County College. Pickerill then enrolled at the University of Birmingham with the intention of studying both medicine and dentistry.

Pickerill at Birmingham

Henry Pickerill entered the University of Birmingham in 1900. His initial qualifications were in dentistry: the LDSRCS (Eng) in 1903 followed by the BDS in 1904. He won several undergraduate dental prizes in the course of his training. Pickerill was the first student to receive the BDS (Birmingham) by examination, but the exam does not appear to have been popular with the student body. To be eligible for the degree, a period of 12 months had to have lapsed after passing the LDS. Of this period, at least six months must have been spent in the dental department of a general hospital approved by the university, and the candidate must have attended and passed examinations in some of the required courses for medical students.[21] Pickerill's contemporaries proved reluctant to put themselves through this additional obstacle course, and were content to enter practice with the LDS. Pickerill was the only BDS graduate at the Congregation of July 1904; the next BDS was not awarded until 1907.

During his fifth year he completed the requirements for the medical course, including medicine, surgery and ophthalmology, and graduated MB ChB in July 1905.[20] Pickerill does not appear to have been an active sportsman at university, but took part in the Queen's College Medical Society, as well as in student politics, and was elected president of the Guild of Undergraduates for the year 1904–05. This would have brought him into contact with civic dignitaries and politicians, providing valuable experience of university administration and politics, which he would later find useful.[20] After his graduation in 1905 he was appointed a clinical demonstrator at Birmingham Dental Hospital and, in 1906, lecturer in dental histology and pathology at the University of Birmingham Dental School.

In 1906 Pickerill read an advertisement for director of a new dental school at a university in New Zealand. He realised it represented exactly what he wanted – the rare opportunity of a full-time academic career. In addition to his part-time appointments as demonstrator and lecturer, he was also working in a dental practice in Hereford. He was undoubtedly well qualified – if somewhat

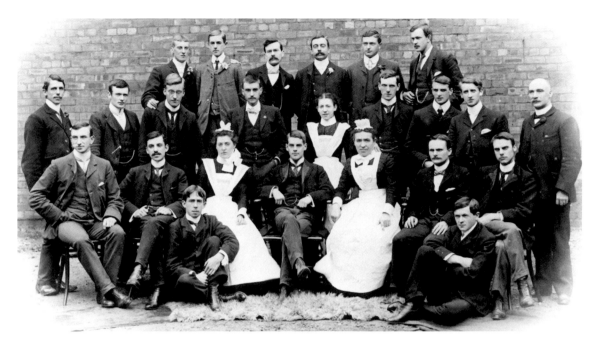

FIGURE 2.5. *Birmingham dental students, 1901. Back Row: AE Wood, FS Machin, AH Proctor, JG Harris, PN Owen, AB Oddie. Third Row: GL Andrews, T Owen, BJ Eccles, FW Broderick, Miss Foddy, HF Marshall, JR Knott (Pickerill's future brother-in-law), HP Pickerill, Mr Cope (Mechanic). Second Row: W Bowater, EV Tomey, Miss Edwards, RW Griffin, Mrs Foddy, AE Nicholls, JL Doubleday. In Front: RJJ Hawkes, RB Edwards.*

(Reproduced with permission of the Hocken Collections, Uare Taoka o Hakena, University of Otago. Pickerill Collection; Accession number: MS-3094/102)

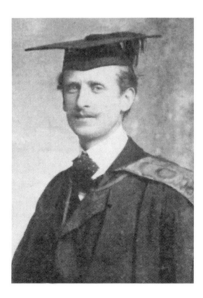

FIGURE 2.6. *Dr HP Pickerill photographed in his University of Birmingham MB ChB gown and mortar board. A graduation photograph taken in 1905.*

(Source: Otago Witness)

University of Otago,
Dunedin,
New Zealand.

SCHOOL OF DENTISTRY.

——

APPLICATIONS, with testimonials, for the position of Director of the School of Dentistry will be received by the Registrar of this University not later than 31st January, 1907.

Salary, £500 per annum.

Duties to begin 1st May, 1907.

Full particulars may be obtained from the undersigned.

W. A. MASON,
Registrar.

FIGURE 2.7. *This advertisement appeared in the October 1906 issue of the* New Zealand Dental Journal *and also in the* British Dental Journal, *where it was seen by Pickerill. It is a masterpiece of brevity and to the point, not something one normally associates with contemporary departments of human resources.*

youthful and lacking in experience – for such a position, and the fact that he had studied medicine as well as dentistry was certainly in his favour. Surprisingly, it seems he embellished his curriculum vitae, since he is usually reported as having attended the University of Oxford – even to the extent of it being repeated in his obituary notices (but not the one in the *British Medical Journal*) almost 50 years later. This solecism appears to have resulted from a memorandum included in his application in which he claims to have received his scientific training at the Universities of Oxford and Birmingham. The Oxford archives have no record of Pickerill ever having attended the university or taken the matriculation examination; the Oxford connection seems to have been confined to a few extension lectures he had attended in Hereford in 1899 before enrolling at Birmingham.[20] It would seem that the tendency of many academic institutions to accept the contents of an applicant's CV at face value is nothing new. The giveaway was the absence of any reference to his college – an omission unlikely to have been made by a member of either of the two ancient English universities – and it is surprising that nobody questioned it; perhaps they were just relieved to get an application from such an obviously well-qualified candidate.

Pickerill moves to Dunedin

Pickerill's application was successful and in February 1907 he was appointed the first Director of the University of Otago Dental School and Hospital, on a salary of £500 per annum, at the age of just twenty-eight years. As it turned out the university had found a first-rate man. Apologising for his youth at his first professorial board meeting, he was advised by Dr Shand, Professor of Natural Philosophy, that there was no need, 'since it is a matter that is only too easily remedied'.[22] Before Pickerill arrived in Dunedin the Dental Hospital, under the Acting Director, OV Davies,[23] assisted by 12 honorary dental surgeons, had opened to the public on 1 July 1907 and was besieged with patients: he therefore took over a going concern. Pickerill took up his duties in September 1907.

Three degree students joined the school at the beginning of the 1908 academic year, and another three in May of the same year.[24]

Davies was an Australian-trained dental practitioner in Dunedin who had played a leading role in the establishment not only of the New Zealand Dental Association, but of the Dental school itself. Unfortunately, Pickerill failed to acknowledge the efforts of Davies and the other members of the honorary staff in getting the school up and running – a discourtesy that was repeated the following year at the official opening ceremony which was attended by the Prime Minister, the Minister of Education and other civic and university dignitaries.[20] Pickerill appears to have been ill-equipped to cope with the less deferential professional culture of New Zealand, and during his tenure as dean was continually in dispute with members of his staff at the school, particularly Davies.

In 1916, when the University Council granted Pickerill leave of absence after he was called away for military service with the NZEF to establish a Jaw Unit in England, once again Davies had to step in as acting dean. The manner in which Davies' appointment was financed, however, was peculiar to say the least. Pickerill proposed that he would personally pay Davies £500 per annum while he was acting dean – an arrangement that was accepted by the University Council, which paid Davies an additional £250 to compensate for his practice expenses. Pickerill in effect employed Davies as a locum during his absence. This was bound to cause difficulties between two men who already had differences, and so it eventually proved.[20]

At the time Davies took over as acting dean, the major unresolved issue was the school's failure to attract sufficient students to make it financially viable: closure was a distinct possibility. With his customary foresight and energy, Davies' solution to the problem was a vigorous publicity and lobbying campaign for the establishment of bursaries to cover university fees and the cost of living in Dunedin.[23] The campaign proved so successful that the government conceded the issue, and by the time Pickerill returned in 1919 the school was thriving and the number of students had risen

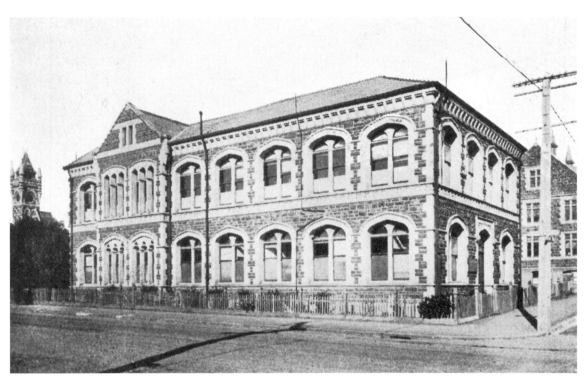

FIGURE 2.8. *The University of Otago Dental School and Hospital at the corner of Castle and Union Streets, opened in 1907. In 1926 the Dental School moved to Great King Street; the building was successively used as the Registry and Law Faculty and is currently the Staff Club.* (From GE Thompson (1919), A History of the University of Otago 1869–1919)

to 33. This does not appear to have improved relations between the two men, and in 1920 Davies left academic dentistry and returned to private practice. As we shall see in Chapter 6, Pickerill's inability to acknowledge the contributions of his closest working associates and collaborators was a recurring theme throughout his life, and a failing that almost certainly led to his eventual professional isolation.

During the period leading up to the First World War, Pickerill undertook research on a wide range of subjects, including the structure of enamel, the nature of saliva and its role in the prevention of dental caries, theories of immunity to dental caries, surgical reconstruction following trauma to the face and jaws, and the treatment of congenital deformities, particularly cleft lip and palate.[25] He wrote two books: *The Prevention of Dental Caries and Oral Sepsis*,[26] for which he received the Cartwright Prize for the quinquennial period 1906–10 from the Royal College of Surgeons of England in 1911; and *Stomatology in General Practice: A textbook of diseases of the teeth and mouth*, published in 1912.[27] He also added the Master of Dental Surgery (MDS) and Doctor of Medicine (MD), both from the University of Birmingham, to his undergraduate degrees. All this activity earned him international recognition and, at the same time, considerably enhanced the prestige of Otago, making it the leading dental school in Australasia.

CHAPTER 3

Gillies is sent to France and becomes a plastic surgeon

THE PEACE THAT EUROPE had largely enjoyed since the Franco-Prussian War of 1870–71 came to an abrupt end on 28 June 1914. On that day, Archduke Franz Ferdinand of Austria, heir to the throne of the Hapsburg Austro-Hungarian Empire, and his wife Sophie, Duchess von Hohenberg, were both assassinated in Sarajevo by Gavrilo Princip, a Serbian nationalist. Austria-Hungary issued a strongly-worded ultimatum to Serbia to punish those responsible and, dissatisfied with the response, declared war on 28 July 1914. Given the politics of the Balkans, there seems little doubt that Austria-Hungary had desired war with Serbia for some time and the assassination provided the appropriate *casus belli*.[1] What followed was a domino effect resulting from the unforeseen consequences of a series of international alliances and treaty obligations, which set in motion the events that were to inadvertently plunge most of Europe into war.

Russia, bound by treaty to protect Serbia against Austro-Hungarian aggression, announced the mobilisation of its army in Serbia's defence. Germany was allied to Austria-Hungary by the Triple Alliance (Italy, the third member joined the Entente in 1915) and, with a bellicose Kaiser intent on dominating Europe, declared war on Russia on 1 August 1914. France, bound to support Russia by the Triple Entente (Great Britain, France and Russia), again found itself at war with Germany. On 2 August 1914, German troops marched into Luxembourg and soon after crossed into Belgium – the quickest route to Paris under the Schlieffen Plan, which had been drawn up in 1905 by Field Marshall Count Alfred von Schlieffen, Chief of the Imperial General Staff, in the event that Germany might be required to fight a war on two fronts – against both France and Russia. The British government, obligated to defend Belgian neutrality under the terms of the Treaty of London (1839), voted for war two days later, on 4 August, much to the surprise of the Germans, who had not anticipated having to fight Britain as well as France and Russia. The Royal Navy was ordered to sea, and on 9 August a British Expeditionary Force (BEF) of six divisions disembarked at Boulogne, Le Havre and Rouen, and was positioned on the left flank of the French Army.

Although the German advance had been held up by the valiant Belgian Army giving the French and British sufficient time to mobilise, by the end of August a series of German victories had forced the Allies into a general retreat south of the River Marne, less than 30 miles from the outskirts of Paris. In one of the decisive battles of the war, the city was saved by a counter-attack launched by the French Fifth and Sixth Armies and the BEF, in what became known as the First Battle of the Marne

(6–10 September 1914), which ended the month-long German offensive. The seemingly invincible German Army was halted and forced to retreat 40 miles back over the Rivers Marne and Aisne to the north of Rheims, where it dug in. This was followed in late September by the 'Race to the Sea', in which the Anglo-French and German armies attempted to outflank each other. By December 1914, a continuous battlefront of trenches, fortifications and barbed-wire entanglements was established, extending from Switzerland to the North Sea (Colour plate 4). The scene was set for the killing fields of the Western Front.

A new kind of surgery

The First World War presented surgeons with a new challenge. No one, including the British Army, was quite prepared for the slaughter that occurred on an industrial scale in Northern France and Flanders from machine guns, explosive shells, high-velocity missiles, and a military strategy that treated the infantry as cannon fodder. Although it would take many days to count the dead and wounded, on the first day of the Battle of the Somme, 1 July 1916, the BEF suffered 60,000 casualties, of whom 20,000 were killed – the largest number of casualties ever suffered in a single day by the British Army.[2,3] Anyone who has counted the names on a village war memorial, or been inside an English parish church, will not find it hard to believe that 60 percent of the junior officers who led the men 'over the top' on that first day were killed. The 10th Battalion, the Prince of Wales' Own West Yorkshire Regiment, for example, lost 23 of its 24 officers and 717 of its 750 men, dead or wounded, during the attack.[3] Field guns and mortars were the main cause of battle casualties; but the stalemate of trench warfare, where the head was exposed, greatly increased the incidence of destructive injuries to the head and face: 15 percent of all soldiers who survived and were evacuated for treatment had received facial injuries, frequently with extensive loss of tissue. Despite the best efforts of surgeons, many soldiers were left hideously disfigured. A new kind of surgery was required.

Plastic surgery was not a development of the First World War. Plastic (from the Greek *plastikos*, to mould or shape) operations date back to the earliest Indian, Egyptian and Greco-Roman records, and many of the plastic operations used early in the war had been tried out during the nineteenth century.[4] Before 1914 there had been some interest in plastic surgery in France and Germany, but apart from John Staige Davis in Baltimore, no one in the English-speaking world saw the need to specialise in the subject. Plastic operations on noses, eyelids, lips and palates were carried out by general surgeons as part of their everyday practice, and the literature was limited to case reports – generally regarded as the lowest form of clinical evidence. In other words, when the war broke out, plastic surgery was in its infancy. Surgeons had little, if any experience in dealing with gunshot injuries to the face involving the widespread destruction of soft tissues, complicated by multiple compound fractures of the jaws. The large number of cases of facial trauma that began to pour into hospitals in the early months of the war enabled surgeons to gain experience in plastic operations, standardise treatment and plan operative procedures with a more predictable outcome. It also became clear that if advances were to be made in the management of facial injuries, close cooperation between surgeons and dental surgeons was essential.

The British Army's last major war with the Boer Republics in South Africa (1899–1902) had in no way prepared army surgeons for the conditions they would face on the Western Front. In addition to differences in the surroundings and soil (in South Africa the veldt was dry, uncontaminated by manure and almost free of pathogenic organisms), the injuries were less severe, with far fewer complications.[5] The rounded bullet of the Boer War period, fired at long distance and travelling at a lower speed, produced much less damage than the pointed bullets of 1914–18, where the majority of wounds were inflicted at close range by a missile travelling at the height of its velocity. Since the centre of gravity of a pointed bullet is further back, it could also tumble through the air and enter the body base first or sideways – particularly in trench

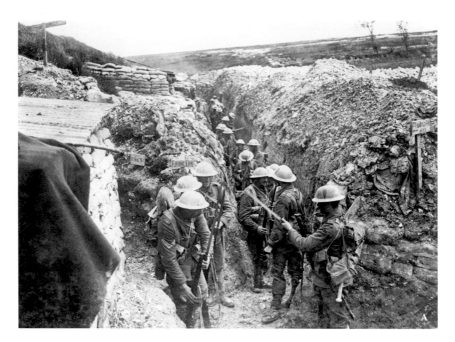

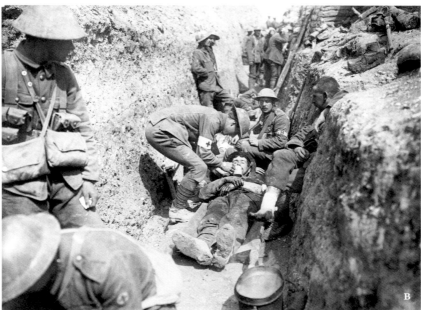

FIGURE 3.1 (A) *Opening day of the Battle of the Somme, 1 July 1916. Prior to the attack on Beaumont Hamel, soldiers of the 1st Battalion Lancashire Fusiliers are fixing bayonets. They are wearing 'fighting order', with the haversack in place of the pack. The officer in the right foreground is wearing other ranks' uniform to be less conspicuous.* (Photographer: Lt Ernest Brooks, IWM: Q 744) (B) *Wounded men of the 1st Battalion Lancashire Fusiliers being tended in a trench in the 29th Division's area near Beaumont Hamel on the morning of the initial assault.* (Photographer: Lt Ernest Brooks, IWM: Q 739)

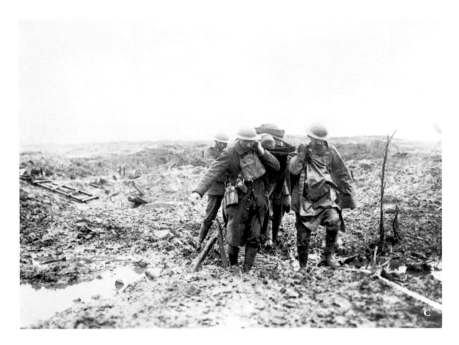

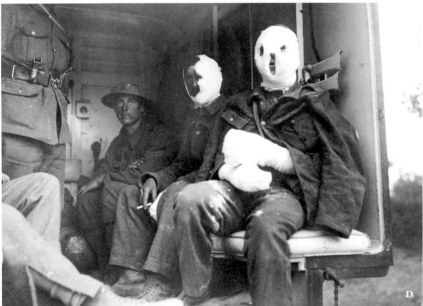

(C) *Stretcher bearers bring in a wounded man over muddy ground at Passchendaele,
6 October 1917.* (Photographer: Lt William Rider-Rider, Canadian official photographer, IWM: CO 2215) (**D**) *Two
heavily bandaged Canadian soldiers being transported in a motor ambulance from
Lieven during the battle of Passchendaele, July 1917.* (Photographer: Lt William Rider-Rider, IWM: CO
1636. By kind permission of the Imperial War Museum, London)

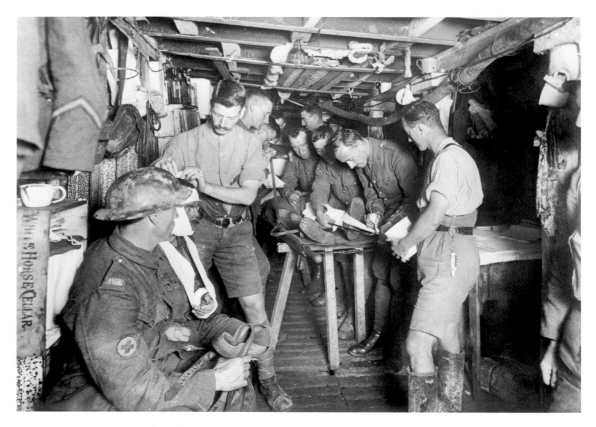

FIGURE 3.2. *Surgeons attending the wounded at an advanced dressing station near Hill 60 on the Ypres Salient, August 1917. Field ambulances or advanced dressing stations were first-aid posts near the front line and were generally very basic. Huts and barns were often taken over and used for resuscitation, emergency treatment and simple surgery.* (Photographer: Australian official photographer, IWM: E (AUS) 672)

warfare, where bullets often passed through the earth of the parapet or struck a sandbag. Dum-dum and other forms of expanding bullet had been outlawed by the Hague Convention of 1899, but terrible wounds were produced by soldiers on both sides cutting off the tips of bullets to enhance their destructive capability – particularly if one of their comrades had been killed by an expanding sniper's bullet.[6] Wounds of the utmost variety were also produced by other forms of missile, all differing in structure and in the way in which they produced injury – including shrapnel shells containing 250–400 round bullets of various sizes and hardness (invented by Henry Shrapnel (1761–

1842), an English artillery officer); high-explosive shells varying in weight from a few pounds to a ton; and bombs of various kinds.[5] When it comes to devising methods for destroying his fellow man, the ingenuity of *Homo sapiens* has no limits.

In the BEF, the wounded passed through a well-organised series of Royal Army Medical Corps (RAMC) ambulance units committed to admitting and evacuating patients as soon as possible.[7] In the early stages, preliminary treatment was restricted to lifesaving first aid at a regimental aid post (RAP) on the front line by the regimental medical officer (RMO), or at an advanced dressing station (field ambulance) in the support line; this largely

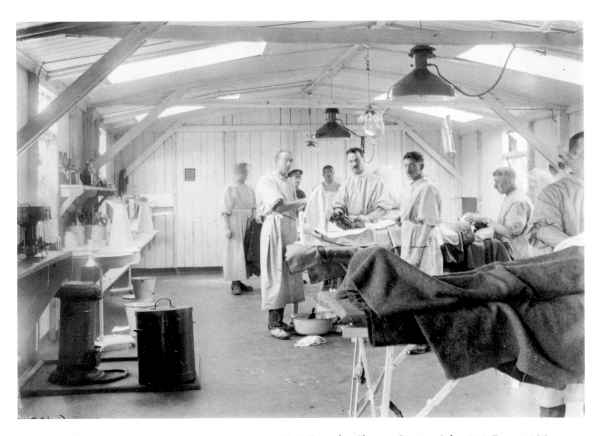

FIGURE 3.3. *Surgery in progress in an operating suite at No 3 Casualty Clearing Station, July 1916. From 16 May 1916 to 6 March 1917 No 3 CCS was at Puchvillers. CCSs (originally called clearing hospitals) were larger, better-equipped hospitals that revolutionised the surgery of war by reducing sepsis and gas gangrene by debridement – the removal of dead and injured tissue, foreign bodies and other contaminants from the wound as soon as possible, before transferring the patient to a base hospital.* (Photographer: HE Knobel; Canadian official photographer, IWM: CO 157. By kind permission of the Imperial War Museum, London)

involved the arrest of haemorrhage, an injection of anti-tetanus serum and, for wounds of the face and jaws, the prevention of suffocation. Casualties were then transported by motor ambulance to a Casualty Clearing Station (CCS) located 6–10 miles behind the front, where dead, injured or infected tissue, foreign bodies and other contaminants were removed.[8] Wounded soldiers remained at the CCS until they could be safely evacuated by ambulance train. These carried up to 400 sick or wounded at a time to a base hospital in the Boulogne area or, if they could not take any more casualties, to Le Touquet or Rouen, and sometimes to Le Havre, 200 miles away.[9]

Die gegenwärtigen Behandlungswege der Kieferschussverletzungen

The Germans were better prepared for war than the Allies. The Balkan Wars of 1912–13 had provided German surgeons with ample opportunity to gain experience in the treatment of maxillofacial injuries: by August 1914, hospitals in Berlin, Strasbourg, Hanover and Düsseldorf were ready to receive face and jaw injuries.[10] In his autobiographical work *The Principles and Art of Plastic Surgery* (1957),[11] Gillies relates how he was inspired to take up facial surgery by a few pictures in a book by the German surgeon Lindemann, a gift from an American dental colleague by the name of Dr CW 'Bobs' Roberts.

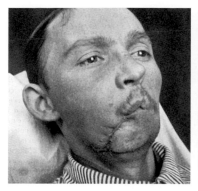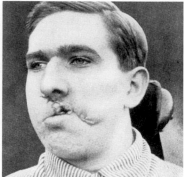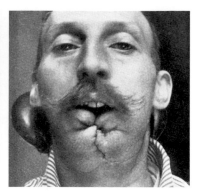

FIGURE 3.4. *Following his arrival in France in 1915 as an ENT surgeon, Gillies was inspired to take up maxillofacial surgery by a few pictures in a book by the German surgeon August Lindemann. This was* Heft I of Die gegenwärtigen Behandlungswege der Kieferschussverletzungen *edited by Christian Bruhn, a small soft-covered volume of 62 pages published in 1915 – Lindemann's contribution consisted of just 16 pages. These three cases were included in the article to illustrate the unsightly deformities produced at field hospitals by bandaging facial injuries without splinting the teeth, or suturing wounds without taking into account injuries to the underlying bone of the jaws.*

At the time Roberts was treating maxillofacial injuries in the Dental Section of the Ambulance Américaine, housed in the Lycée Pasteur at Neuilly-sur-Seine and suggested to Gillies he might like to take up this type of work.

Given that Gillies arrived in France in 1915, the book was almost certainly Heft (Issue) I of *Die gegenwärtigen Behandlungswege der Kieferschussverletzungen* (Contemporary treatment methods of gunshot injuries of the jaws), a small, soft-covered volume of 62 pages that first appeared in April 1915. Edited by Professor Christian Bruhn, the book was based on experiences at the jaw hospital in Düsseldorf, with contributions from Friedrich Hauptmeyer, August Lindemann[†], Max Kühl and Bruhn himself, a dentist by training. Lindemann's entry consisted of 16 pages, entitled *Zur Deckung grösserer Defekte der Weichteile bei Kieferschussverletzungen*. (On the covering of larger defects of the soft tissues after gunshot injuries of the jaws).[12] Non German-language readers may be excused for concluding the cases shown in Lindemann's article were examples of the surgery being performed at Düsseldorf, whereas in fact the aim was to illustrate the deformities produced by poor surgical techniques at field hospitals. These included immediate wound closure; bandaging facial injuries without splinting the teeth; and stitching up wounds without taking into account injuries to the underlying bones of the jaws (Figure 3.4). The results may not have been pretty, but surgeons at Feldlazarette (German field hospitals), like their Allied counterparts, were often called upon to treat hundreds of patients under the most primitive conditions; and early closure, which was later shown to reduce the incidence of wound infection, probably saved many lives (see Chapter 4 for further discussion).

Die gegenwärtigen Behandlungswege der Kieferschussverletzungen eventually extended to 10 parts under the editorship of Bruhn – usually found bound together in a single volume dated 1916–17. Heft IV–VI, published in 1916, are of interest because they contain a report by Lindemann of 97 cases in which he had carried out bone grafts on jaws. All the operations were performed under local anaesthesia and of the 97 cases the union was primary in 86. In the absence of a surface wound, Lindemann's policy was to expose the mandible via an external incision to minimise infection from the mouth, and graft the defect with a piece of bone with periosteum attached, usually from the tibia.[13,14]

Presumably in a culture where duelling scars were regarded as a badge of honour, the patients were less concerned about the appearance of facial scarring, something that would certainly have offended Gillies' aesthetic sense – the restoration of appearance was as important to Gillies as the restoration of function; indeed, he regarded the two as inseparable.

Gillies meets Auguste Charles Valadier

At the outbreak of war, Gillies, who was 32, offered his services to the British Red Cross Society (BRCS). In January 1915 he was sent as a general surgeon to Boulogne, where he met Auguste Charles Valadier[†] – a Franco-American dentist who played an important role in establishing a dental service in the British Army. Valadier was a fascinating character and much of what we know about him comes from four articles. The first, 'The mysterious AC Valadier' by Robert Ivy[†] (1971), unearthed a good deal of information about Valadier's early life and career, but was written in a rather patronising style.[15] The contributions of McAuley[16] and Cruse[17] are more measured, but more information is now available courtesy of the Internet, which has resolved several questions regarding Valadier's early career, as well as the maxillofacial unit at Boulogne under his command.

It is generally agreed that Auguste Charles Valadier was born in Paris on 26 November 1873, the son of Charles Jean-Baptiste Valadier and his wife Marie Antoinette Valadier (née Parade), and that he emigrated to the United States as a child with his parents.[15–17] However, Valadier is referred to interchangeably in the literature as both Auguste and Charles, creating the impression they were one and the same person. Ordinarily this would not be a problem, but in his application to join the RAMC in 1914, Valadier describes himself as an oral surgeon and lists his qualifications as follows: College of Physicians and Surgeons, Columbia University, 1895; Philadelphia Dental College, 1901; New York Medical University, 1903; Faculté de Médecine de Paris, 1912.[18] In the absence of supporting documentary evidence, there has always been doubt as to whether Valadier had actually been a medical

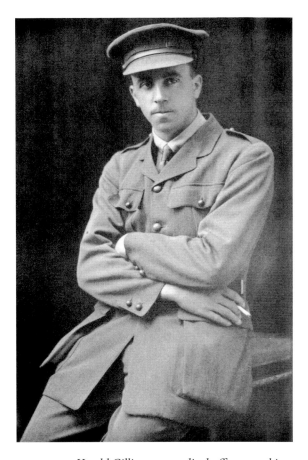

FIGURE 3.5. *Harold Gillies as a medical officer, working with the Red Cross in France, 1915. A cigarette was often used as a prop in photographs of the period. When Gillies gave up smoking at the age of 66, he calculated that in 48 years he had smoked 448,000 cigarettes.* (Courtesy of Brian Morgan and the Antony Wallace Archive, British Association of Plastic, Reconstructive and Aesthetic Surgeons, Royal College of Surgeons of England)

student and completed medical training.

Reports in the *New York Times* reveal that a student by the name of Charles Auguste Valadier had a very distinguished undergraduate career at Columbia College in New York City, graduating Bachelor of Arts with honours in 1892.[19] He then spent three years studying medicine at the College of Physicians and Surgeons, the medical school of Columbia University. The 1900 edition of *Officers and Graduates of Columbia University: Originally* the College of the Province of New York known as King's College: General Catalogue 1754–1900, published online in 2007, records that in 1895 Charles Auguste Valadier was awarded the degree of Doctor of Medicine (MD), and, as if that wasn't challenging enough, a Master of Arts as well (AM 1895). Charles Valadier was clearly talented academically. The following year, according to the Yale University Library online catalogue, he published a small volume of 78 pages entitled Questions and Answers on Physiology … for the use of medical students. Charles Auguste Valadier (1871–1909) is also recorded on the Yale website as the author of Materia Medica, a larger work of 360 pages published by JT Dougherty of New York in 1898. His death at the age of 38 is recorded on page 165 of the 1916 edition of Officers and Graduates of Columbia University with the following entry: 'Charles Auguste Valadier AB '92; AM and MD '95, deceased 1909'. The report of his death and date of birth were unforeseen, but the possibility that it might have been a case of mistaken identity could not be ruled out (the present author suffered such a fate in 1989 with his entry in the Roll of Graduates of the University of Otago).

It is possible to access applications for United States passports online and this uncovered an application from Auguste Charles Valadier, and three more in the name of Charles Auguste Valadier. In his application (No 13446) dated 10 June 1896, Auguste Charles Valadier solemnly swore he was born in Paris on 26 November 1874; that his father had become a naturalised citizen of the United States in 1881; that he had lived in New York from 1880 and followed the occupation of builder (which came as a surprise). On 28 June 1900, Charles Auguste Valadier, born in Paris on 12 January 1871, whose father became a naturalised citizen of the United States in 1881, applied for a passport (No 29091) giving his occupation as physician: in a letter to the Department of State following rejection of the application, he is referred to by his lawyers as Dr CA Valadier. The signatures of the applicants on both forms appear quite different; moreover, Auguste was 5 feet 11½ inches

tall, with a dark complexion, while Charles was 5 feet 10 inches tall, and fair.

The website of the Church of Jesus Christ of Latter-day Saints also records that Auguste Charles Valadier married Marion Stowe on 4 February 1899 in Manhattan and that Charles A Valadier married Regina Karschmaroff on 28 February 1899 also in Manhattan. It is therefore difficult to avoid the conclusion that Charles Auguste Valadier MD was the elder brother of Auguste, who had somewhat embellished the truth about his connection with Columbia University. Why Valadier felt it necessary to falsify his CV is unclear, but given the circumstances and the likelihood that nobody would check the Columbia records, he probably felt it would enhance his chances of being accepted by the RAMC. His association, if any, with New York Medical University is unknown.

There is, however, no question that in 1898 Auguste Charles Valadier gave up being a builder and enrolled as a dental student at Philadelphia Dental College (now part of Temple University), and in 1901 he received a DDS degree.[15] After passing the examinations for licensure in the states of Pennsylvania and New York, he practised as a dentist in New York City for a number of years at West 42nd and East 59th Streets. In 1910, 'on the death of her other son who had practised medicine in Paris',[16] Auguste Valadier (McAuley refers to him as Charles) was persuaded by his widowed mother to return to France, where she rented an apartment for him at 22 Place Vendôme. Two years later, when the Faculté de Médecine of the Université de Paris had granted him a Diplôme de chirugien dentiste, Valadier established a fashionable practice at 47 Avenue Hoche in the 8th arrondissement of Paris.

Valadier joins the RAMC

On the outbreak of hostilities in 1914, Valadier approached the French authorities with an offer of assistance. However, the French did not have an organised dental corps at the time, and since he was forty years old and a US citizen he was faced with either becoming a private in the French Army or serving with the Foreign Legion.[20] Understandably

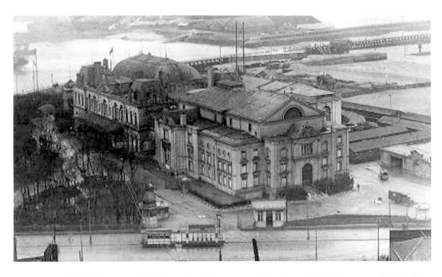

FIGURE 3.6. *The Municipal Casino, Boulogne-sur-Mer, Pas de Calais, occupied by No 13 General Hospital BEF from October 1914 to February 1919. Used largely as an evacuation hospital, in November 1917 it was taken over by the staff of American Base Hospital No 5 (Harvard) AEF under Dr Harvey Cushing and turned into a surgical unit. The casino also housed Sir Almroth Wright's Research Laboratory where Wright, Alexander Fleming and Leonard Colebrook studied the bacteriology of septic wounds.* (From Yanks in the King's Forces.[21] US National Archives Photograph: 111-SC-44196)

not being attracted by either choice, Valadier wrote to the BRCS offering his services without remuneration, subject to acceptance by the RAMC. In September 1914 he was sent to Abbéville, and in October was accepted for duty with the British Army by Sir Arthur Sloggett, Director-General of Medical Services in France and assigned to No 13 General Hospital, BEF – a base hospital at Boulogne-sur-Mer – with the temporary rank of local lieutenant. Valadier thus became the first dental surgeon to officially provide treatment for British soldiers in France. Unusually for a time when photographs of military personnel in uniform were commonly taken for the historical record, the only known photograph of Valadier appears to be the rather grainy one unearthed by Robert Ivy in the 1901 Class Year Book of the Philadelphia Dental College.

Before hutted hospitals were built, base hospitals were often located in substantial prewar buildings such as seaside hotels or casinos. There

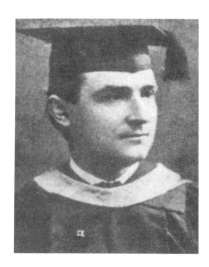

FIGURE 3.7. *Dr Auguste Charles Valadier. Graduation photograph, Philadelphia Dental College (DDS, 1901), the second-oldest dental school in the USA and since 1907 part of Temple University.* (From Ivy (1971), Plastic and Reconstructive Surgery)

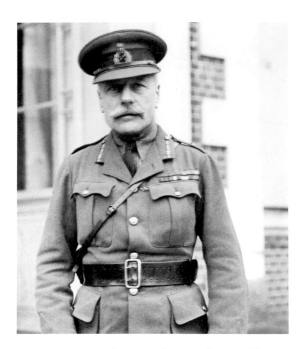

FIGURE 3.8. *General Sir Douglas Haig (later Field Marshall Lord Haig) Commander of the British Expeditionary Force in France and Belgium from December 1915 to the end of the war. Haig suffered severe toothache during the Battle of the Aisne, October 1914, and his timely treatment by Valadier led to the incorporation of dental officers into the British Army.* (By kind permission of the Imperial War Museum London: IWM Q 23659)

were two types of base hospital: stationary (200 beds) and general (500-plus beds). Both types were in reality clearing hospitals performing emergency operations and evacuating patients to England as soon as possible. They differed only in size; eventually any distinction between the two was abandoned and each hospital was encouraged to expand as its site permitted.

At the time provisions for dental treatment in the British Army were negligible; there were no facilities for treatment at the front, and no dental surgeons accompanied the BEF to France.[20] So little thought had gone into the provision of dentistry for the army that qualified dental practitioners were serving in the combatant ranks: the casualties listed in the *British Dental Journal* were a grim

reminder of the fate of many. Tradition has it that requests to the War Office for dental officers date from October 1914, when General Sir Douglas Haig, Commander of the BEF's First Army Corps, suffered severe toothache and there were no British dentists available to relieve the pain; Valadier is almost certainly the 'dental surgeon from Paris' whose timely treatment of Sir Douglas led to the decision to incorporate dental officers into the army. Twelve dental surgeons were subsequently sent to France in November 1914 with temporary commissions in the RAMC, and the number increased to twenty in December. However, it was not until 1916 that dental officers were attached to CCSs at the front, and another five years before an Army Dental Corps was formed.

No 13 Stationary Hospital, Boulogne-sur-Mer

By the time Gillies arrived in France, Valadier had convinced the British authorities of the need for special facilities to treat face and jaw injuries, usually described in the literature (including by Gillies himself) as a 50-bed unit attached to the 83rd (Dublin) General Hospital in Wimereux, a seaside town 3 miles north of Boulogne – the only problem is that at the time No 83 General did not exist. Valadier's unit was initially established at No 13 General and then, with the development of specialised units in the Boulogne hospitals, was transferred to No 13 Stationary. This had been established in October 1914 by the RAMC in a large shed used for storing sugar on the Gare Maritime, an ideal site for transferring patients from ambulance trains arriving from the battlefront directly to hospital, or to a hospital ship bound for Dover and other ports in England. During the early months of the war the resources of the RAMC and the Army Nursing Services were stretched to the limit. Ian Hay (nom de plume of Major-General John Hay Beith) describes the chaotic situation in *One Hundred Years of Army Nursing* (pp. 89–90):[22]

> *One of the most important, and possibly the best remembered hospitals of those very early days was No 13 Stationary Hospital – a group of converted*

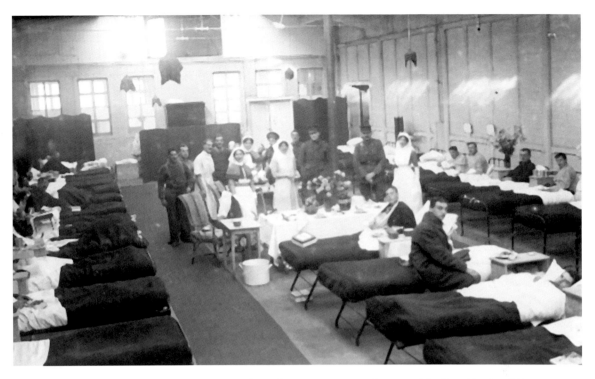

Figure 3.9. *A ward at No 13 Stationary Hospital, Boulogne-sur-Mer. At the time of the First Battle of Ypres, October 1914, when casualties were pouring into Boulogne at the rate of 2500 per day, the RAMC commandeered a large shed used for storing sugar and other merchandise on the Gare Maritime and converted it into a base hospital. No 13 Stationary, where Valadier established the first face and jaw unit in the BEF, remained at Boulogne from October 1914 to September 1915.* (Photograph kindly provided by Sheila Brownlee, whose grandmother Ruby Cockburn (in the centre of the picture) worked as a British Red Cross nurse at No 13 Stationary during 1914–15)

sugar-sheds on the quay at Boulogne. The great doors at one end admitted the casualties as they arrived, while those at the other end discharged cases fit to travel straight into the Gare Maritime, whence they were evacuated to England. Here is the scene, as described by one of the sisters: 'What an indescribable scene! In the first huge shed there were hundreds of walking wounded cases: as long as a man could crawl he had to be a walking case. All were caked with mud, in torn clothes, hardly any caps, and with bloodstained bandages on hands, arms and legs. Many were lying asleep in the straw that had been left in the hastily cleared sheds, looking weary to death.'

Hay continues:

Then there were the stretcher cases, for whom beds were being brought in and partitions run up, to form some sort of a surgical ward. The beds as soon as they arrived were occupied by badly wounded men who had to be put into them as they were, clothes and all, until such time could be found to cut off the clothing, wash the patient and dress his wounds. Doctors, nurses and orderlies almost submerged under the endless stream of casualties from the Marne, Aisne, and Ypres fronts, laboured without ceasing, almost without sleep, to meet the demands made upon them … It was not until Maud McCarthy, Matron-in-Chief of the BEF, arrived and took personal control that order began to emerge from the confusion.

No 13 Stationary is renamed No 83 (Dublin) General Hospital

No 13 Stationary, known as the 'Sugar Store Hospital', remained on the quay until September 1915 when, under pressure from the army postal authorities, the sheds were evacuated and it was reestablished as a hutted hospital on the road leading to Wimereux. In May 1917 the name of No 13 Stationary was changed to No 83 (Dublin) General Hospital. This coincided with the arrival of a group of surgeons from Ireland, 'Dublin' being introduced into the title because the group in question had come over under an agreement made by Sir Alfred Keogh, Director-General of the Army Medical Service, with the Royal Colleges in Dublin, which had undertaken to supply medical men for a base hospital in France for three-month periods.[23] The group was led by Sir William Taylor (1871–1933), who had been elected president of the Royal College of Surgeons in Ireland in 1916, and one gets the impression the name change had been a quid pro quo on Keogh's part and distinctly unpopular with the existing staff. But that was not the only problem.

As explained by Lieutenant Colonel Stephen in his comprehensive history of Boulogne as a military medical base, with few exceptions the medical officers at Boulogne had been private practitioners before the war, and many had given up their practices and enrolled for service from the very beginning. Considerable resentment was created by the arrival of the Dubliners, who had been able to remain at home and carry on their private practice for nearly three years. To add insult to injury, during their period of service they were appointed as majors and lieutenant colonels in the numbers to which general hospitals were entitled, and then, because of their lack of experience in the treatment of war wounds, were obliged to work as understudies of the existing staff.

In reality, the disappearance of No 13 was nominal only, 'as the CO (a major) of No 13 remained in command … and the ophthalmic and jaw surgery departments which had reinforced the reputation built up by No 13 as the Sugar Store Hospital, continued their work under their original officers'.[23] Valadier's unit, for example, continued to use notepaper headed 'Oral Surgical Department, No 13 Stationary Hospital, BEF' for the rest of the war (Colour plate 5). The Official War Diary of Dame Maud McCarthy makes several references to Valadier's unit at No 13 Stationary in 1915 and 1916 and at No 83 General in 1917; her entry for 25 July 1917, for example, includes mention of a group of visiting dignitaries who were 'shown Major Valadier's wonderful jaw wards'.[24]

Valadier had provided much of the equipment at his own expense (in addition to his practice earnings, his mother had died in 1915, leaving him a considerable estate), as well as a dental laboratory in which the technicians from his Parisian practice made the appliances used to treat jaw fractures. As Gillies was to acknowledge 40 years later (p. 6), 'The credit for establishing the first British plastic and jaw unit, which so facilitated the later progress of plastic surgery, must go to the remarkable linguistic talents of the smooth and genial Sir Charles [sic] Valadier.'[11] By 1917 he and his staff had treated more than 1000 maxillofacial injuries.[25] Valadier's services were entirely gratuitous until October 1918, when it was decided to issue him the pay and allowances of a Major of Infantry.

Initially, Valadier seems to have conducted all the surgical operations by himself, but it was decided he should be assisted by a trained surgeon and Gillies, with his expertise in ENT surgery, was assigned to the role – not that ENT surgeons were better trained for maxillofacial surgery than anybody else at the time. How long Gillies remained with Valadier is not known, but the experience was the turning point in his career, when he realised that a new approach was required if traumatic facial wounds were to be successfully treated. When the opportunity for leave came in June 1915 he arranged to meet the famous surgeon Hippolyte Morestin† from Martinique, at the time considered the premier facial surgeon in Europe, who was performing reconstructive surgery at the Val de Grâce Military Hospital in Paris. Gillies later described his meeting with Morestin (p. 7):

I stood spellbound as he removed half a face distorted with a horrible cancer and then deftly turned a neck flap to restore not only the cheek but the side of the nose and lip, in one shot. Although in the light of present-day knowledge it seems unlikely that this repair would have been wholly successful, at the time it was the most thrilling thing I had ever seen. I fell in love with the work on the spot.[11]

Gillies felt 'a tremendous urge to do something other than the surgery of destruction'. On a subsequent visit to Morestin the following year, however, he was refused entry to the operating theatre. Apparently the Entente Cordiale did not extend to the unlimited sharing of surgical expertise.

Maxillofacial surgery at No 13 Stationary Hospital

Valadier published several papers during the war, including some with Captain H Lawson Whale[†], an ENT surgeon who joined him in July 1916. Lawson Whale had been in France with the BEF since 1914 and been awarded the Mons Star – the BEF's first major battle of the war. He had gained considerable experience in treating face and neck injuries at the Val de Grâce Hospital in Paris with James Dundas-Grant (1854–1944), as well as at the 53rd General Hospital in Boulogne. He was a staunch supporter of Valadier and his work, and while with the unit he translated *Injuries of the Face and Jaw* by Martinier and Lemerle into English.[26] When Lawson Whale was posted to the British Section at the Queen's Hospital, Sidcup, in 1918 (he is one of the officers sitting on the grass in Figure 5.6) he was replaced by Captain Frederick J Cleminson[†] who, like Gillies and Lawson Whale, was another Cambridge-educated ENT surgeon. The standard of treatment shown in these articles was clearly the equal of their German and Allied contemporaries.[27,28] (See Whale, *Injuries to the Head and Neck* (1919) for other examples of the plastic surgery practised in Valadier's unit.)[29]

The first report from the unit, which was published in the *British Journal of Surgery* in July 1916, dealt with the management of fractured jaws.

In the report, Valadier demonstrates how fractures may be immobilised using wires ligated to the teeth, as well as by splints of various designs. For example, in the case of a displaced unilateral maxillary fracture, aluminium cap splints with hooks had been cemented to the teeth of both jaws and the fracture reduced by means of elastic traction. There is also an example of an open Kingsley splint made of vulcanite with wire whiskers exiting the mouth (identical to the extraoral traction or headgear used in contemporary orthodontic treatment), designed to reduce maxillary fractures by attaching the whiskers to a head appliance by means of elastics. The most interesting, however, are two cases involving fractures of the mandible with bone loss, in which Valadier was clearly practising what is now known as distraction osteogenesis (Figure 3.10).

The concept is not new: a woodcut dated 1517 shows a leg brace with a screw mechanism used by the Teutonic knights to straighten legs; and there is the case of St Ignatius of Loyola, whose left leg was shattered by a French cannonball at the Battle of Pamplona in 1521 and stretched back to its normal length with weights on a rack – a device at the time more commonly identified with the Inquisition. A crude method was described in 1905 by Alessandro Codivilla (1861–1912) for limb lengthening,[30] but modern distraction osteogenesis is generally acknowledged to date from the 1950s, when the Russian orthopaedic surgeon Gavriel Ilizarov developed an osteotomy technique for managing orthopaedic limb deformities.

In both of Valadier's cases – one of which is illustrated with study models and X-rays – the lower jaw was shot away completely from second premolar to second premolar. The two ends of the mandible were allowed to come together by wiring, and subsequent X-ray examination showed that a bony callus was forming. An impression of the lower teeth was taken, and an expansion screw attached to a vulcanite plate was used to slowly push apart the fractured ends of the mandible, thereby distracting the callus and stimulating new bone formation; after four weeks a retention appliance was inserted (Figure 3.10(B)). Three

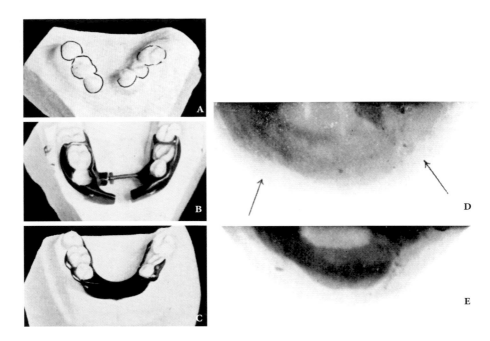

FIGURE 3.10. *One of Valadier's distraction osteogenesis cases. (A) Study model taken at the time a skiagram (the name used at the time for an X-ray or radiograph) showed that a callus was forming between the bone ends. (B) Split vulcanite plate with expansion screw to slowly separate the fractured ends of the two halves of the lower jaw (mandible). After 4 weeks a retention appliance was inserted and 3 weeks later a larger screw inserted. (C) Plate to retain the expansion and allow for strengthening of the callus prior to insertion of a partial denture. (D) Callus formation between the bone ends at 7 months. (E) At 10 months: callus is remodelling to form new bone. Skiagrams produced a positive image of hard and soft tissues and not the negative image of contemporary radiographs.* (From Valadier (1916), British Journal of Surgery)

weeks later another appliance with a larger screw was inserted and expanded until the desired width had been achieved, which was then retained (Figure 3.10(C)). Valadier used this technique on several patients, and there is little doubt that he had a better understanding of the dynamics of bone growth and regeneration than most, if not all, of his surgical and dental colleagues.

Gillies' biographer, Reginald Pound, put McAuley in touch with Private Philip Thorpe of the King's Liverpool Regiment. Thorpe had been wounded on 5 June 1918 by a shell fragment which had cut away most of his lower lip and a large fragment of the anterior (front) part of the mandible. He was admitted to No 83 General Hospital, which he describes as a collection of wooden huts on the

Boulogne–Wimereux road. The deficiency in the bone of Thorpe's lower jaw had been treated by Valadier in the same way, and the expansion was finally retained with a lower denture. In a letter to McAuley dated 29 May 1965, Thorpe notes that this was not a serendipitous discovery:

Only on two occasions did I see Major Valadier display any excitement or emotion. The first time was when he had examined an X-ray plate of my jaw. He suddenly put down the plate, grabbed the ward sister round the waist and pranced up and down the ward shouting 'We've done it, we've done it.' It transpired that in view of my youth he had been hoping that he could induce the bone to grow and so save having a bone graft. By drawing the two ends of the bone towards each other, reducing

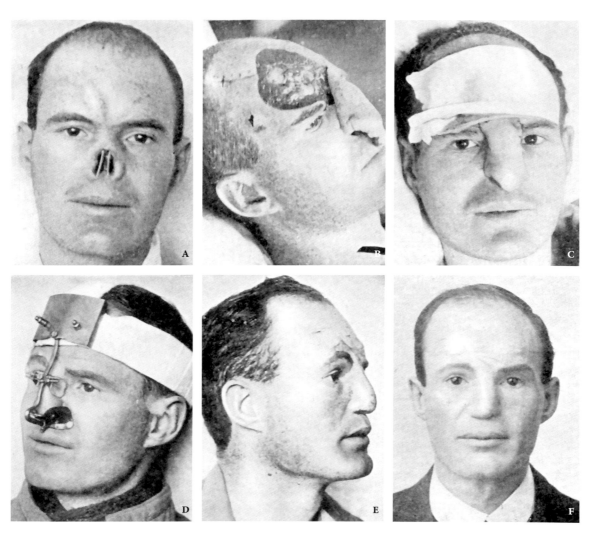

FIGURE 3.11. *Case of Private W. Nose reconstruction by rotated forehead flap; surgery by Captain H Lawson Whale. (A) Healed condition. Oiled vulcanite plates have been inserted to discourage adhesions between the turbinals and remains of the nasal septum. A strip of costal cartilage from the 8th rib destined to form the bridge of the nose has been inserted into the forehead under the periosteum. (B) The cartilage-bearing flap has been turned down. (C) The columella has been attached to the philtrum and the pedicle divided higher up. The size of the new nose has been deliberately exaggerated. (D) Various operations have been performed to shape the nose. The patient is wearing a prosthesis designed by Valadier which serves the double purpose of maintaining compression on the nasal bridge and checking stenosis of the nostrils. (E) Patient on discharge. The forehead has been repaired with a full thickness Wolfe-Krause graft. The patient wears two small oval vulcanite rings at night to prevent shrinkage of the nostrils. (F) Twenty months after the last operation and 29 months after the wound. The patient has dispensed with night-time wear of the rings in his nostrils.* (From Lawson Whale (1919), Injuries to the Head and Neck. This case was also included in Valadier & Whale (1917), British Journal of Surgery 5, 151–71)

the gap from two and one half inches to one and
a quarter inches and by holding them firm in that
position by means of a splint he had kept hoping,
but had said nothing to anyone. The x-ray had
shown a thin white line stretching across the gap,
and he realised that he had succeeded, for the first
time in Medical (or should it be Surgical) history.[31]

It is interesting to note that distraction techniques have only been applied to maxillofacial surgery since the early 1990s, and although used to correct upper and lower jaws that have failed to grow properly, the fundamental principles remain the same.

Figure 3.11 shows the sequence of operations required to reconstruct the nose, where the nasal bones and anterior part of the septum are missing. The case was originally reported by Valadier and Whale in the *British Journal of Surgery* (1917) while Gillies was still at Aldershot, and was later included by Whale in *Injuries to the Head and Neck* as an example of a total rhinoplasty; it has the most complete series of clinical photographs in the book. However, unlike *Plastic Surgery of the Face*, which appeared the following year, the report by Valadier and Whale lacks the planning diagrams and the clarity of Gillies' surgical notes, making it difficult to follow exactly what was done (see Figure 5.8 for comparison). It is not clear, for example, whether a lining membrane was provided for the new nose. Nonetheless, the result is as good as those achieved later at Sidcup, and was holding up after 20 months: the patient wrote to Whale to report he was in very good health and never felt anything was the matter with his nose (p. 175).[29]

Valadier's legacy

Posterity has not been kind to Valadier, a man clearly ahead of his time who made significant contributions to the advance of maxillofacial surgery that were conspicuously ignored by his colleagues. He was an outsider, and appears to have been admired and disliked in equal measure by his contemporaries. Success breeds jealousy, and it is not hard to imagine some lesser souls, such as Dr Ferdinand Brigham at the First Harvard Surgical Unit,[15] being envious of his flamboyant character, fluent French and German, chauffeur-driven Rolls-Royce and successful Parisian practice. He also had friends in high places, including General Sir Arthur Sloggett, Director-General of Medical Services, who appointed him to the RAMC; as well as Field Marshall Sir John French, Commander-in-Chief of the British Army, who recommended to the War Office in October 1915 that Valadier be granted the honorary rank of major while serving with His Majesty's Army in the field.[32] Valadier was also mentioned in dispatches three times, and was appointed CMG as early as June 1916, with strong personal support in a letter from General Sir Douglas Haig:

> *I cannot speak too highly of the excellent and*
> *most valuable surgical work on the jaw performed*
> *gratuitously by this gentleman for all ranks of the*
> *British Army. He has performed a large number of*
> *operations on the jaws that require a high degree*
> *of surgical skill, with the most excellent results*
> *and which had not hitherto been attempted by the*
> *profession. I strongly recommend that he be given*
> *some tangible recognition of his services.*[33]

He was made a Knight of St John of Jerusalem in 1917, and was awarded the Croix de Chevalier de la Legion d'Honneur (the Knight's Cross) by the French government in 1919.

Valadier also had a long-standing dispute with the authoritative academic personage of Frank Colyer over the question of whether teeth in the region of a fracture should be extracted. This probably didn't help Valadier's reputation in some quarters: he was in favour of retaining the teeth if at all possible, while Colyer advocated their removal to minimise sepsis. As usual, dogma got in the way of rational clinical practice. (The controversy was still unresolved by the beginning of the Second World War, until the introduction of penicillin in 1943 made such arguments largely redundant.) Many erroneous and unsubstantiated statements have been made about Valadier and his career, and in later years Gillies, while he gave Valadier full credit for establishing the first British maxillofacial unit in France, could not resist making somewhat condescending comments about him. As Reginald Pound points out in *Gillies: Surgeon Extraordinary* (p. 23), Gillies perhaps owed more to Valadier's experience and skill than he was prepared to admit.[11]

Valadier may not have been a particularly nice man – he abandoned his first wife and three-year-old son in 1903, and spent three months in Ludlow Street Jail in New York City after she sued him for separation (the divorce was a particularly acrimonious one, judging by the court reports in the *New York Times*)[34] – but there is little doubt he was an innovative and talented maxillofacial surgeon. His drift into relative obscurity – RH Ivy's 'mysterious AC Valadier' – was due to the fact that, like most of his wartime contemporaries, he went back into practice after the Armistice and, unlike Gillies in London and Kazanjian[†] in Boston, did not train a cohort of devoted acolytes to perpetuate his name. Interestingly, Colyer and Valadier were both knighted in 1920 for their military service during the war (in the case of Valadier, conferred in 1921 after he obtained British citizenship) – the only two dental surgeons to be so honoured. Gillies had to wait until 1930 for his KBE.

The First Harvard Surgical Unit

Valadier's maxillofacial unit at Boulogne-sur-Mer may have been the first to be established in France with the backing of the British Army, but it was soon followed in July 1915 by the dental surgeons attached to the First Harvard Surgical Unit, a few miles down the road at Dannes-Camier. It seems to have been largely forgotten today, but throughout the First World War, Harvard and other American universities had volunteer medical personnel serving in surgical units attached to the BEF in France.[35-37] Although the United States was officially neutral, many Americans supported the Allied cause; and the sinking of the Cunard ocean liner RMS *Lusitania* off the southwest coast of Ireland by the German submarine *U-20* on 7 May 1915 with the loss of 1195 lives, 128 of them American, did much to harden US public opinion against Germany. However, it was the sinking of the RMS *Laconia* on 25 February 1917 by the

submarine *U-50* that provided the catalyst for the United States Congress declaring war on the Imperial German Empire on 6 April 1917.[38]

Canadian-born Sir William Osler, at the time Regius Professor of Medicine at the University of Oxford and an influential figure in Anglo-American medicine, proposed that leading American and Canadian universities should provide medical services for the Anglo-French armies close to the battlefront. On 3 April 1915 he wrote to Abbot Lawrence Lowell, the president of Harvard: 'Do you think that Harvard University would offer to staff a British war hospital for 1040 beds?' Under the terms of the Geneva Convention of 1864 a neutral nation was permitted to send sanitary and medical aid to a belligerent nation without breaking the neutrality of the persons in that service, provided the nation to which the aid was sent notified its enemy. It was under this clause that American citizens went to treat the wounded of the BEF and the French Army.[37]

On 26 June 1915, Harvard sent the first surgical unit to England. The War Office assigned it to the 22nd General Hospital at Dannes-Camier, a few miles south of Boulogne near Etaples. The unit (the first of three) consisted of 32 surgeons, three dentists and 75 nurses. As they were not British subjects, they were given temporary honorary commissions in the RAMC. Conditions were primitive: the hospital was situated in a field and, except for a few huts made of wood and cement where surgery was performed, the wards, officers and staff were housed in tents.[39] Devotees of *M*A*S*H* will have no difficulty in imagining what it must have been like.

Dr Varaztad Kazanjian, who was head of the Prosthetic Department at Harvard Dental School when war broke out, was appointed Chief Dental Officer to the unit. He chose as his assistants Ferdinand Brigham and Frank Cushman – both final-year dental students. Initially the assignment was for three months, but it eventually stretched to January 1919 when the Harvard Unit was retired. Because of the lack of dentists in the British Army at the beginning of the war, Kazanjian and his team were soon in demand, not only for routine

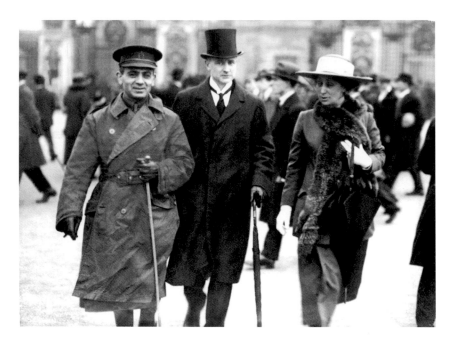

FIGURE 3.12. *Major Varaztad H Kazanjian RAMC with Mr and Mrs W Warwick James outside the gates of Buckingham Palace, following his investiture by King George V as a Companion of the Most Distinguished Order of St Michael and St George, 15 March 1919. The CMG, awarded to Kazanjian for his wartime service, was the highest honour that could be bestowed by the Crown on someone who was not a British subject.* (Published with the kind permission of Harvard Medical Library in the Francis A Countway Library of Medicine, Boston, Massachusetts. Kazanjian Archive: Series V, M-18)

dentistry but also for managing fractured jaws and mouth wounds, which at the time were being treated by general surgeons. Kazanjian was able to combine his knowledge of maxillofacial prosthetics and occlusion of the teeth in treating jaw fractures, and he acquired a considerable reputation as a surgeon, being dubbed by the British press with their weakness for hyperbole, the 'Miracle Man of the Western Front'.[37] Given the standard of care available during the early months of the war this is likely to have been a fairly accurate description.

For Kazanjian the treatment of the external wound was always secondary to that of the fractured jaws; only when the jaw fragments had been correctly aligned would facial and/or plastic surgery be performed.[40,41] Kazanjian's talent at the time lay in what can best be described as maxillofacial orthopaedics rather than soft-tissue facial reconstruction, and later in the war cases requiring major plastic surgery were sent to Gillies at Sidcup. Gillies and Kazanjian enjoyed a harmonious and respectful professional working relationship; indeed, Gillies tried to recruit Kazanjian to Sidcup. During its time at Dannes-Camier, the Harvard Unit treated 3000 cases of maxillofacial wounds and Kazanjian was awarded the CMG for his service to the Crown. As Gillies was to write later in the preface to *Plastic Surgery of the Face*:

> *The work of Valadier and Kasanjian* [sic] *in France has been of great service in the improvement of the treatment of jaw wounds. I am indebted to the former for many photographs of the original conditions, and to both for the stimulation of their work and for much kindly encouragement.*[42]

CHAPTER 4

The Cambridge Military Hospital, Aldershot

O**N HIS RETURN FROM** France, Gillies lobbied the army medical authorities – including Sir Alfred Keogh, Director-General of the Army Medical Service, and Sir William Arbuthnot Lane† – for permission to establish a unit for the treatment of injuries to the face and jaws. Lane, who features prominently in Gillies' wartime career and was the consultant surgeon to whom he was immediately responsible, had been asked by Keogh to take over the Aldershot Command and its twin hospitals, the Cambridge and the Connaught, as director of the Army Surgical Service. Permission for a face and jaw unit was granted and in January 1916 Gillies, by now a captain in the RAMC, was posted by the War Office to the Cambridge Military Hospital at Aldershot in Hampshire 'for special duty in connection with plastic surgery'. The Cambridge had been built on a hill to Florence Nightingale's 'pavilion' specifications, with a long central corridor and airy wards with plenty of sunlight to reduce cross-infection. It had opened its doors for the admission of patients in 1879 and was named after Prince George, 2nd Duke of Cambridge (1819–1904), Commander-in-Chief of the British Army.[1]

When Gillies arrived the hospital was already overflowing with patients, but two wards were reluctantly cleared for his patients. The ward sister was Catherine Black, a nurse from the London Hospital who, on the outbreak of war, volunteered for Queen Alexandra's Imperial Military Nursing Service (QAIMNS) and was sent to Aldershot. In her autobiography *King's Nurse, Beggar's Nurse*,[2] she describes her first meeting with Gillies (p. 85):

I had not been more than a few weeks at the Cambridge Hospital when there strolled into my ward, which was crowded to the last bed with acute medical cases, a good-looking young officer with the casual, free and easy manners of the Colonial, who introduced himself as Captain Gillies: 'I'm looking for a ward for my jaw cases … ' he explained. 'This is the very thing for them. We'd better move them into it directly … these poor fellows can be transferred to other wards …' He spoke as airily as though finding places in an already overcrowded hospital for thirty men, all of them seriously ill, and getting them transported there was a matter of a few minutes. He was evidently not taking into consideration the ways and means of it, just taking it for granted that it would be done. And it was. This I discovered was very typical of him. There was no such word as impossible in his vocabulary. He would not admit defeat.

Gillies was clearly pleased with the description of him as a young officer with the casual, free and easy manners of the Colonial; he repeated it (modestly leaving out the good-looking bit) many years later in *The Principles and Art of Plastic Surgery*,[3]

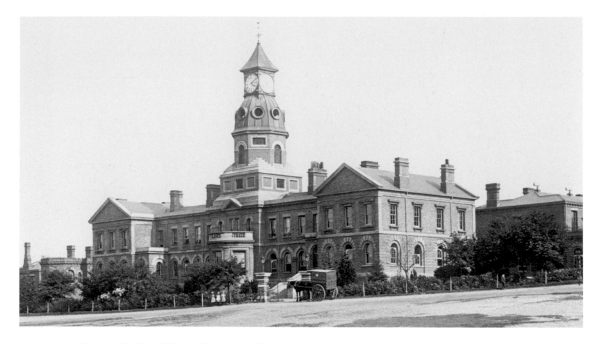

FIGURE 4.1. *The Cambridge Military Hospital, Aldershot, in 1891. It opened for patients on 18 July 1879 – and closed in 1996. The building, set on Gun Hill, was constructed of yellow brick with a neoclassical front dressed with Bath stone. Six pavilion ward blocks projected south from the long central corridor. The building is dominated by the massive clocktower, around 109 feet high, which is visible for miles around and which originally housed the Sevastopol Bell, one of a pair from the Church of the Twelve Apostles (the other went to Windsor Castle), brought back as trophies from the Crimean War in 1856.*[1] (Courtesy of the Francis Frith Collection, Aldershot)

although he neglected to acknowledge where it came from. Sister Black goes on to say (pp. 86–87):

> *In all my nursing experiences those months at Aldershot in the ward for facial wounds were, I think, the saddest. Sadder even than the casualty clearing stations to which I went afterwards, for there death was swifter and more merciful, and it is not so hard to see a man die as to break the news to him that he will be blind and dumb for the rest of his life. And that was something we had to do so often in that silent ward where only one in ten patients could mumble a few words from the shattered jaws, for the facial wounds were in many respects the most serious of the War casualties. Despite all that could be done for them, they were responsible for a terribly high mortality rate. The risks for gangrene were enormous and one had always to be on the watch for sudden haemorrhages.*

Gillies' suggestion to the War Office that all wounded face and jaw patients at advanced dressing stations should be labelled for Aldershot was received without enthusiasm, so to make sure the unit had sufficient patients he bought £10 worth of labels at a bookshop in The Strand, addressed them to himself and took them back to the Chief Medical Officer in Whitehall. To his surprise, within a few weeks soldiers with facial injuries began arriving with the labels pinned to their uniforms.[3] With the British offensive planned for the summer of 1916 approaching, Lane warned Gillies he foresaw a huge influx of casualties and assigned him a further 200 beds. However, even that number proved hopelessly inadequate – in the fortnight following the Battle of the Somme, which began on 1 July when British and French armies attacked the German positions along a 25-mile front, 2000 arrived at Southampton, all neatly

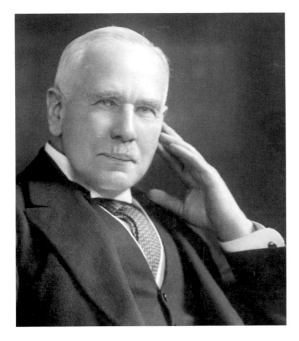 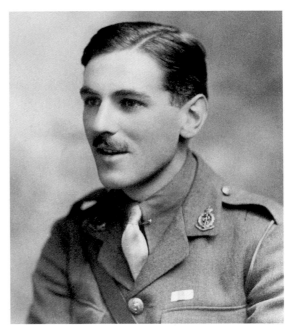

FIGURE 4.2. (LEFT): *Sir William Arbuthnot Lane, Bart, CB, ca 1910. His friends and students called him 'Willie'; however, on being created a Baronet in 1913, he felt compelled to adopt his rather more formal middle name Arbuthnot, and was known as Sir Arbuthnot Lane. Lane was a powerful supporter of Gillies and was the driving force behind the establishment of the Face and Jaw Unit at Aldershot, and subsequently the Queen's Hospital at Sidcup in Kent.* (Published with the permission of Getty Images/Hulton Archive)

FIGURE 4.3. (RIGHT): *Captain William Kelsey Fry MC, RAMC. The medal ribbon is the Military Cross (three equal parts of white, purple, white) awarded to Kelsey Fry, 'For conspicuous gallantry and devotion to duty at Festubert between 16th and 18th of May 1915, while carrying out his work under heavy fire. He himself was wounded while attending others.' Supplement to the* London Gazette, *24 July 1915.* (Photograph and citation courtesy of his son, Dr Ian Kelsey Fry)

labelled. Gillies and his team were overwhelmed. Given the crowded atmosphere of Aldershot and the absence of a convenient convalescent home for patients to recuperate between operations, it was clear that larger, purpose-built facilities were needed. The result was the transfer of the unit to the Queen's Hospital at Sidcup in August of the following year.

An interdisciplinary approach

One of the features of the Aldershot and Sidcup units was the combined approach to the treatment of facial injuries between the surgeons led by Gillies, and a dental department staffed with Captains Leonard King and Alexander Fraser. King was later transferred to Valadier's unit at No

13 Stationary Hospital, Boulogne-sur-Mer, and was replaced by Captain William Kelsey Fry, who had been invalided home from France after being wounded for the second time. Kelsey Fry[†] had a good war. Soon after completing his medical and dental studies at Guy's Hospital, he joined the RAMC as a regimental medical officer (RMO) with the 1st Battalion, the Royal Welch Fusiliers.[4] The regiment had originally been raised in the border counties of Wales as the 23rd Regiment of Foot in 1689 to help William of Orange fight his father-in-law, the deposed Catholic King James II, and his French allies in Ireland.

The duty of an RMO was to establish a regimental aid post in whatever shelter could be found as near to the firing line as was considered safe, where he was expected to remain and await the arrival of the sick and wounded. However, bravery under fire was highly valued in the RAMC, and many RMOs accompanied the men forward during an attack as a matter of course, exposing themselves to considerable danger.[5] In the course of the war 743 RAMC officers (as well as 6130 warrant officers, NCOs and men) lost their lives, the majority of them RMOs, who were either killed in action or died of their wounds.[6] By mid-1917 the numbers of RMOs had been depleted to such an extent that Arthur Balfour, the Foreign Secretary, on a special mission to the United States in April 1917 made an appeal for medical manpower. The call was answered, and during the last year of the war 1427 American doctors were loaned to the British, over 1200 serving with combatant troops; by the summer of 1918 the situation was so acute that the majority of battalion medical officers in the BEF were Americans, thus contributing in large measure to the maintenance of RAMC services. One hundred and eighty-seven American RMOs attached to the BEF were awarded the Military Cross, including William Chapin, author of *The Lost Legion*, a record of their experiences and a tribute to the men who volunteered to serve in the King's Army in France.[7]

Kelsey Fry was an RMO in this tradition and during the first two years of the war had shown great physical courage: in May 1915 he was awarded the MC during the Battle of Festubert for continuing to dress the wounded under heavy fire, despite being handicapped by a shrapnel wound through the elbow. Earlier he had been mentioned in dispatches for attending, and then carrying the body of Lieutenant William Gladstone out of the trenches on 13 April 1915, with the help of Corporal Welsh. Gladstone was a tall man and had been shot through the forehead by a German sniper, a wound that proved to be fatal. This incident, as described by Major Dickson, is mentioned in Viscount Gladstone's memoir of his nephew (pp. 123–24):

When Lieutenant Fry came to Will a few minutes after he was shot, his men had already bandaged his head so well the doctor would not disturb him.

Thinking that Will had a chance of life, and it being impossible to get him along the twisty trench, the doctor called for volunteers to get out of the trench and run the risk of taking him back across the open – the distance at that spot between the German and British trenches being only one hundred yards. Corporal Welsh stood to his medical chief, and these two carried Will some three hundred yards across the open in full view of the German trenches followed by some bearers. There can be no doubt that this was a dangerous and most gallant act done in the hope of saving Will's life. Lieutenant Fry is noted for his bravery and is loved by all.[8]

Earlier in the month, Gladstone had written in a letter to his mother (dated 3 April) that he was recovering from an attack of rheumatism thanks to some Thermogene (a medicated wadding) given to him by the doctor. He goes on to say (pp. 116–17):

The doctor, by the by (Lt Kelsey Fry) is a man everyone here swears by; he is very competent, and the sort of doctor who always does the right thing for some reason or other, and puts his man on his legs again. He is a man of extraordinary bravery and has earned the VC they all say … [8]

Students of Siegfried Sassoon – who also served as a subaltern with the 1st Battalion, the Royal Welch Fusiliers – may be interested to know that in *Memoirs of an Infantry Officer*,[9] the doctor referred to on a number of occasions by Sassoon was Kelsey Fry. For example (p. 71):

Early in the afternoon the Doctor bustled up from Battalion Headquarters to tell me that my MC had come through … Homeliness and humility beamed in Barton's congratulations; and the little doctor, who would soon be dressing the wounds of moaning men, unpicked his own faded medal-ribbon, produced a needle and thread, and sewed the white and purple portent on to my tunic.

Kelsey Fry was injured again at Delville Wood (Devil's Wood) during the Somme offensive in August 1916 and was invalided home, the sole survivor of a field dressing station that had received a direct hit from a 5.9-inch shell, killing five wounded men and five stretcher-bearers, including two who had been awarded the DCM. The Delville Wood incident is also referred to in *Memoirs of an Infantry Officer* in a letter from a fellow officer named Dottrell (Joe Cottrell, the Battalion Quartermaster)[10] to Sherston while the latter was convalescing in England (p. 138):

The old Batt is having a rough time. We were up in the front a week ago and lost 200 men in three days. The aid-post, a bit of a dug-out hastily made, was blown in. At the time it contained 5 wounded men, 5 stretcher-bearers, and the doctor. All were killed except the Doc. who was buried in the debris. He was so badly shaken when dug out that he had to be sent down, and will probably be in England by now. It is a hell of a place up here.

The doctor mentioned in the book as Captain Munro was James Churchill Dunn DSO, MC and Bar, DCM, the Medical Officer attached to the Second Battalion – reckoned by Frank Richards to be the best fighting officer in the regiment.[11] With Sassoon, Robert Graves, Richards and Dunn – who edited and wrote about the exploits of the 2nd Battalion in *The War the Infantry Knew*[12] – the Royal Welch Fusiliers were endowed with more than their fair share of literary soldiers.

Kelsey Fry had clearly made his mark with the regiment, and it was during his time as an RMO that he had become interested in jaw injuries – and the tragic mortality that could follow their unskilled management in the field. Regimental aid posts and CCSs soon discovered that if patients with facial injuries were laid on their back, there was a strong likelihood that the tongue would obstruct the airway and they would choke to death. Having served two years at the front and survived two narrow escapes, the Army Medical Service appears to have decided that Kelsey Fry was more use to the war effort alive than dead, and after a period of convalescence they transferred him to the face and jaw unit at Aldershot. At his first meeting with Gillies he is reputed to have said, 'I'll take the hard tissues. You take the soft.'[3] Given the sheer volume of casualties, in practice the distinction was of necessity blurred. And in any event a significant

number of the surgeons at Aldershot and Sidcup were doubly qualified in medicine and dentistry and the specialty was generally referred to simply as maxillofacial surgery. It is only since the Second World War and the trend towards subspecialisation that plastic surgery and what is now called oral and maxillofacial surgery have gone their separate ways – and largely along the lines originally proposed by Kelsey Fry.

The iconography of plastic surgery

Art has always played a leading role in the iconography of war. Until the Crimean and American civil wars, the pictorial representation of battle was largely dependent on the work and imagination of artists and to some extent it still is, especially for action scenes of fighting and aerial combat. Who can fail to be moved by Lady Butler's magnificent, heavily dramatised painting *Scotland for Ever*, depicting the charge of the Royal Scots Greys at Waterloo, particularly those with Scottish genes?

Gillies, who was an enthusiastic amateur artist, believed that plastic surgery was a form of art and that the activities of the plastic surgeon demanded the vision and insight of the artist.[13] Since plastic surgery was a new specialty, he was particularly conscientious about keeping comprehensive written and pictorial records, using both photography and portraiture for teaching, publication and research, the benefits of meticulous record keeping clearly paying off when he came to write *Plastic Surgery of the Face* in 1920. The artistic theme was given considerable impetus from the very beginning by the contribution of Henry Tonks[†],[14-16] who recorded much of the plastic surgery being carried out at Aldershot and later at Sidcup. Tonks was too old for active service (he was 52 at the beginning of the war), but was eager to assist the war effort. In January 1915 he was at the village of d'Arc-en-Barrois in the Haute Marne, helping in a Red Cross Hospital for French soldiers (Colour plate 7). After returning to England, in January 1916 he was appointed to a temporary commission as a lieutenant in the RAMC and sent to Aldershot, where he was discovered by Gillies working behind a desk in the adjutant's office. One of Tonks' friends wrote to an acquaintance that she had seen Tonks 'as nice as ever' but looking in his uniform like the great Duke of Wellington as he would have 'if degraded to the rank of a subaltern'.[14]

Gillies recruits Henry Tonks

Tonks had originally trained as a surgeon, qualifying MRCS in 1886 and FRCS in 1888. His transition from a surgical to an artistic career in his late twenties was a most unusual one, particularly as he was regarded by Sir Frederick Treves as the best medical student of his year at the London Hospital. After Tonks had obtained his surgical fellowship, Treves was instrumental in arranging for him to be appointed Senior Medical Officer at the Royal Free Hospital. Tonks had always been interested in art, and he started taking lessons in his free time with Frederick Brown at the Westminster School of Art.

Brown was an inspiring teacher with the ability to exert a considerable influence on all his pupils, not least of all Tonks, who for the rest of his life never ceased in his admiration for the master's character, artistic gifts and skilful teaching.[14] By the time Tonks left the Royal Free to accept the position of demonstrator in anatomy to the London Hospital Medical School, he had given up any notion of becoming a surgeon – he was distressed by any human suffering and would spare no effort to alleviate it, leading Treves to reluctantly conclude that Tonks did not have the right temperament to be a surgeon.[14] This must have come as a great personal disappointment to him as Tonks' mentor.

Tonks finally left medicine for good in 1892, when Frederick Brown was appointed Slade Professor of Fine Art at University College London and offered Tonks the post of Professor of Drawing, starting salary £150 per annum. Much to the displeasure of his father, Tonks accepted, and was to remain at the Slade for nearly 40 years, succeeding Brown as Slade Professor and director in 1918. By all accounts an attractive and impressive figure (he was 6 foot 4 inches tall), if somewhat austere and demanding (with a reputation for reducing female students to tears), Tonks used his knowledge of anatomy to teach life drawing and became an

important and inspiring teacher: as a draughtsman he was arguably better qualified to represent the work of the British Army Medical Services than any other artist at the time.[15] His pupils in the 1890s included such celebrated artists as Augustus John, William Orpen and Wyndham Lewis and, in the decade leading up to 1914, Stanley Spencer, CRW Nevinson and Paul Nash.[17] All went on to produce striking and often controversial images of the war: Nevinson's 1917 painting *Paths of Glory*, showing two dead British soldiers lying face down in the mud in a barbed-wire-strewn wasteland, was famously censored by the War Office.

It also seems likely that Gillies was well aware of the publicity value of having someone with Tonks' reputation and standing in the art world involved, through his association with the Slade and the New English Art Club (NEAC) – the London equivalent of the Salon des Refusés, founded in 1886 for British artists wishing to exhibit their work outside the stuffier confines of the Royal Academy[17] – not to mention a circle of friends that included such well-known artistic figures as John Singer Sargent, Walter Sickert and Philip Wilson Steer. Tonks and Sargent were later sent to France as official war artists in June 1918, where Tonks painted *An Advanced Dressing Station in France* (Colour plate 8).

Joseph Hone's biography *The Life of Henry Tonks*[14] includes a letter (p. 127) written by Tonks in April 1916 to his friend, the influential painter, art critic and museum administrator Dugald Sutherland MacColl (1859–1948). MacColl had also taken art lessons from Frederick Brown, and, like Tonks, was a regular exhibitor at the NEAC.

I am doing a number of pastel heads of wounded soldiers who had their faces knocked about. A very good surgeon called Gillies who is nearly a champion golf player is undertaking what is known as the plastic surgery necessary. It is a chamber of horrors, but I am quite content to draw them as it is excellent practice. One poor fellow has the DCM, a large part of his mouth has been blown away, he is extraordinary and contented. I hope Gillies will make a good job of him. You bring up flaps from wherever is convenient. I may be going abroad. I

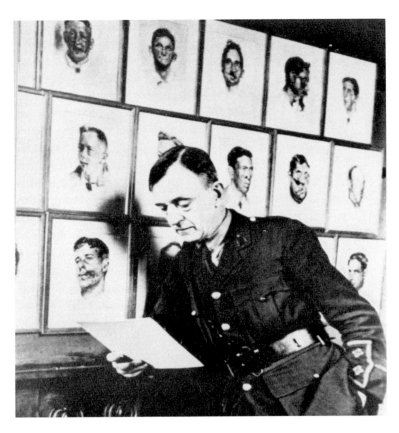

FIGURE 4.4. *Henry Tonks FRCS in the uniform of a lieutenant in the RAMC, with a display of his pastels. Tonks had trained as a surgeon before giving up medicine to become a teacher at the Slade School of Art, University College London. He recorded the plastic surgery carried out by Gillies (whom he thought 'a very good surgeon') and his team at Aldershot and Sidcup, including 72 pastel sketches housed in the Hunterian Museum at the Royal College of Surgeons of England.*

put down my name when I was not satisfied with my work here; now I might just as well stop, as I am faint use here.

Unlike the other artists attached to plastic and maxillofacial units at the time, who commonly used watercolour to document facial injuries, Tonks chose pastel as his medium. Seventy-two of these are housed in the Hunterian Museum at the Royal College of Surgeons of England and may be viewed online under Tonks at www.surgicat.rcseng.ac.uk. As Diana Orpen, a former student, recalled in her personal memoir of Henry Tonks,[18] 'Not long before his death in 1936 this great but alarming man said to me, "The only drawings that I ever made and am not ashamed of are the ones I made for Harold Gillies in the 1914–18 war."' Although Tonks' drawings are beautifully executed and justifiably acclaimed as representing the complete fusion of artist and anatomist, one cannot help feeling that his innate compassion and use of pastel softened the stark reality and despair captured by black and white

photography. Tonks' contract with the War Office terminated at the end of 1916 and he resigned his commission, continuing his association with Gillies in a civilian capacity. For the record, this suggests that the photograph in Figure 4.4 was taken at Aldershot in 1916, not in 1917 at Sidcup as usually reported (see also Figure 5.4).

Lately, Tonks' First World War pastels have undergone something of a renaissance among the academic art community, with several exhibitions of his work and scholarly articles.[19] For those who work directly with patients it is interesting to discover how others regard Tonks' images, particularly the extent to which their purpose has been intellectualised. Whether they occupy an ambiguous middle ground between portraiture and medical illustration, or raise uncomfortable questions regarding the nature of subjectivity and the ethics of viewing, depends on one's background: practical-minded clinicians are likely to take a more utilitarian view than those with an artistic temperament, and regard them as pictorial representations of soldiers with facial trauma. Unfortunately, when printed in black and white, Tonks' pastels lose much of their impact and appear little different from Sydney Walbridge's clinical photographs – the likely reason why only five were included by Gillies in *Plastic Surgery of the Face* (1920).

Masks for facial disfigurement: 3rd London General Hospital

At the beginning of the war many of the major facial defects at Aldershot and other hospitals were not reconstructed by plastic surgery, but were masked by external prostheses.[20,21] Facial masks were used in cases involving extensive tissue loss, or where the patient had decided against further surgery, but very few examples remain. The leading exponent of this technique in the United Kingdom was Francis

Derwent Wood, a sculptor who was working at the 3rd London General Hospital in Wandsworth as head of the splint-making department. Disturbed by the reaction of relatives to disfigured soldiers, and the suicides of the soldiers themselves, he requested permission to open a workshop for constructing facial masks. This was granted and the Masks for Facial Disfigurement Department, predictably nicknamed 'The Tin Noses Shop', came into being. The 3rd London General, which occupied an impressive Scottish baronial pile erected in 1859 as the Royal Victoria Patriotic Asylum (an orphanage for the daughters of former servicemen who had fought during the Crimean War), was one of a number of public buildings earmarked by Sir Alfred Keogh for use as an auxiliary hospital in the event of hostilities. It was requisitioned by the War Office on 5 August 1914 – the day after the declaration of

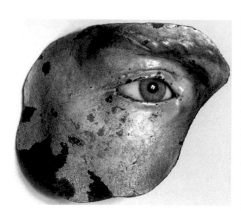

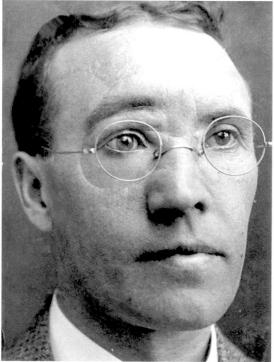

FIGURE 4.5. *In cases involving extensive tissue loss, or where the patient had decided against further surgery, major facial defects were not reconstructed by plastic surgery, but masked by external prostheses – commonly referred to as 'tin faces' by the soldiers. The painted mask on the left was made by Archibald Lane, a dental technician at the Queen's Hospital, Sidcup, and secured in position by spectacles.* (Reproduced courtesy of the Gillies Archive, Queen Mary's Hospital, Sidcup)

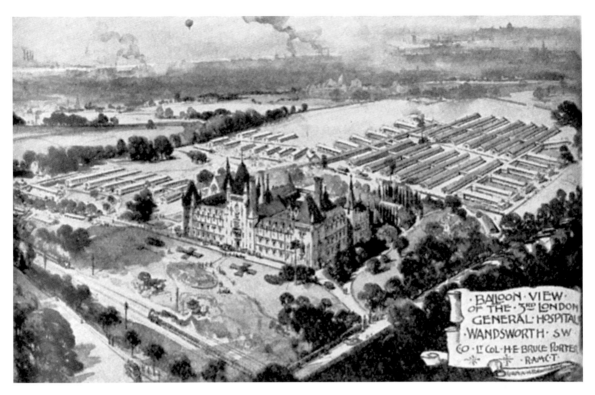

FIGURE 4.6. *The 3rd London General Hospital at Wandsworth, southwest London. Wash-drawing by Albert Henry Fullwood (1863–1930). Fullwood worked as an RAMC orderly at the hospital from April 1915 until November 1917, before being sent to France as an official war artist with the Australian Imperial Force.* (From The Gazette of the 3rd London General Hospital, *November 1916*)

war. The surgical and medical staff were supplied by the Middlesex, St Mary's and University College Hospitals, and with the addition of huts in the extensive grounds, 3rd London General grew into one of the largest hospitals in the country with up to 2000 beds.

To provide sufficient orderlies for the hospital, the commanding officer, Lieutenant Colonel HE Bruce Porter CMG, RAMC(T), had the brilliant idea of recruiting members of the Chelsea Arts Club who were either too old or otherwise unfit for military service. In addition to Wood, the hospital thus acquired an eclectic assortment of artists, sculptors, writers and journalists among its RAMC orderlies. Some were very distinguished artists with an Australian background, such as Tom Roberts and Arthur Streeton (both of whom were of the Heidelberg School and painted en plein air in the Impressionist tradition), George Coates, and

Henry Fullwood, who produced the aerial view of the hospital in Figure 4.6. Roberts, who joined the hospital in 1915 at the age of 53, worked as a porter and eventually became the sergeant in charge of the dental department, while Streeton and Fullwood were later appointed official war artists attached to the Australian Imperial Force (AIF) and sent to France as honorary lieutenants. Richard Nevinson, who had served in France as an ambulance driver in 1914, also spent time at the 3rd London General as an RAMC orderly before returning to the Western Front in 1917 as an official war artist.

Another bright idea of Lieutenant Colonel Porter, and an enduring legacy of his decision to enlist members of the Chelsea Arts Club as orderlies, was *The Gazette of the 3rd London General Hospital Wandsworth* – a journal published monthly from October 1915 until July 1919, price threepence, containing articles, cartoons and

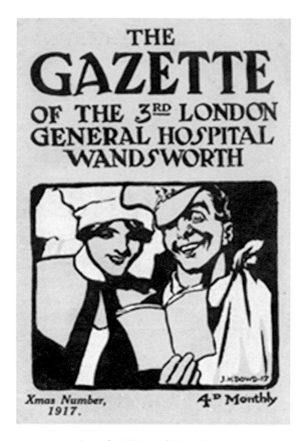

FIGURE 4.7. *Cover by JH Dowd,* Punch *cartoonist and illustrator of children's books, who was an RAMC orderly at the hospital.*

drawings contributed by the staff and patients. Nevinson contributed several illustrations in his Futurist–Vorticist style after he had left; others included JH Dowd, RB Ogle, HM Bateman and J Hodgson Lobley. The editor was a journalist by the name of Ward Muir. *The Gazette* is a unique and particularly rich source of information which, together with Muir's *Observations of an Orderly* (1917) and *The Happy Hospital* (1918),[22] provides a matchless insight into life at an auxiliary military hospital in England. The 3rd London General closed in August 1920 and in the six years of its existence treated over 62,000 patients from all over the British Empire.

As Wood explained in *The Lancet*,[23] his work began when the surgeon's work was complete. He attempted, using his skill as a sculptor, to make a man's face as near as possible to what it had been like before he was wounded. A plaster-of-Paris cast was made of the face and was then electroplated to produce a copper mask. This was coated with a thin layer of silver, and then hand-painted in oil-based enamel to match the flesh tones of the patient. Wood's prosthetic reconstructions were in the tradition of the French military surgeon Ambroise Paré (1510–1590), whose outstanding surgical treatise *Les Oeuvres de M. Ambroise Paré* (1575) contains illustrations of artificial noses, eyes and ears made of gold or silver and then enamelled. Influenced by the work of Wood, in November 1917 an American sculptor from Massachusetts by the name of Anna Coleman Ladd (1878–1939) opened the American Red Cross Studio for Portrait-Masks at the Val-de-Grâce Military Hospital in Paris. There is no record of the number of masks created by Wood, but in Ladd's case the number is unlikely to have been much more than a hundred.[24] The masks were uncomfortable and difficult to secure in place. Eventually it was the soldiers' own attitude to the masks that put an end to them: 'Can't you give us something we can wash and shave and won't fall off in the street?'[20] The challenge was accepted, and massive grafts of soft tissue and bone – which were not previously thought possible – were soon found to be practicable.

John Bagot Glubb

One former patient who did not share Ward Muir's description of the 3rd London General as the 'Happy Hospital' was John Glubb (1897–1986).[25] On 24 November 1915 Second Lieutenant John Bagot Glubb left for France at the age of 18 to join the 7th Field Company, Royal Engineers; he was to serve at Ypres, on the Somme, at Arras and Cambrai. On the evening of 21 August 1917, while out on his horse, he was severely wounded in the face at Hénin near Arras by a German long-range shell. The wound was plugged by an RAMC orderly, which stopped the bleeding, and after some days at No 20 CCS at Ficheux in the Pas-de-Calais, Glubb was taken to Rouen where he was marked with one of Gillies' labels – 'Cambridge Hospital, Aldershot',

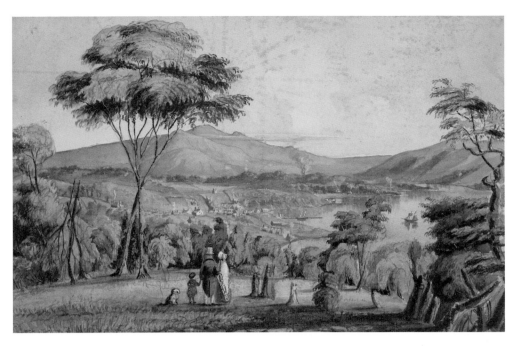

PLATE 1. *Dunedin from Little Paisley. The weaving industry in Paisley was in recession through much of the 1840s and many came to Otago where part of Dunedin became known as 'Little Paisley'. Contemporary paintings such as this, reminiscent of Nicolas Poussin, created the impression Dunedin was an arcadian paradise; the reality was somewhat different.* (Watercolour by Edward Immyns Abbot, 1849. Courtesy of the Hocken Collections, Uare Taoka o Hakena, University of Otago, accession number 14,414)

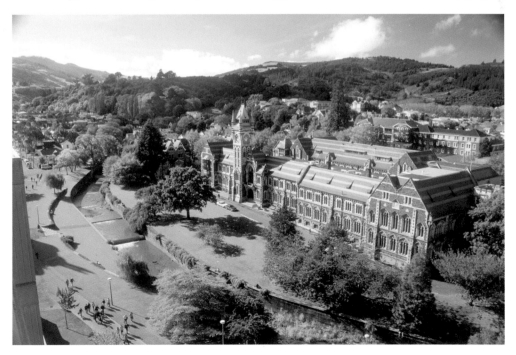

PLATE 2. *Contemporary view of the University of Otago Clocktower complex adjacent to the Water of Leith (Leith Stream). Southward extensions carried out by Edmund Anscombe (1874–1948) in 1912 and 1922, constructed in local materials such as Leith andesite and Port Chalmers bluestone with white Oamaru limestone facings consistent with the original Gothic design, helped reinforce Dunedin's image as the 'Edinburgh of the South'.* (Photograph courtesy of Fotosearch.com: J41-400962)

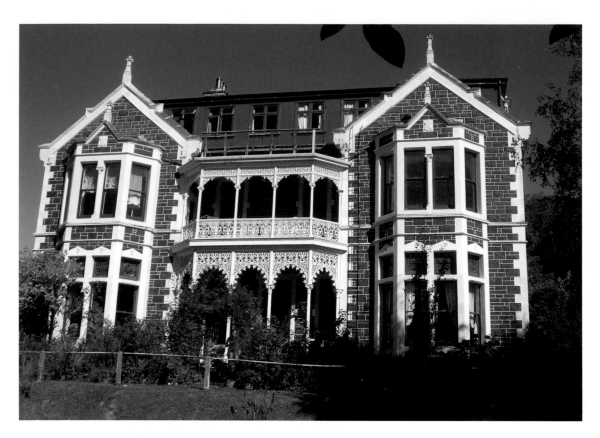

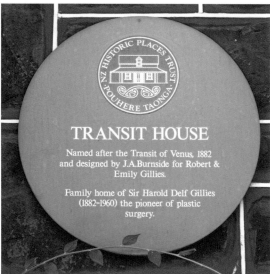

NZ HISTORIC PLACES TRUST · POUHERE TAONGA ·

TRANSIT HOUSE

Named after the Transit of Venus, 1882
and designed by J.A.Burnside for Robert &
Emily Gillies.

Family home of Sir Harold Delf Gillies
(1882–1960) the pioneer of plastic
surgery.

PLATE 3. *'Transit House', 44 Park Street, Dunedin, home of Robert and Emily Gillies, viewed from the eastern aspect. Robert Gillies, a keen amateur astronomer, had an observatory installed in a revolving dome in the roof. The Transit of Venus was observed in 1882, the year the house was built – hence the name. From 1940 to 1980 the building, renamed Dominican Hall, was used as a hall of residence for Catholic female university students. Unfortunately, the Sisters replaced the roof with an ugly dormitory.*

(Photograph 2007, courtesy of Harriet Meikle)

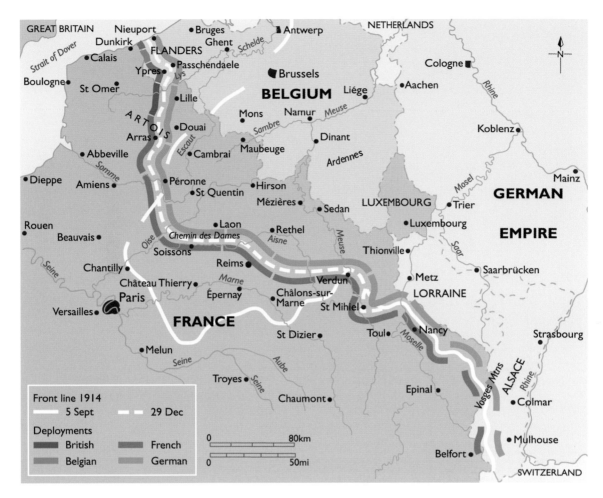

GREAT BRITAIN

Strait of Dover

NETHERLANDS

Nieuport • •Bruges Ghent •▲Antwerp
Dunkirk Schelde
•Calais FLANDERS
Ypres• •Passchendaele Brussels BELGIUM Liége
Boulogne• St Omer Lys •Aachen Cologne■
•Lille Mons •Namur Meuse Rhine
ARTOIS •Douai Sambre Dinant Koblenz•
Arras• •Cambrai Maubeuge
•Abbeville Escaut Ardennes Mosel
•Dieppe Amiens• Somme •Péronne •Hirson Mainz
•St Quentin Mézières• LUXEMBOURG GERMAN
Rouen• Laon• •Rethel •Sedan •Trier EMPIRE
Beauvais• Chemin des Dames Aisne Meuse •Luxembourg
Oise Soissons• Reims• Thionville• Saar
Seine Chantilly• Marne Verdun •Metz •Saarbrücken
Château Thierry• Épernay Châlons-sur- LORRAINE
Paris• Marne St Mihiel• •Nancy
Versailles• FRANCE St Dizier• Toul• Strasbourg
Moselle
•Melun Seine ALSACE
Seine Aube •Epinal Rhine
Troyes• Colmar
Chaumont• Vosges Mtns
•Mulhouse
Belfort•
SWITZERLAND

Front line 1914
——— 5 Sept   - - - 29 Dec
Deployments
■ British   ■ French
■ Belgian   ■ German

0   80km
0   50mi

PLATE 4. *Map of the Western Front. By the end of August 1914, a series of German victories had forced the Anglo-French armies into a general retreat south of the River Marne, less than 30 miles from Paris. The city was saved by a counter-attack by the French Fifth and Sixth Armies and the BEF in the First Battle of the Marne (6–10 September 1914), which forced the German army to retreat 40 miles back over the Rivers Marne and Aisne to the north of Rheims. This was followed by the 'Race to the Sea' in which both armies tried to outflank each other – by December 1914 a continuous battlefront of trenches, fortifications and barbed wire entanglements was established from Switzerland to the North Sea.* (Graphic by Allan Kynaston)

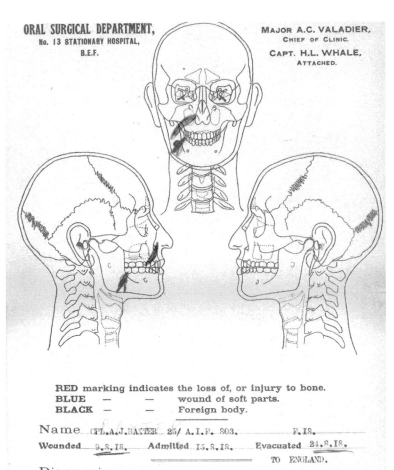

ORAL SURGICAL DEPARTMENT,
No. 13 STATIONARY HOSPITAL,
B.E.F.

MAJOR A.C. VALADIER,
CHIEF OF CLINIC.

CAPT. H.L. WHALE,
ATTACHED.

RED marking indicates the loss of, or injury to bone.
BLUE   —   —   wound of soft parts.
BLACK   —   —   Foreign body.

Name (PL.A.J.BAXTER 25/ A.I.F. 803.   F.IS.
Wounded 9.8.18.   Admitted 15.8.18.   Evacuated 24.8.18.
                                        TO ENGLAND.

Diagnosis:

Entry wound over right cheek. X-Ray shows fracture right mandibular angle with F.B. (shell fragment) at site of fracture.
Operation 16.8.18. F.B. removed via mouth. Deep groove on dorsum of tongue stitched. Face wound excised and sutured. Tube drain through stab at left mandibular angle. 22.8.18. Face sutured mucous membrane trimmed in mouth.

PLATE 5. *Chart for recording head and neck injuries used by Major AC Valadier and Captain HL Whale in the Oral Surgery Department at No 13 Stationary Hospital, BEF. In this patient, admitted on 15 August 1918, a shell fragment (black) is lodged in the angle of the jaw at the site of a fracture (red); there is also a facial flesh wound (blue).* (Courtesy of the Army Medical Services Museum Archives, Keogh Barracks, Aldershot)

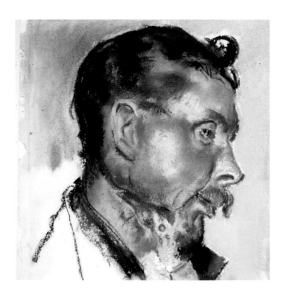

PLATE 6. Portrait of a Serviceman (detail) *by Henry Tonks. Pastels on paper, 27.1 cm x 21.3 cm (RCSSC/P 569.49). Gillies used this sketch as the frontispiece in Volume I of* The Principles and Art of Plastic Surgery *(1957).* (Reproduced with the kind permission of the Hunterian Museum at the Royal College of Surgeons of England)

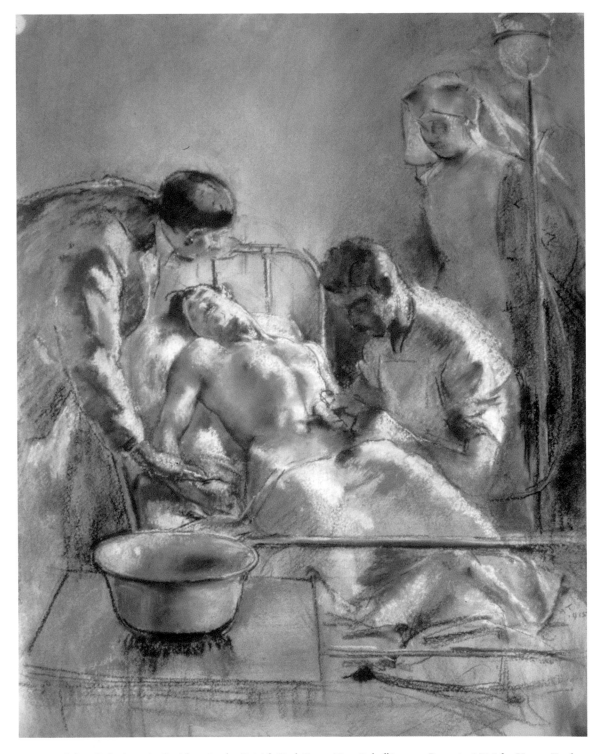

PLATE 7. Saline Infusion: An Incident in the British Red Cross Hospital, d'Arc-en-Barrois, 1915 *by Henry Tonks.*
Pastels on paper, 67.9 cm x 52 cm. Imperial War Museum (IWM ART 1918). At the outbreak of war, Tonks,
although he was fifty-two, was eager to help and in January 1915 was in the village of d'Arc-en-Barrois in the
Haute-Marne, working as a volunteer in a hospital for French wounded. (By kind permission of the Imperial War Museum, London)

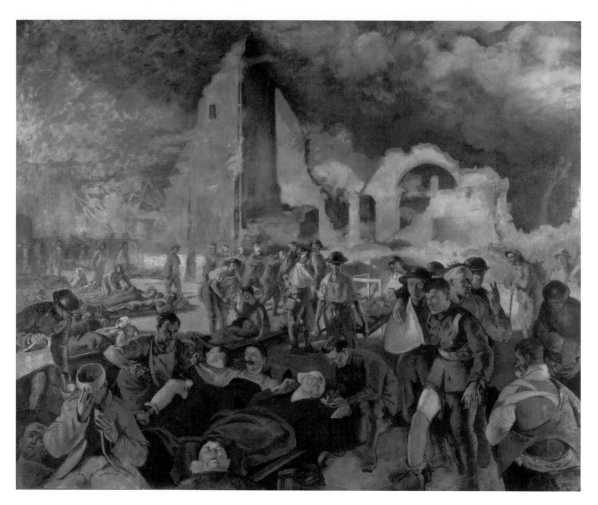

PLATE 8. An Advanced Dressing Station in France *by Henry Tonks. In June 1918 Tonks and John Singer Sargent were sent as official war artists to France, attached to the Guards Division at Arras. Tonks was commissioned to record the work of the RAMC and produced this painting from studies made while stationed near Berles-au-Bois, a commune in the Pas de Calais. 'The advanced dressing station was an incredible sight in time of battle, a kind of organized confusion, by this I mean an apparent confusion because they were beautifully run and I pride myself that it gives a reasonable account of modern war.'* (IWM: ART 1922. Reproduced with the kind permission of the Imperial War Museum, London)

FACING: PLATE 10.
LEFT: Portrait of Private Walter Ashworth *by Henry Tonks, 1916. Pastels on paper, 27.3 cm x 20.9 cm (RCSSC/P569.50).* RIGHT: *Tonks' planning diagram of the proposed operation. Ink and pencil on paper, 28.8 cm x 20.5 cm (RCSSC/P 569.51).* (Reproduced with the kind permission of the Hunterian Museum at the Royal College of Surgeons of England)

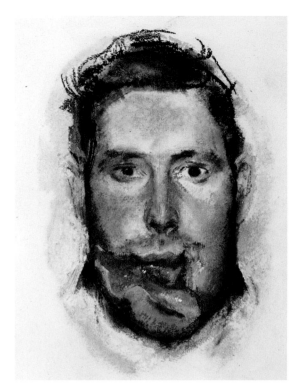
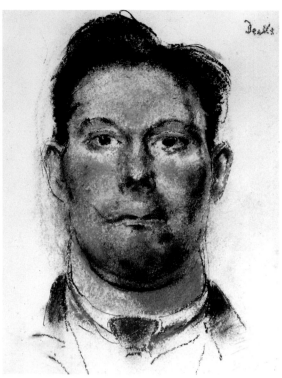

ABOVE: PLATE 9. Portrait(s) of Private Charles Deeks *by Henry Tonks. Deeks, a twenty-five-year-old private in the King's Own Royal Lancaster Regiment, had received facial wounds from a machine-gun bullet on 1 July 1916.* LEFT: *Pastels on paper, 26.8 cm x 20 cm (RCSSC/P 569.1).* RIGHT: *Pastels on paper, 28.5 cm by 20.8 cm (RCSSC/P 569.2).* (Reproduced with the kind permission of the Hunterian Museum at the Royal College of Surgeons of England)

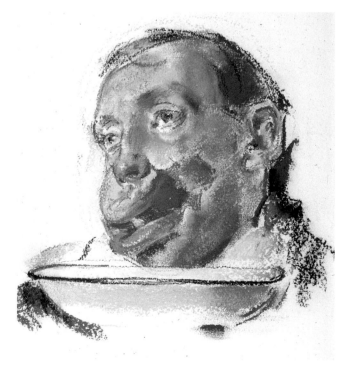
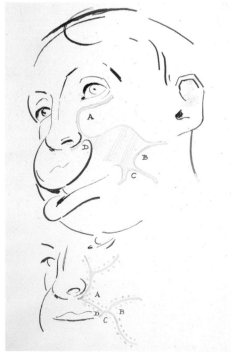

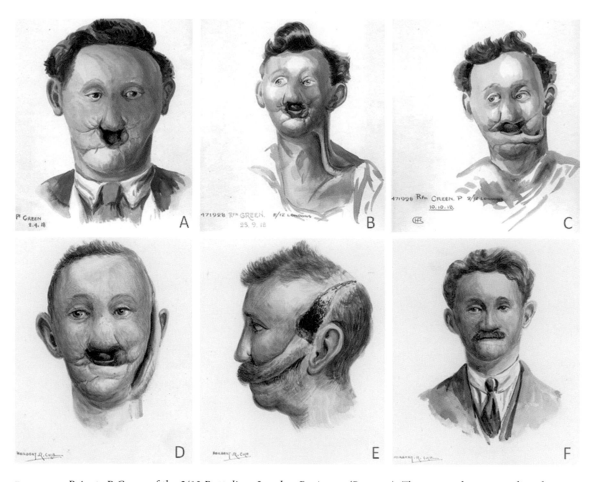

PLATE 11. *Private P Green of the 2/12 Battalion, London Regiment (Rangers). The watercolours recording the sequence of operations were painted by Herbert Cole and demonstrate a maturing of his painting technique following lessons at the Slade School of Art, University College London. The final watercolour corresponds to a photograph dated 28.12.19.* (The top three watercolours are from the Macalister Archive in the Gillies Archive, Queen Mary's Hospital, Sidcup; the bottom three are in the Hocken Library, Uare Taoka o Hakena, University of Otago, Pickerill papers, Reference number MS-1620/013, reproduced with permission.)

and repatriated to England. However, on the boat he was advised that since Gillies' unit was no longer at Aldershot, he was to be transferred to the 3rd London General. Glubb describes his arrival (pp. 193–94):

Arrived at Wandsworth. I was trundled down long passages on a wheeled stretcher and into another ward. A VAD gave me a wonderful drink of cocoa. Later on a sister came and dressed my wound which was incredibly putrid and evil-smelling. My pyjamas were soaked in this putrescent discharge as well as my bandages. Its smell hung over me like a cloud. I had not been bandaged or cleaned since we left Rouen.

I lay for three months in my bed in Wandsworth, during which my wound remained septic, and received no medical attention. About once a week, we were all carried down long passages and lined up on our stretchers outside the doctor's door. We were then carried in, one at a time. The doctor would say to the ward sister, 'Temperature normal? Bowels open? No complications? Right. Take him away and bring in the next.' No doctor ever looked at our wounds or removed our bandages. Presumably there were not enough doctors.

Glubb was being charitable. Desperate to escape, he sent numerous applications to all and sundry via his mother, requesting a transfer to another hospital, and considering his father was a general in the Royal Engineers, why it took so long is something of a mystery. Eventually, however, in November 1917 he was moved to Sidcup where he came under the care of Gillies and Kelsey Fry. As he recalls:

Here things were very different. My broken and septic teeth were extracted and my wound cleaned. The problem then was how to reunite the broken fragments of my lower jaw bone, which were still hanging loosely in my mouth. The solution adopted was to set the broken bones of the lower jaw and then cement it to the upper jaw, which thereby acted as a splint to hold the pieces of the lower jaw in position. As I had lost almost all of my front teeth in both jaws, I was able to push small pieces

of food into my mouth between my gums. While I was at Sidcup I received the notification that I had been awarded the Military Cross … As most of my lower jaw had gone, I was shown an album of photographs of handsome young men and asked to choose the chin I would like to have!

Glubb declined to have his chin reconstructed (as later photographs show), since it would have required additional months in hospital and he was keen to get back into action. After a period of convalescence he was passed fit by a medical board and in June 1918 returned to the front for the last few months of the war. Unfortunately, his Sidcup medical records have not survived. Better known as 'Glubb Pasha', in 1930 he became an officer in the Arab Legion, and in 1939 its commanding officer. He retired in 1956 as Lieutenant-General Sir John Glubb KCB, CMG, DSO, OBE, MC, after his dismissal by King Hussein of Jordan, who wished to distance himself from the British. Glubb was affectionately known by the Bedouin as *Abu Hunaik* – 'Father of the Little Jaw'.

While he was languishing at Wandsworth, it is difficult to understand how Glubb managed to avoid being seen and treated in the Dental Department by the hospital's dental staff, which included William Warwick James[†], a distinguished, doubly qualified dental surgeon with an FRCS (see Figure 3.12). In addition to his private practice, James was on the honorary staffs of the Royal Dental Hospital, the Middlesex Hospital and the Hospital for Sick Children, Great Ormond Street. During the war he worked in the Maxillofacial Unit at the 3rd London General Hospital, where he demonstrated considerable skill in repairing facial injuries and, together with his surgical colleague Zachary Cope (Sir Vincent Zachary Cope, 1881–1974), carried out many successful bone grafts of the mandible. In 1940, with BW Fickling[†], he wrote *Injuries of the Jaws and Face*,[26] based on what remained of the clinical case records from the 3rd London General that had not been destroyed by the Ministry of Pensions when the hospital was closed down in 1920. (Since it is rare for one generation to appreciate what the next might regard as being of historical interest, it is perhaps naïve to assume that medical records would be treated any differently.) Warwick James and Fickling were also able to contact and re-examine as many as 50 of the unit's former patients, and this provided valuable evidence regarding the best approach to the treatment of jaw fractures (see Chapter 10). In view of the high standard of maxillofacial surgery available at the hospital during the war, one can only conclude the size of the hospital and the attitude of some of the medical staff meant that patients sometimes got lost in the system.

The treatment of infected wounds

Unlike the British Army's previous war in South Africa, fought largely on the veldt – open spaces covered in grass or low scrub, on soil that was practically sterile – in Northern France and Flanders bullets, shrapnel and other missiles carried bacteria into the tissues from contaminated clothing and soil. The centuries-old heavily manured fields with their rich microbial flora provided an ideal medium for growth of the spore-forming anaerobic *Clostridium* species (*C tetani* and *C perfringens*, formerly *C welchii*) that caused tetanus and gas gangrene, the two most serious complications of wounds. Tetanus was prevalent at the beginning of the war, but the practice of injecting anti-tetanus serum at the earliest opportunity markedly reduced the number of fatalities. Gas gangrene, however, was a much more intractable problem. The RAMC had never experienced it before and had no idea how to treat it. Soldiers with contaminated wounds died in droves from gas gangrene, particularly after the Battle of the Marne in 1914, when difficulties were encountered in rapidly evacuating the wounded. Even amputation often failed to halt progression of the disease.[27] As the American surgeon George Crile, operating three years later at No 17 CCS during the Third Battle of Ypres, recorded in his autobiography for 3 August 1917 (p. 302):

I operated all day and all night. Our dump ran as high as eighty waiting. At one time we were thirty-six hours behind the list waiting on the stretchers for operation. Many of those acquired gas gangrene

while waiting. Each day of delay was marked by the noise of saws in the waiting room. Many were lost on account of the 'gas gangrene of delay.'[28]

In the early months of the war, controversy regarding the surgical management of wounds soon arose. It revolved around two questions: first, the extent to which strong antiseptics should be applied; and second, the merits of early (primary) closure versus delayed (secondary) closure of wounds. Joseph Lister had revolutionised the treatment of open fractures with the use of carbolic acid to sterilise wounds,[29] and the Listerian tradition of antisepsis was firmly adhered to by the RAMC. The old chemical antiseptics such as carbolic acid, hydrogen peroxide and 2 percent iodine in spirit were widely used in military hospitals for cleansing infected wounds, but while these killed some of the bacteria, they were also toxic and irritating to the tissues. Overall the results were disappointing. The introduction in 1915 of the hypochlorite-based antiseptics Eusol (Edinburgh University solution of lime)[30] and Dakin's solution[31] represented an improvement, but hypochlorous solutions rapidly lost their antiseptic power. This problem was surmounted by Alexis Carrel, who devised a technique for continuously irrigating wounds via a system of rubber tubing; however, since open wounds required dressing several times a day, prolonged use of antiseptics with delayed wound closure placed heavy demands on an already stretched nursing service.

Because of differences in wound management between British and French surgeons, a meeting of the Inter-allied Surgical Conference was held at the Val-de-Grâce Hospital in May 1917 to discuss best practice. Belgian surgeon Antoine Depage (1862–1925) and French surgeon Samuel-Jean Pozzi (1846–1918) had both worked closely with Carrel and, together with other French surgeons, had reintroduced the practice of debridement plus irrigation with Dakin's solution. This allowed them to close wounds between the fourth and twelfth day post-injury – 'delayed primary closure' – which reduced the failure rate for soft-tissue injuries from 10 percent to 3 percent.[32] Surgeon-General Sir Anthony Bowlby, consulting surgeon to the BEF, was impressed by these results, and accepted the method for use in all RAMC hospitals. However, in a review of the background leading up to the acceptance of primary wound closure which he published in the *British Medical Journal*,[33] Bowlby failed to acknowledge the work of Colonel Sir Henry Gray (1870–1938) and other BEF surgeons. This earned him a reprimand from Gray, who pointed out that the foundations of excision and primary wound closure had been successfully established in an unostentatious manner by himself and others as early as November 1914.[34] (Perhaps of more interest to the lay reader than this controversy is that Pozzi conducted a 10-year affair with Sarah Bernhardt, who called him Docteur Dieu; had his portrait painted by John Singer Sargent in 1881; and was murdered in his consulting rooms by a deranged patient, who shot him four times in the abdomen before committing suicide.[35])

Sir Almroth Wright and Captain Fleming were not persuaded

Sir Almroth Wright and Alexander Fleming, who were working in the bacteriology laboratory at No 13 General Hospital in Boulogne, were not persuaded about the use of antiseptics. Fleming's experiments had shown that not only could the bacteria causing tetanus, gangrene and other infections be cultivated from samples of clothing taken from wounded men, but also that chemical antiseptics did not have an appreciable effect in sterilising wounds. In fact, Fleming had shown in a series of elegant test-tube experiments that antiseptics in the presence of serum not only favoured the growth of bacteria, but also killed the leucocytes (white blood cells, including neutrophils, macrophages and lymphocytes) that play a key role in host immunity, thereby compromising the patient's ability to fight infection.[36] Their recommendation was to surgically remove as much dead and damaged tissue as possible and, instead of antiseptics, to irrigate the tissues freely with hypertonic saline (5% NaCl) to stimulate the body's natural defences, followed by immediate closure of the wound.[37] (This approach, it has to be said, sounds remarkably similar to that reported by Gray

in 1915.) Needless to say the RAMC was reluctant to adopt such iconoclastic advice, even from such an important medical scientist as Wright, who had developed an anti-typhoid vaccine before the Boer War.[38] (Sir Almroth Wright, an outspoken advocate of mass immunisation and opponent of women's suffrage, was reputed to be the model for the unscrupulous Sir Colenso Ridgeon in George Bernard Shaw's 1906 play *The Doctor's Dilemma* – not Sir William Arbuthnot Lane, as is sometimes reported.)

If the patient survived these first few critical days before arriving at one of the maxillofacial units in the Boulogne area (or if they were lucky enough to have a 'Blighty One' and be sent to England), wound infection, the destruction of soft and hard tissues, plus the retention of foreign bodies such as tooth fragments and shrapnel presented maxillofacial surgeons with formidable reconstructive problems. Other complicating factors included limited suction in operating theatres, the difficulties of administering general anaesthetics to patients with facial trauma, a lack of stored blood for transfusion, and no antibiotics. There were also virtually no forms of resuscitation, and no special instruments.[39] Transport and communication were problematic too – the evacuation of casualties from France to England took an average of about 10 days (provided they didn't get lost on the way). In the circumstances, it is surprising the results turned out as well as they did. One thing maxillofacial surgeons had in their favour, however – an advantage not shared by other surgeons – was the rich supply of blood of the head and neck, which aided the survival of damaged tissues.

Early plastic operations at Aldershot

In two papers published in 1917, and later included in *Plastic Surgery of the Face*, Gillies reported on the outcome of some of the soldiers who had been treated at Aldershot.[40,41] These cases are of particular interest because they were treated within the first few months of the establishment of the unit, most of them following the Battle of the Somme, and the deformities are comparatively minor by later Sidcup standards. At the time, Gillies and his colleagues were operating under extremely difficult conditions. Overnight surgeons were dealing not with minor injuries but with the prospect of having to reconstruct half a face. The operations were therefore performed during the experimental phase of facial reconstruction, when many of the elementary principles that were eventually adopted were being worked out through trial and error.

The first article, 'Mechanical supports in plastic surgery', published by Gillies with Captain Leonard King in *The Lancet* (17 March 1917), emphasised the importance of close cooperation between dentist and surgeon in treating injuries to the face and jaws. The most common cause of failures in plastic surgery, in their opinion, was the failure to provide a suitable substructure.[40] The cases chosen to illustrate the value of combined work were mainly examples of prosthetic appliances that had been used to fill large bony defects, particularly of the maxilla (upper jaw) and, to a limited extent, the mandible (lower jaw). The use of rib grafts of cartilage and bone, or bone from the tibia and the iliac crest, to reconstruct major osseous defects of the mandible was yet to become routine.

The problem of tissue loss

Lacerations involving the soft tissues could be accurately reapproximated or joined with minimal scarring. However, with more extensive tissue loss the temptation was to cover the gap by pulling adjacent tissue together with straight advancement flaps, when in reality what was needed was the introduction of new tissue. Gillies' second paper, published in the May 1917 edition of the *St Bartholomew's Hospital Journal*, illustrates the problems that could be encountered with advancement flaps.[41]

In Case 1 the loss of tissue comprised: (1) the nasal bones, underlying portion of the nasal septum, frontal spine and the nasal processes of both maxillary bones; (2) the skin covering this area, and (3) the right eye. There was a small opening into the nose about half an inch square, surrounded by scar tissue and granulations (Case 268 in *Plastic Surgery of the Face*, pp. 218–19). The first operation, on 4 June 1916, involved excision of the scar tissue and the submucous resection of

a piece of the perpendicular plate of the ethmoid, which was swung forward to form a bridge and sutured to the nasal septum with catgut. Two sliding lateral flaps from the cheek were cut, undermined and sutured over the bridge with fine interrupted silk sutures (Figure 4.8). Primary healing with a good cosmetic result occurred, apart from a slight breakdown at the angle of the right eye. However, the bridge of the nose gradually sank as the cartilage was not strong enough to support the contracting skin flaps. At the second operation (3 September 1916) a piece of rib cartilage was cut and inserted under the skin and periosteum, with its lower end resting on the cartilage of the lower part of the septum; two months later this end had slipped, producing a slight deformity.

In Case 2, Gillies discussed existing methods for treating surface depressions of the face caused by loss of the underlying bone, including fat grafts, cartilage grafts and foreign (alloplastic) materials such as celluloid, ivory or wax. In his experience fat grafts were unpredictable – after primary union, aseptic fat necrosis often set in about the tenth day, and he had found celluloid plates to be unsatisfactory because they acted as a tissue irritant, stimulating a foreign-body reaction in the patient. The method described in the article used a flap of temporal muscle, which was elevated from the bone, passed under the bridge of skin and sutured to the deep tissues to make up the contour. The long-term result was likely to have been equally unsatisfactory. Cases such as these undoubtedly contributed to one of Gillies' commandments: 'It may be laid down as a guiding maxim that the replacement should be as near as possible in terms of tissue loss – bone for bone, cartilage for cartilage, etc, etc.' However, he was not above ignoring his own advice when it suited him.

The soldier in Case 3 is of particular interest because there is not only a complete record of the surgery that was performed, but also before and after pastel portraits and planning diagrams drawn by Henry Tonks (Colour plate 9). Charles Deeks, a twenty-five-year-old private in the King's Own Royal Lancaster Regiment, had received facial wounds from a machine-gun bullet on 1

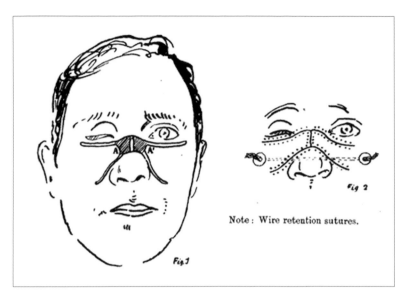

Note: Wire retention sutures.

FIGURE 4.8. *Case 1. Planning diagram drawn by Henry Tonks: Two sliding flaps were cut from the cheek, undermined and sutured over a bridge formed by a piece of the perpendicular plate of the ethmoid that had been sutured to the nasal septum. Tension in the sutures inevitably led to a breakdown of the wound. At Sidcup, nasal wounds like this were usually treated with rotational forehead flaps.* (*From Gillies (1917),* St Bartholomew's Hospital Journal)

July 1916 – the first day of the Battle of the Somme (Case 5 in *Plastic Surgery of the Face*, pp. 130–31). X-rays showed that the body of the right side of the mandible had been fractured in the region of the first molar tooth and the symphysis (midline), with the intermediate fragment of bone being displaced. At the first operation (11 September 1916), the scars were excised on both sides. On the right side the two surfaces of the cheek were drawn together and the mucous membrane from inside the mouth brought out to form a new angle. On the left side a combined skin and mucous membrane flap was swung towards the mouth in both the upper and lower lips. The result of this operation was satisfactory except that the movement of the lower jaw began to stretch the line of union of the flaps on the right cheek and the wound partially broke down near the corners of the mouth (Figure 4.9(C)); this was limited by fitting a closely applied chin splint and attaching it over the head.

A second operation (31 October 1916) involved the revision of scar tissue to raise the corner of the mouth on the right side. In a third operation (1 January 1917) part of the right scar which had

broken down was re-excised, and local fat flaps were turned in from above and below. These were sutured together with catgut and the skin sewn with fine interrupted horsehair sutures. A small mucous membrane correction was made on the left upper lip and the left lower lip was raised at the corner by making a horizontal incision through the whole thickness of the lip and sewing it up perpendicularly. The dental work was carried out by Captain FE Sprawson RAMC.

Another example of the problems associated with the closure of large soft-tissue defects with advancement flaps is Case 14 in *Plastic Surgery of the Face* (pp. 62–63). Private Walter Ashworth was another soldier who had received an extensive gunshot wound to the face at the Battle of the Somme, with destruction of the cheek and lips and loss of supporting bony structures, particularly involving the upper jaw (Colour plate 10 and Figure 4.10(A)). The fractures of the jaws were successfully reduced and his upper jaw (maxilla) was fixed with a bar attached to a headcap (Figure 4.10(B)). The first plastic operation was performed three months later, on 4 October 1916, when

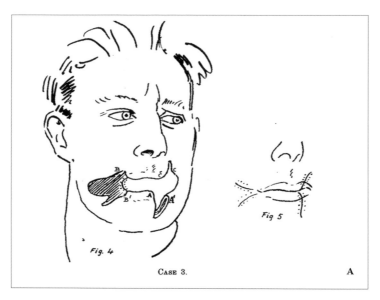

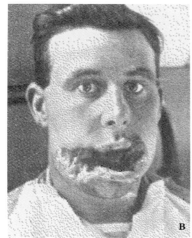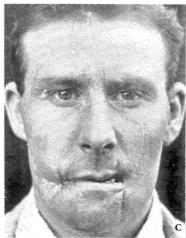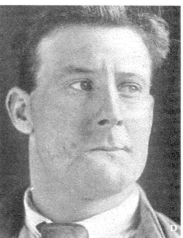

FIGURE 4.9. *Case 3. Private Charles Deeks.* (A) *Planning diagram drawn by Henry Tonks. On the right side the two surfaces of the cheek were sutured together and mucous membrane from inside the mouth used to form a new angle; on the left a combined skin and mucous membrane flap was swung towards the mouth in both the upper and lower lips.* (B) *On admission 3.7.1916.* (C) *After the first operation 11.9.1916. The result was satisfactory except that movement of the lower jaw began to stretch the line of union of the flaps on the right cheek and the wound partially broke down near the corners of the mouth; this was limited by fitting a closely applied chin splint and attaching it over the head. A second operation (31.10.1916) involved the revision of scar tissue to raise the corner of the mouth on the right side. In a third operation (1.1.1917), part of the right scar which had broken down was re-excised, and local fat flaps turned in from above and below. A small mucous membrane correction was made on the left upper lip and the left lower lip was raised at the corner by making a horizontal incision through the whole thickness of the lip and sewing it up perpendicularly.* (D) *After the third operation 1.1.1917.*

(*From Gillies (1917), St Bartholomew's Hospital Journal*)

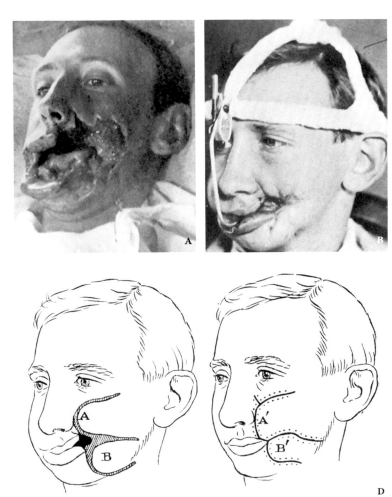

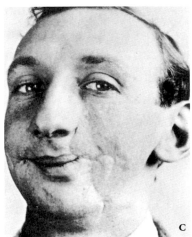

FIGURE 4.10. *Private Ashworth.*
(A) *Condition a few days after being wounded on 1.7.1916. After successfully reducing the fractures of the jaws, his upper jaw (maxilla) was stabilised with a bar attached to a headcap.* (B) *The healed condition three months later 4.10.1916 when the first plastic operation was carried out at Aldershot.* (C) *The healed condition in September 1917.*
(D) *Planning diagrams showing the excision of scar tissue and flaps A and B cut and sutured.* (From Gillies (1920), Plastic Surgery of the Face)

healing had apparently diminished the loss of tissue (Figure 4.10(D)). However, excision of the scar produced a very extensive gap. To meet this difficulty, two large swinging (rotating) flaps were made. The larger one (A) comprised the remains of the soft tissues of the cheek and was defined by means of an incision extending from the side of the nose and carried outwards beneath the eye to the malar prominence. The lower flap (B) was outlined by an incision carried down from near the corner of the mouth to below the mandible in the submaxillary region. These two thick flaps were widely undercut and swung towards each other – the upper flap completed the gap above the level of the mouth, while the lower one was sutured along its lower border. Because of the large deficiency of

mucous membrane it was not possible to complete the mouth to its original size and some sacrifice was made in the length of the lips. Relaxation sutures were inserted to retain the untouched part of the lower lip to the large cheek flap, and drainage was provided at a suitable spot. The result of this operation was satisfactory in that it produced a result that satisfied the patient, although it left him with a whimsical, one-sided expression (Figure 4.10(C)). But as Gillies was to comment 40 years later in *The Principles and Art of Plastic Surgery*, 'Double cheek advancement flaps produced a moderately reasonable result, but his mouth contraction was tight and his dental efficiency poor. His original tissue loss was too great to be closed without the introduction of new tissue.'

CHAPTER 5

The Queen's Hospital, Sidcup: Birthplace of modern plastic surgery

Written in collaboration with Andrew N Bamji

FOLLOWING THE BATTLE OF the Somme, it became clear that the 200 beds allocated to Gillies at Aldershot were inadequate for treating the unprecedented number of casualties arriving with major head wounds. However, lack of accommodation was not the only problem. Many of the patients suffered from depression and were acutely aware of their disfigured condition, refusing to return home until they were convinced everything possible had been done for them. Convalescence between operations was the answer, but the War Office refused to allow a military patient to leave hospital until he could be returned to the trenches. It was Gillies' attempt to have some of these patients placed in a convenient convalescent home that led indirectly to the move to Sidcup.[1] A committee that included Sir William Arbuthnot Lane approached Sir Charles Kenderdine, one of the founders and organisers of Queen Mary's Hospital, Roehampton, for guidance in the search for suitable premises.[1,2] Kenderdine advised a much more ambitious scheme than they had originally envisaged, and suggested that Frognal House at Sidcup in Kent, which had recently been inherited by Hugh Marsham-Townshend, might be available for sale. Frognal House and the extensive grounds would provide a suitable site for a new hospital, and its close proximity to the main railway line from Dover to London was an added advantage.

This advice was followed and Sir Charles Kenderdine undertook the organisation of the scheme along the same lines as Roehampton, which had been founded in 1915 as a centre for the rehabilitation of amputees. A general committee was formed with Kenderdine as honorary secretary and treasurer, and a public appeal for funds was launched. Generous donations were immediately forthcoming from Red Cross societies in the United Kingdom, Australia, Canada and New Zealand, the Order of St John of Jerusalem, the National Relief Fund, War Office, Admiralty and many other organisations and individuals, including the Queen's Special Fund. The project was greatly helped by the personal interest of Queen Mary, who acted as patron and commanded that on completion it should be named the Queen's Hospital, Sidcup. The Frognal Estate was leased and construction of the new hospital began in February 1917; it was completed in five months. Frognal House and about 90 acres, including the new hospital buildings, were then purchased by the National Relief Fund for £16,000, and handed over to three trustees – Viscount Chilston, Sir Arthur Stanley and Laurence Brock (representing the National Relief Fund) – for use as a hospital for pensioners of the war.[2]

The first patients were admitted in August 1917, and the cases that were being treated at Aldershot

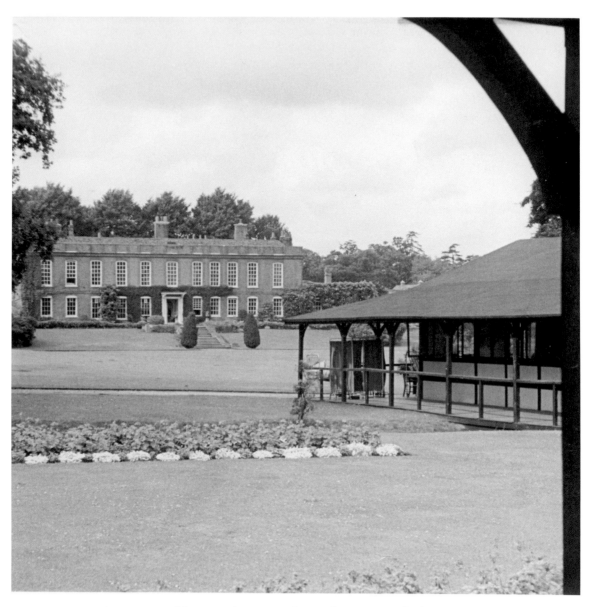

FIGURE 5.1. *Frognal House viewed from Ward IA. Frognal, a Jacobean mansion built in the early eighteenth century, was the birthplace and residence of Thomas Townshend, 1st Viscount Sydney, after whom the capital of New South Wales, Australia, was renamed (from Port Jackson) in 1785. Viscount Sydney was Secretary of State in the first Pitt government.* (Reproduced courtesy of the Gillies Archive, Queen Mary's Hospital, Sidcup)

were immediately transferred to Sidcup. Sir Alfred Keogh was so impressed with the hospital on his first visit that he decided it should be the Central Military Hospital for facial and jaw injuries not just for the United Kingdom, but for all the expeditionary forces. The scheme was immediately enlarged, and from August 1917 to March 1920, when it was taken over by the Ministry of Pensions, the hospital together with its auxiliary hospitals functioned under the War Office as a Central Military Hospital.

A British Empire Hospital

Sir William Arbuthnot Lane had been asked by Keogh to act as consulting surgeon to the new hospital. This put him in a powerful position to determine its future direction – consulting surgeons set the scope and standard of the clinical and scientific work of a military hospital, as well as the surgical policy to be followed by the administration.[3] In other words, unlike in contemporary civilian hospitals, the quality of the work rested with the consultants – and Lane was not averse to a little empire-building. He envisaged making Sidcup the largest and most important hospital for maxillofacial surgery in the world, and had singled out Gillies as the man to lead it. In a letter to Gillies on 6 September 1917, Lane wrote: 'I want to make Sidcup the *biggest* and *most important* hospital for jaws and plastic work in the world and you consequently a leader in this form of surgery,' and, in another letter: 'The larger the hospital, the bigger the men associated with it, the stronger will be your position. We must work together to this end.'[4]

Lane's fundamental aim was that it should be a British Empire Hospital, to which all casualties with facial wounds would be sent from every theatre of the war. The hospital was eventually divided into four sections – British, Australian, Canadian and New Zealand – each staffed by its own officers. This was achieved with some difficulty, requiring a good deal of persuasion and arm-twisting from Lane, as well as the personal intervention of Queen Mary, because each of the sections had wanted to remain with its own hospital. In addition to the Empire

contingents, with the entry of the United States into the war in April 1917 and the eventual arrival of their wounded, teams of American surgeons and dentists were attached to the hospital for specialised training.[2] (The names of the surgeons, dental surgeons and other officers who held appointments at Sidcup from 1917 until its closure in 1929 are listed in Appendix II.)

The hutted hospital erected in the grounds of the estate was based on a layout suggested by Gillies and designed by AB Hayward and DC Maynard. Frognal House itself, a Jacobean mansion built in the early eighteenth century, accommodated the medical and nursing staff. The spacious wards, with twenty-six beds in each, radiated from a large, covered, horseshoe-shaped wooden ramp connected at the ends by the central administration block. Within the perimeter of the horseshoe were the operating theatres and dental, physiotherapy, photographic and X-ray departments. There was also a museum, known as the Sir Alfred Keogh Museum, which was under the direction of Henry Tonks, assisted by Sidney Hornswick (who later taught at the Slade), and Lieutenant JW Edwards, a sculptor who made the plaster casts on which Gillies and the other surgical teams worked up their cases.[1] At the time, Tonks was teaching at the Slade three days a week and then hurrying down to Sidcup to 'paint a nose'. The total sum spent on buildings and equipment was about £149,000. There were 600 beds available at Frognal itself, together with convalescent beds at satellite hospitals in the immediate vicinity at Swanley (Parkwood, 200 beds), Bromley (Oakley, 60 beds), Chislehurst (Abbey Lodge and The Gorse, 40 beds each) and Bickley (Southwood, 40 beds). When the Sir John Ellerman Hospital at Regent's Park in London was added in July 1918, The Queen's Hospital had upwards of 1000 beds at its disposal.

The British Section took two-fifths of the patients, while the remaining three sections took one-fifth each. When the Americans arrived for surgical training in 1918 they were attached in equal numbers to the existing sections. The hospital was under the command of Lieutenant Colonel JR Colvin, a retired Indian Army Service Corps officer

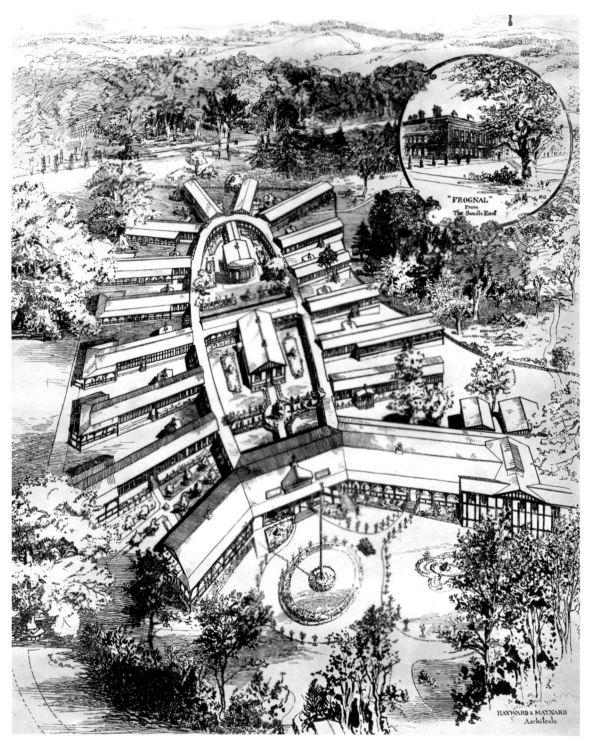

"FROGNAL"
From
The South East

HAYWARD & MAYNARD
Architects

FIGURE 5.2. *Architectural drawing by Hayward and Maynard of the proposed Queen's Hospital at Frognal in Kent for the treatment of facial and jaw injuries, showing the distinctive horseshoe layout.* (Reproduced courtesy of the Gillies Archive, Queen Mary's Hospital, Sidcup)

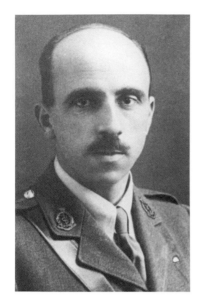
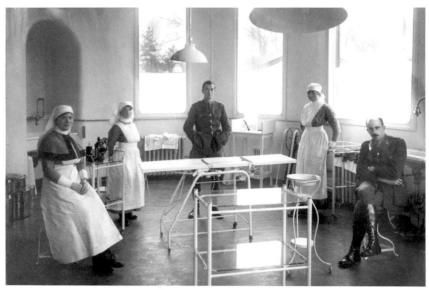
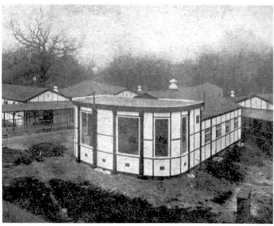
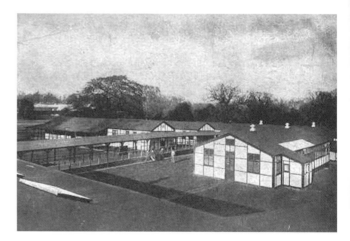

FIGURE 5.3. *The Queen's Hospital, Sidcup.* CLOCKWISE FROM TOP LEFT: *Major HD Gillies, RAMC; Gillies with the theatre staff: in the middle is Lieutenant R Wade, Gillies' anaesthetist; Exterior view of the plastic surgery theatre; Dental workshop and surgeries.* (Reproduced courtesy of the Gillies Archive, Queen Mary's Hospital, Sidcup)

and a skilful administrator. Colvin did not know any medicine, which he claimed was a positive advantage from an administrative point of view.[5] Evidence of recent hospital management suggests this is not necessarily the case.

The first to arrive were the members of the British Section, shown in Figure 5.4. Dominating the photograph (dated November 1917) is the towering presence of Henry Tonks, who by this time had returned to civilian status. The line-up

includes the unmilitary figure of Major HD Gillies FRCS, Chief Medical Officer; Capt JL Aymard MRCS, LRCP, Gillies' principal assistant, a South African ENT surgeon who had trained at Guy's Hospital; Lieutenant G Seccombe Hett FRCS[†], another ENT surgeon whose work particularly on nasal reconstruction was regarded by Gillies as outstanding;[6] and Lieutenant R Wade MRCS, LRCP, senior anaesthetist, who later contributed an entry on the subject in *Plastic Surgery of the Face*. Several

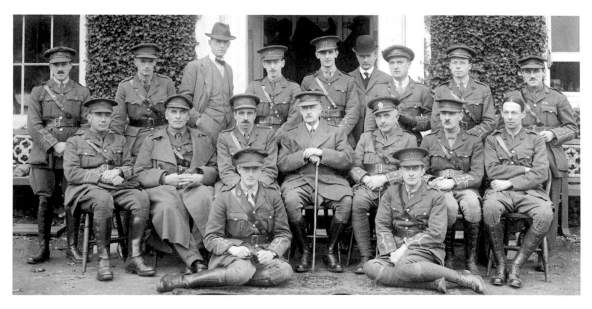

FIGURE 5.4. *The Officers, the Queen's Hospital, Frognal, Sidcup, Kent, November 1917. Back Row: Capt EG Robertson, Lieut R Wade, Mr Henry Tonks, Capt EW Lowe, Capt AL Fraser, Mr T Pope, Capt Andrew Jupp, Lieut HC Malleson, Capt W Kelsey Fry MC. Front Row: Capt TC Clayton, Capt JL Aymard, Major HD Gillies (Chief Medical Officer), Lt-Col J Colvin (Commandant), Major JC Duff (Quarter-master), Capt CF Rumsey, Lieut G Seccombe Hett. In Front: Lieut R Montgomery, Lieut HM Johnston. Photograph by Sydney S Walbridge.* (Reproduced with the permission of Brian Morgan FRCS, Antony Wallace Collection, British Association of Plastic, Reconstructive and Aesthetic Surgeons)

dental surgeons are also present: Captains W Kelsey Fry MC, MRCS, LRCP, LDS, Officer-in-charge of the Dental Department; AL Fraser MRCS, LRCP, LDS; CF Rumsey MRCS, LRCP, LDS; EW Lowe LDS; A Jupp LDS and Lieutenant HC Malleson MRCS, LRCP, LDS. Sir Francis Farmer and JF Colyer later joined the staff as consulting dental surgeons. The RAMC officers' uniform of Sam Browne belt, riding breeches, field boots and spurs was a legacy of the medical corps' role as a mounted service with mobile horse-drawn field ambulances; in the early part of the war field ambulances were still horse drawn and each medical officer was entitled to a horse, groom and servant.

The Australian Section was commanded by Lieutenant Colonel HS Newland[†]. He was the most senior-ranking officer of the four section commanders and had been awarded the DSO in 1917 for outstanding service in the Middle East and the Western Front. Newland had qualified FRCS (Eng) in 1900 and, in addition to 15 years'

experience as a general surgeon in London and Adelaide, had built up considerable expertise in treating war casualties. A veteran of the ill-fated ANZAC Gallipoli campaign of 1915 in the Dardanelles, he followed this with periods in Egypt; as a surgical specialist at No 3 Australian General Hospital at Brighton treating infected fractures; and at various casualty clearing stations in Flanders at the time of the Allied offensive in July 1917 known as the Third Battle of Ypres or Passchendaele. Newland was posted to Sidcup in October 1917 and performed his first operation in January 1918.[7] Although his work as a plastic surgeon at Sidcup gave Newland his international reputation, on his return to Adelaide in 1919 it was to general surgical practice, not plastic surgery.

The officer commanding the Canadian Section was Major CW Waldron[†]. He had tried to enlist in the Canadian Army Medical Corps (CAMC) at the outbreak of the war, but found there were nearly 400 applicants ahead of him. To circumvent this problem

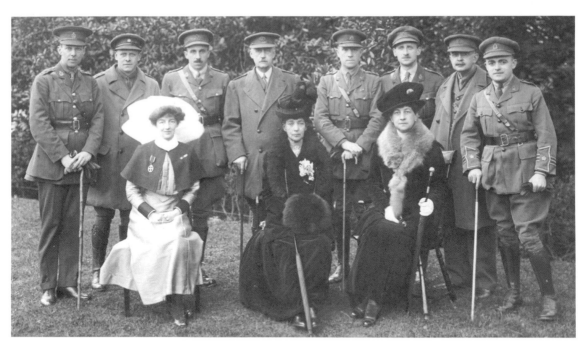

FIGURE 5.5. *Queen Alexandra's visit to the Queen's Hospital, Sidcup, 30 April 1918. Back Row: Capt G Seccombe Hett, Major JW Blencowe (Chaplain), Major HD Gillies (Officer-in-Charge, British Section), Lieut-Col JR Colvin (Commandant), Lt-Col HS Newland, DSO (O-in-C, Australian Section), Major HP Pickerill (O-in-C, New Zealand Section), Major Sir Francis Farmer (Consultant Dental Surgeon), Major CW Waldron (O-in-C, Canadian Section). In Front: Mrs R Barber (Matron), Queen Alexandra, Grand-Duchess George.* (Photograph by Sydney S Walbridge.

Reproduced with permission of the Hocken Collections, Uare Taoka o Hakena, University of Otago. Pickerill papers; reference number: MS-1620/021)

he purchased his own ticket to London and, with letters of recommendation from influential friends, including Sir William Osler and a fraternity brother of Waldron's who was the executive officer for the Surgeon-General of the CAMC, was commissioned as a lieutenant on 28 December 1915. Waldron was doubly qualified, and his training in otolaryngology and maxillofacial pathology at Johns Hopkins was the ideal background. He was delegated to organise a Canadian service for facial injuries, first at the Westcliffe Canadian Eye and Ear Hospital at Folkestone in Kent, and subsequently at the Ontario Military Hospital, Orpington, just 6 miles up the road from Sidcup. With the transfer of the Canadians to Sidcup, it soon became obvious from the volume of casualties that Waldron could not manage on his own, so he sent for his Toronto colleague, Captain Fulton Risdon[†]. At the end of the war Waldron and Risdon returned to Canada where they continued

the postwar care of war casualties until 1920, first at Sainte-Anne-de-Bellevue in Quebec and later at the Toronto Military Orthopaedic Hospital (later called the Christie Street Veterans' Hospital; it was demolished in 1981).

The New Zealand Section was commanded by Major HP Pickerill. After arriving in England in March 1917, he had been posted to No 2 New Zealand General Hospital at Walton-on-Thames in Surrey to establish a unit for the treatment of facial and jaw injuries. Pickerill's career up until the First World War had been spent largely in academia as Dean of the University of Otago Dental School. He had received no formal surgical training and did not have a surgical fellowship. During the nine months spent at Walton-on-Thames, his clinical practice had been limited to treating facial fractures, bone grafting the jaws and repairing intraoral soft tissues. With the transfer of the unit to Sidcup in

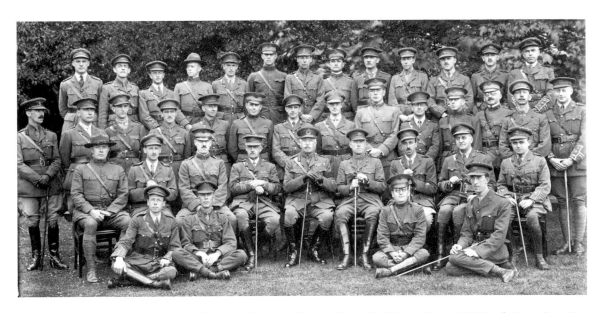

FIGURE 5.6. *Visit of HRH the Duke of Connaught to the Queen's Hospital, Sidcup, 4 June 1918. Back Row: Capt K Russell, Capt EO Watson, Capt G Johnson, Capt TM Terry, Lieut R Wade, Capt EF Lafitte, Capt G Seccombe Hett, Major WJ Scruton, Capt CF Rumsey, Capt V Macdonald, Capt EG Robertson, Capt GM Hicks, Capt EF Risdon. Second Row: Capt P Ashworth, ADC, Capt JC Clayton, Capt AL Fraser, Capt W Kelsey Fry, MC, Capt GC Birt, Lieut JJ Ogden, Capt JM Turner, Capt R Montgomery, Capt HW Brent, Lieut HM Johnston, Major RP McGee, Capt JM Waugh, Capt AWL Campbell, Capt B Mendleson. Front Row: Major TC Stellwagen, Major HP Pickerill, Major GM Dorrance, Lt-Col JR Colvin, HRH the Duke of Connaught, Lt-Col HS Newland, DSO, Major HD Gillies, Major A Wheeler, Major CW Waldron. In Front: Capt HC Malleson, Capt HL Whale, Lieut EJ Kelly, Lieut JW Edwards. Photograph by Sydney S Walbridge.* (Reproduced with permission of the Hocken Collections, Uare Taoka o Hakena, University of Otago. Pickerill papers; reference number: MS-1620/013)

January 1918, he was able to carry out major plastic operations to reconstruct the soft tissues of the face and in the process established a considerable reputation as a plastic and reconstructive surgeon. Pickerill's wartime career is discussed in detail in Chapter 6.

Despite not being the senior ranking officer at Sidcup, Gillies had overall responsibility. This raised a few military eyebrows, but his position as Chief Medical Officer was based on his experience as a maxillofacial surgeon, not on his rank. The concentration of cases in one hospital proved to be a factor of prime importance in the improvement of treatment methods. In the preface to *Plastic Surgery of the Face*, Gillies wrote that each of the sections and the officers serving with them joined heartily in friendly rivalry and healthy competition, to the great benefit of the poor 'mutilés'. The reality was

somewhat different, however – hardly surprising given the personality, ambition and self-confidence required to become a successful surgeon. As we will see later, the question of who had first carried out a certain operative procedure was the usual cause of friction.

The size of the surgical staff in the photograph of the visit in June 1918 of HRH the Duke of Connaught (Figure 5.6) gives some idea of the amount of work that was undertaken; there were six operating theatres running to capacity daily. Seated in the front row are the officers in charge of the sections: the officers standing are the surgical, dental and anaesthetic officers on the staffs of the four sections. There are 10 US officers (surgical and dental) in the photograph – distinguishable by their uniforms (with the high collars) or hats. Of course there were many others, both before and after,[5] including Ferris N Smith, Vilray P Blair[†], who was Chief Consultant in Maxillofacial Surgery to the American Expeditionary Force (AEF), George M Dorrance, Eastman Sheehan and Read P McGee. All became well-known plastic surgeons, but at the time (apart from Ferris Smith, who had joined the RAMC in 1916) they had little experience in the type of plastic and maxillofacial surgery being performed at Sidcup.

Each of the units was self-contained and autonomous, but there was a common record office open to all, which enabled surgeons to keep abreast of the latest developments in operative techniques. During the busiest period of the hospital, from August 1917 to June 1921, a total of 11,752 major operations were carried out, of which over 8000 were for maxillofacial injuries.[2]

Plastic Surgery of the Face

Gillies' wartime experiences provided the material for his classic book of 408 pages and 844 illustrations entitled *Plastic Surgery of the Face*, published in 1920.[8] The *British Medical Journal* described it as 'one of the most notable contributions made to surgical literature in our day'; the *British Dental Journal* said that 'for recent advances in plastic surgery, the world is indebted to the author of this book as greatly as anyone'. When it is compared with the leading maxillofacial surgery textbook of the day – *Surgery and Diseases of the Mouth and Jaws* by Vilray Blair[9] – it is not hard to see why it made such a dramatic impact.

Up until the First World War, the scope of plastic and maxillofacial surgery consisted largely of treating surgical conditions involving the head and neck, such as fractures, cleft lip and palate, temporomandibular joint disorders, deformities of the jaws, infections and malignancies. Blair, a general surgeon in St Louis with a special interest in surgery of the face and jaws, had been appointed to head the subsection of Plastic and Oral Surgery at the Office of the Surgeon-General to the Army in 1917; his book had been revised for distribution to AEF hospitals and surgeons in France as a training manual.[10] The third edition had been updated to include the latest war data on gunshot injuries to

the face and jaws, including soft and hard tissue repair, but the additions are modest by comparison with Gillies' book, and did not include photographs of patients under treatment. Pre-, progress-, and post-operative photographs illustrating the various surgical procedures required to reconstruct the face on actual patients are the outstanding feature of *Plastic Surgery of the Face*, highlighting the value of clinical photography. Line diagrams are a very useful adjunct to explaining surgical technique, but are a poor substitute for a photograph of the real thing.

A much more impressive competitor was *Plastic Surgery: Its principles and practice*,[11] which had appeared a year earlier, in 1919. It was a scholarly work of 770 pages, with extensive references and 864 illustrations covering all parts of the body. The author, John Staige Davis[†], was the first surgeon in the United States to limit his practice exclusively to plastic surgery. The anonymous reviewer in the *British Journal of Surgery* (1919, Volume 7, Issue 28, pp. 556–57) was unimpressed by much of this, however, complaining the bibliography was voluminous and somewhat unnecessary and that numerous methods were described diagrammatically without good records of operative results on actual cases. A clue as to the identity of the reviewer is suggested by the comment, 'It is a pity also that the tubed pedicle was not annunciated before the book was written, as the English method of tubing the pedicle of a flap has solved almost 70 percent of the difficulties inherent in transplanting skin from a distance.' (In defence of Staige Davis' scholarship, one has to say that both of Gillies' books are irritatingly devoid of references.)

Plastic Surgery did not have the same spectacular impact as *Plastic Surgery of the Face*, and Staige Davis seems to have been peeved at being upstaged by Gillies and others treating facially mutilated war casualties. As he wrote in 1926, 'With few exceptions, the group of men assigned to plastic work during the World War were those who had previously confined their practice to eye, ear, nose or throat surgery, or to dentistry, and few had a general surgical training. The majority of them, I venture to say, had never done a plastic operation and were ignorant of the literature on the subject.'[12] The implication was that it had been necessary for this group of neophyte plastic surgeons and dentists to reinvent the wheel. Although there was a certain element of truth in much of this, Davis mellowed somewhat with the passage of time, conceding twenty years later that some good things had come out of the Great War. A greater source of vexation for Davis was the powerful figure of William Halsted (1852–1922), Chief of Surgery at Johns Hopkins, who continually blocked any attempt by Davis to start a plastic surgery service or residency programme at the hospital.

Plastic Surgery of the Face is not a textbook: it is an instruction manual showing how to surgically reconstruct traumatic injuries of the head and neck. The seeds of modern maxillofacial surgery may have been sown in various base hospitals in France and at Aldershot, but it was at Sidcup that many of the principles of contemporary plastic surgery became established and eventually adopted worldwide. Admittedly that is an exclusively Anglo-centric point of view – French and German surgeons could no doubt make equally compelling claims. Nevertheless, *Plastic Surgery of the Face* established Gillies' reputation as arguably the most distinguished plastic surgeon of his generation and the doyen of twentieth-century plastic surgery. As Staige Davis had been at pains to point out, various plastic techniques such as rhinoplasty and skin flaps date back to antiquity, but it was under Gillies at Sidcup that these procedures evolved, became standardised, and led to the foundation of plastic surgery as we understand it today: plastic surgery had passed from trial and error to a specialty based on reasonably sound surgical and biological principles.

Kelsey Fry, in addition to writing a chapter on prosthetic appliances in the book, was awarded the Cartwright Prize for the quinquennial period 1916–20 by the Royal College of Surgeons of England for his essay on the treatment of jaw injuries, as well as publishing several articles arising from the work at Sidcup.[13] Looking at the mutilated faces of servicemen staring out from Sidney Walbridge's numerous black and white photographs makes one realise how heartbreaking it must have been, not only for these men and their families, but also for the people responsible for trying to put them together again.

The tubed pedicle flap

As we have seen in the previous chapter, the major problem faced by surgeons in maxillofacial units was that primary closure of major gunshot wounds was unsatisfactory: areas of tissue loss could only be successfully reconstructed by the introduction of new tissue – local rotational and transposed flaps of various types for wound closure and soft tissue repair – and bone grafts from the ribs, tibia or iliac crest to reconstruct osseous defects of the jaws. Two of Gillies' major surgical innovations at Sidcup were the tubed pedicle flap and the epithelial outlay technique for reconstructing eyelids – which brings us to the famous case of Able-Seaman Vicarage.

Able-Seaman William Vicarage had received terrible facial burns in a cordite explosion on HMS *Malaya* at the Battle of Jutland (31 May 1916). The explosion had destroyed his nose, lips, eyelids, ears and neck, leaving extensive scarring (Figure 5.7(A)). His hands had also been burned and – as would happen to many airmen in World War II – had contracted into frightful deformities. As Gillies wrote later, 'It required very considerable moral courage to attempt an operation such as could in any way radically cure the condition.'[8] It was in the course of operating on Vicarage that Gillies, while raising two skin flaps from the chest and noting their tendency to curl, had the inspiration of stitching them into tubes to create tubed pedicles. The advantage of tubed pedicles was that they created a cylinder of living tissue with a good blood supply that was closed to infection – the cross-vessels are cut, but the longitudinal circulation increases. They were also far less liable than conventional pedicle flaps to contract or degenerate, and were much more portable. After three weeks, one end could be divided without fear of sloughing.

Who first developed the principle of the tubed pedicle was a matter of acrimonious dispute between Gillies and his colleague Captain Aymard. On 18 October 1917 Aymard had raised a tubed pedicle flap from the chest to reconstruct a nose, and two months later in an article in *The Lancet* claimed this to have been the first.[14] To set the record straight, Gillies, in a letter to the editor of

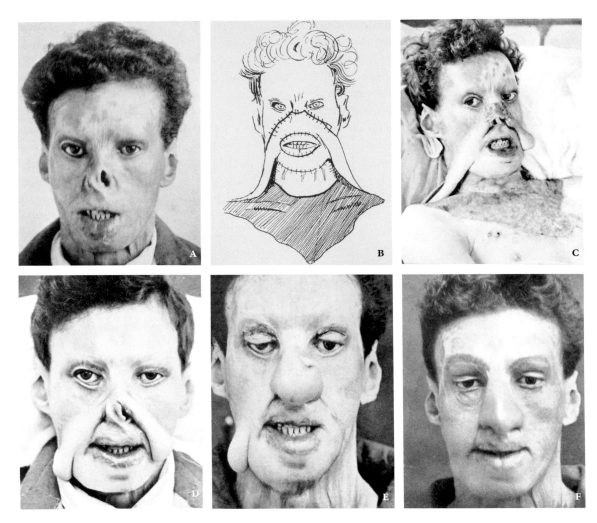

FIGURE 5.7. *The famous case of Able-Seaman Vicarage. William Vicarage had received terrible facial burns in a cordite explosion on HMS Malaya at the Battle of Jutland involving destruction of the nose, lips and eyelids – and the ears and neck were also burnt. It was in the course of operating on Vicarage 18 months later at Sidcup that Gillies had the inspiration, while raising two skin flaps, of stitching them into tubes to create tubed pedicles. (A) The healed condition. (B, C) Tubed pedicles raised to the face. (C) Left pedicle divided following the onset of gangrene at the tip of the nose. (D) Both pedicles divided. (E) After change to epithelial outlay and rhinoplasty; note lymphoedema of the nose at this stage. (F) Cartilage from another man was inserted into the bridge of the nose to give it more definition and prominence. No grafting from the patient of the raw area of the chest was attempted, but three small skin grafts from another patient were laid on the granulations without success.* (Case 338 in Gillies (1920), Plastic Surgery of the Face. pp. 356–59)

The Lancet published in 1920, pointed out that the operating books, surgical records and ward sisters' report books all showed that the first tubed flap was performed by him on 3 October 1917.[15] Furthermore, the tubed pedicles progressed so well that the second-stage operation – division of the pedicle towards its base for use on the face – was performed (on his behalf by Lieutenant HC Malleson) on 17 October 1917, and legend has it that Aymard was actually present at the operation. In any case it later turned out that the tubed pedicle flap had, like all good ideas, been invented independently by Vladimir Filatov in Odessa[16] and Hugo Ganzer in Berlin[17] – as Gillies found out to his great disappointment on his visit to the United States in 1920. Gillies can, however, be credited with making this valuable procedure universally popular – it was enthusiastically adopted by the other surgeons at Sidcup and elsewhere.

At the first operation on 3 October 1917, 18 months after the original injury, a large 'Masonic-collar' skin flap with double-tubed pedicles was raised from the chest and split to encircle the mouth (Figure 5.7(B)). The lower border of the incision was sutured to the mucous membrane of the lower lip, while the upper border was carried round over the tip of the nose. The upper lip was not replaced, as the scar tissue was not so marked there. In order to keep the flap free from tension, the neck was kept flexed with a plaster apparatus. Unfortunately, the portion of the flap that went over the bridge of the nose was under the greatest tension and any movement of the head tended to tear the stitches. This affected the blood supply to the tip of the nose, and gangrene supervened. On 16 October 1917 (a day earlier than the date mentioned by Gillies in his letter to the editor of *The Lancet*) the left pedicle was therefore severed under local anaesthesia with Novocaine (Figure 5.7(C)), and the right pedicle a fortnight later, followed by three months' rest.

At the next operation on 19 February 1918 the left pedicle was partly detached from below and swung around to form a flap of skin sufficient for rhinoplasty (Figure 5.7(E)). At the same time, both upper eyelids were reconstructed by the epithelial outlay procedure (described below). Three months later (30 May 1918) epithelial outlays were applied to both lower lids, the secondary pedicle of the rhinoplasty divided and trimmed, and the right pedicle opened and spread over the right cheek, where it was sewn after the excision of scar tissue. On 6 March 1919 cartilage from another man was inserted into the bridge of the nose to give it more definition and prominence; trimming and alterations were made in the right ala (Figure 5.7(F)) and two full-thickness (Wolfe) skin grafts were taken from the scalp to make eyebrows. During the course of Vicarage's treatment there was no attempt made to graft skin from elsewhere on his body to the raw area on his chest. Three small skin homografts from another patient were laid on the raw granulation tissue, but without success.

The epithelial outlay operation

The first successful operations to provide an epithelial lining for deepened hollows or wounds were carried out by JF Esser, a Dutch plastic surgeon, who wrapped a Thiersch graft around a mould of dental composition with the deep surface outwards, which he inserted into a surgically prepared pocket and sutured firmly into place.[18] Prior to the Esser technique, surgically prepared pockets both inside and outside the oral and nasal cavities that were not lined with epithelium readily became infected and shrank through cicatrisation (scar formation) of the suppurating wound surfaces. The need to apply pressure to the grafted tissues in these situations was a problem and led to the construction of many weird and wonderful appliances by the dental technicians.

Scar tissue had caused Vicarage's eyelids to contract and turn inside out (everted). This posed a risk to his eyesight and forced him to sleep with his eyes open. Gillies adapted the Esser inlay technique to restore the function and appearance of Vicarage's eyelids – a method he referred to as the 'epithelial outlay' technique (Figure 5.8). An incision was made skirting the lid edge and the lid dissected freely until closure could be achieved without tension. A closely fitting stent mould, covered with

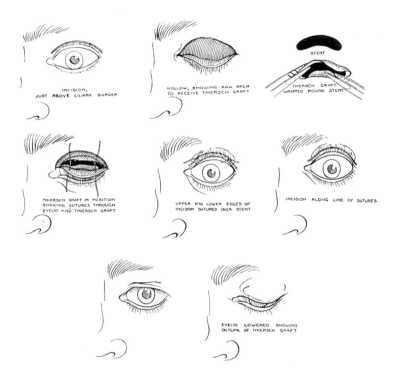

FIGURE 5.8. *Stages in the epithelial outlay operation to reconstruct the upper eyelid. This operation was used extensively by McIndoe and others during the Second World War to reconstruct the eyelids of burned airmen at the Queen Victoria Hospital, East Grinstead, and other hospitals – see Chapter 8.* (From Gillies (1920), Plastic Surgery of the Face, p. 17)

a Thiersch graft, was buried in the resulting cavity. The edges of the incision were then sewn over this with horsehair, the sutures taking up the edges of the skin graft. After about eight days the stent was removed and, according to Gillies, the lid fell easily into position.[19]

The word stent has a curious etymology. Nowadays most people think of a stent as a tube used to keep a coronary blood vessel open, but the term has been adapted to mean different things to different medical disciplines.[20] Charles Stent (1807–1885) was an English dentist who, in 1865, added plasticisers and inert fillers to gutta percha to produce 'Stent's Impression Compound', a material which could be easily softened and moulded in warm water. Although Esser used Stent's compound to produce his moulds, it would appear that Gillies was the first to use Stent's name as a noun when he wrote in a footnote on page 10, 'The dental composition used for this purpose is

that put forward by Stent, and a mould composed of it is called a Stent.'[8]

Rhinoplasty: reconstructing the nose

Rhinoplasty is among the most ancient of plastic operations, dating back to the renowned Indian surgeon Susruta (ca 6th century BC) who, in *Suśruta Samhitā*,[21] described the technique of forehead flap rhinoplasty to reconstruct noses that had been amputated from thieves and unfaithful wives by their irate husbands. Gaspare Tagliacozzi (1545–1599), Professor of Surgery at the University of Bologna, describes restoration of the nose and parts of the lips and ears using skin flaps taken from the upper arm, in his treatise *De Curtorum Chirurgia per Insitionem*, published in 1597.[22,23] Most of Tagliacozzi's patients were soldiers, so his surgery also treated physical violence. Nowadays any operation on the nose is commonly referred to as a rhinoplasty, but a 'reconstructive rhinoplasty'

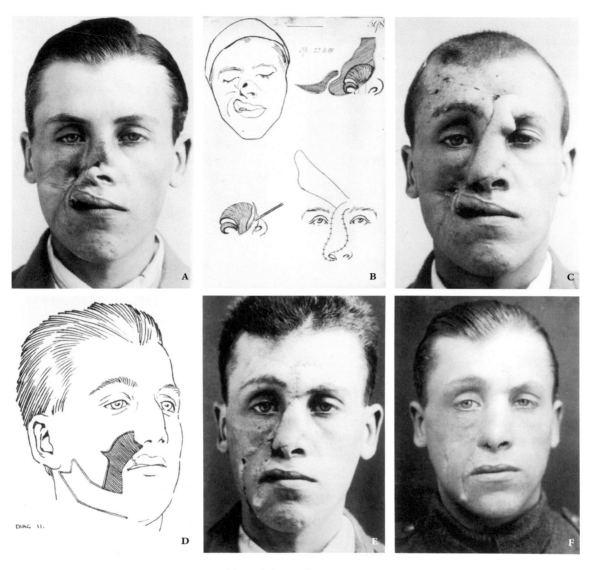

FIGURE 5.9. (A) *Sergeant Beldam of the Machine Gun Corps suffered a major loss of the upper lip and adjacent cheek with destruction of the lower part of the nose apart from the columella and left ala.* (B, C) *At the first operation (22.6.1918) an incision was made in the skin over the upper portion of the nose (referred to as Flap A, but not labelled in the preoperative sketch) and reflected skin inwards to provide an epithelial lining. This incision also freed the remains of the columella and right ala so they could be brought into a normal position. Another flap lying inside the scar line was reflected inwards to line the right ala, followed by a rhinoplasty using a frontal flap.* (D, E) *The second operation (15.8.18) involved correction of the ectropion of the upper lip by excising the scar tissue and reconstructing the upper lip and cheek with a rotated pedicle flap.* (F) *The right eyebrow is raised slightly due to scarring of the forehead donor site.* (*Case 598 in Gillies (1920),* Plastic Surgery of the Face. *pp. 240–43. Diagrams are by Lieutenant Daryl Lindsay.*)

is distinct from operations performed to improve the function or cosmetic appearance of the nose (perfected in Berlin during the early part of the twentieth century by Professor Jacques Joseph).

Although Vicarage's nose had been reconstructed using part of the left tubed pedicle raised from his chest, most noses at Sidcup were restored by the 'Indian method' of Susruta, using a rotating forehead flap. Sergeant Beldam of the Machine Gun Corps, aged twenty, had been wounded on 28 November 1917 and admitted to Sidcup on 7 March 1918 from Queen Mary's Military Hospital at Whalley in Lancashire. According to the case notes, he had lost a major part of the tip of the nose and the right ala, with the remaining two-thirds of the nose excepting the left ala and columella undamaged. Complications included ectropion (eversion) of the upper lip at the right corner, and a depressed scar into the floor of the right antrum (Figure 5.9).

At the first operation, on 22 June 1918 (Figure 5.9(B),(C)), an incision was made in the skin over the upper portion of the nose (referred to as flap A, but not marked on the pre-operative sketch) and reflected skin-inwards to provide an epithelial lining. This incision also freed the remains of the columella and right ala so they could be brought into a normal position. Another flap (flap B) lying inside the scar line was reflected inwards to line the right ala; to quote Gillies, 'Omission to provide a lining membrane for mucous cavities has in the past been the supreme cause of plastic failure.'[8] Flap B was followed by rhinoplasty with a flap turned down from the right frontal region to reconstruct the nose.

The second operation (15 August 1918) involved correcting the eversion of the upper lip by cutting away the scar tissue and reconstructing the upper lip and cheek with a rotating pedicle flap (Figure 5.9(D),(E)). One year later, on 8 August 1919, under local anaesthetic, cartilage was implanted into the nose to raise the bridge – and removed 10 days later. A further attempt to raise the bridge of the nose (28 July 1920) was carried out, again under local anaesthetic. The columella was divided at its root and turned up, and a piece of rib cartilage from a Private Jordan was inserted from bridge to tip; scar tissue on the right cheek was also excised. Progress was reported as being very satisfactory on 24 September 1920, and the patient was discharged from the army and the hospital on 25 January 1921.

The planning diagrams for Beldam's operations were drawn by Lieutenant Daryl Lindsay[†], a medical artist attached to the AIF. Early in 1918 Lindsay had been sent down to Sidcup at the request of Colonel

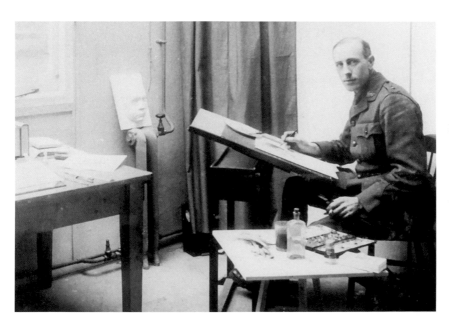

FIGURE 5.10. *Lieutenant Daryl Lindsay, medical artist attached to the Australian Imperial Force, working on an illustration in the studio at Sidcup. (Courtesy of the Gillies Archive, Queen Mary's Hospital, Sidcup)*

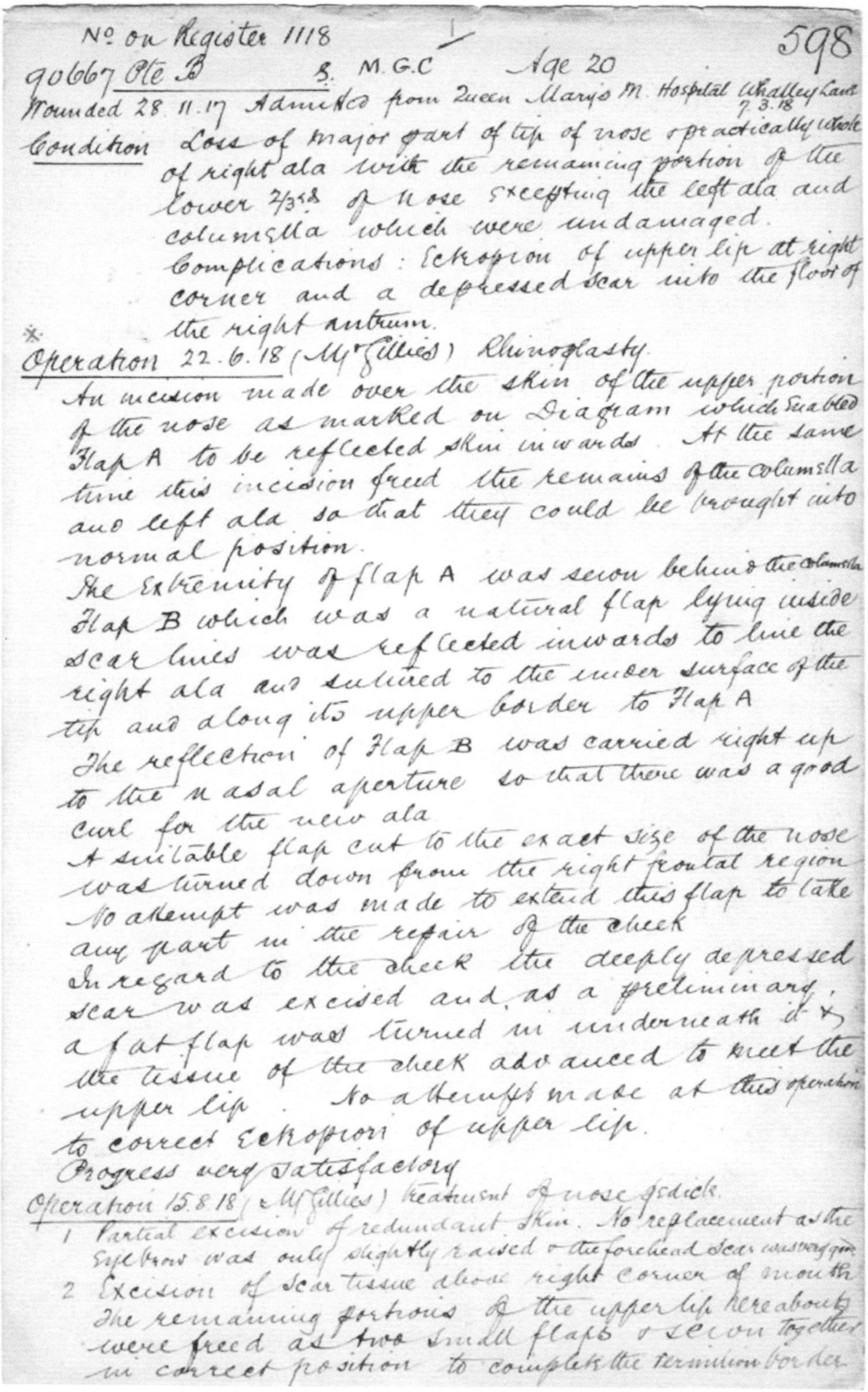

No. on Register 1118   598

90667 Pte B   B. M.G.C   Age 20

Wounded 28.11.17 Admitted from Queen Mary's M. Hospital Whalley Range 7.3.18

Condition Loss of major part of tip of nose & practically whole of right ala with the remaining portion of the lower 2/3rds of nose excepting the left ala and columella which were undamaged.

Complications: Ectropion of upper lip at right corner and a depressed scar into the floor of the right antrum.

Operation 22.6.18 (Mr Gillies) Rhinoplasty.

An incision made over the skin of the upper portion of the nose as marked on Diagram which enabled Flap A to be reflected skin inwards. At the same time this incision freed the remains of the columella and left ala so that they could be brought into normal position.

The extremity of flap A was sewn behind the columella Flap B which was a natural flap lying inside scar lines was reflected inwards to line the right ala and sutured to the under surface of the tip and along its upper border to Flap A

The reflection of Flap B was carried right up to the nasal aperture so that there was a good curl for the new ala

A suitable flap cut to the exact size of the nose was turned down from the right frontal region No attempt was made to extend this flap to take any part in the repair of the cheek

In regard to the cheek the deeply depressed scar was excised and, as a preliminary, a fat flap was turned in underneath it & the tissue of the cheek advanced to meet the upper lip. No attempt made at this operation to correct ectropion of upper lip.

Progress very satisfactory

Operation 15.8.18 (Mr Gillies) treatment of nose & chk.
1 Partial excision of redundant skin. No replacement as the eyebrow was only slightly raised & the forehead scar unsagging
2 Excision of scar tissue above right corner of mouth The remaining portions of the upper lip hereabouts were freed as two small flaps & sewn together in correct position to complete the vermilion border

FIGURE 5.11. *First page of Sergeant Beldam's hospital notes.* (*Courtesy of the Gillies Archive, Queen Mary's Hospital, Sidcup*)

Newland, who urgently wanted someone who could do medical diagrams. In his autobiography *The Leafy Tree* (1965) Lindsay devotes a chapter to his experiences during the war and his time at the Queen's Hospital:[24]

> As a surgeon [Gillies] was a wizard with the scalpel and it fascinated me to see the precision and artistry he brought to his craft. I am pleased to think that some of my surgical diagrams were used in his book on plastic surgery … But to me the most interesting of them all was Henry Tonks.
>
> My first meeting with Tonks was at Sidcup where he was putting in a day a week doing diagrams and drawings for Harold Gillies. I was struggling with a drawing and became aware of being overlooked by a tall, hatchet-faced man, who looked like a cross between a Roman emperor and a wedge-tailed eagle. He asked me what I was doing and I said: 'Trying to draw.' He said: 'I'm glad you said "trying" which is the best that can be said of it; but I think I may be able to help you' … Thanks to the kindness of Henry Newland, I was allowed to go to the Slade one day a week to study under Tonks.

Transplantation immunity

These two cases – Beldam and Vicarage – illustrate how little was known about transplantation immunity at the time of the First World War. Three small skin homografts had been applied to the raw area of the chest donor site of Able-Seaman Vicarage without success, and both patients had cartilage homografts inserted into the bridge of the nose to give it more definition. (It's not hard to see from the post-operative photographs why Gillies had a reputation for producing somewhat patrician noses!)

Surprisingly, given its importance, the systematic study of transplantation immunity did not begin for another twenty years – until early in the Second World War, when the War Wounds Committee of the Medical Research Council asked Peter Medawar to investigate why homografts of human skin were rejected. Medawar, together with Thomas Gibson at Glasgow Royal Infirmary, first investigated the fate of skin autografts and first- and second-set homografts in a patient with severe burns and concluded that a humoral mechanism was responsible for rejection.[25] At the time, the focus of immunology was on humoral immunity and antigen–antibody relationships; the function of lymphocytes and cell-mediated immunity was unknown.

Medawar then returned to Oxford to make the first detailed histological study of homograft rejection in a rabbit skin-graft model. In a deceptively simple series of experiments he found that although all the ingredients of inflammation were present within the host tissues, the reaction was atypical and lymphocytes took the place of poly-morphonuclear leucocytes. Medawar concluded that the elimination of foreign skin was due to a process he called 'actively acquired immunity'; the most direct demonstration of this was the accelerated rejection of second-set homografts.[26,27] This occurred in patients who had received skin grafts on two separate occasions from the same donor, usually a relative. Medawar and his co-workers subsequently showed that transplantation immunity was due to tissue antigens expressed by cells of the lymphocyte series.[28] In 1960 the Nobel Prize for physiology or medicine was shared by Sir Peter Medawar and Sir Frank Macfarlane Burnet for the discovery of acquired immunological tolerance.

In *Plastic Surgery of the Face* Gillies wrote that for large cosmetic purposes, cartilage stands unrivalled as a transplant material, and he stubbornly continued to use cartilage, including heterografts of bovine cartilage, for contour filling and support purposes throughout his surgical career, even though these grafts were ultimately destined to fail.[29] Unlike skin grafts, cartilage homografts and heterografts have the potential to survive for up to several years; the gel-like proteoglycan-rich extracellular matrix confers some degree of protection from the host and enables nutrients to reach the cells, so that cartilage cells (chondrocytes) can remain viable for long periods. However, chondrocytes, like all cells, possess transplantation antigens and are immunogenic,[30,31] so that as the cartilage matrix is slowly broken down by phagocytic action and the cells become exposed and collapse, and resorption of the explants is just a matter of time.[32] Gillies and Kristensen, in their series of 144 ox cartilage grafts, reported a resorption rate varying from 5 to 70 percent after an average period of about one year;[29] and Gibson and Davis noted that the histology of excised bovine cartilage implants all showed signs of resorption after 18 months.[33,34] It is interesting to note that because of the frequent failure of both cartilage autografts and homografts in a series of 40 patients reported by Rainsford Mowlem in 1941, he had abandoned using cartilage for restoring nasal contour, preferring instead to use autogenous bone from the iliac crest – a method first carried out, as far as he was aware, by Gillies in 1932.[35]

Armistice 1918

After the Armistice the Canadian, Australian and New Zealand Sections together with their staff and patients returned home. Gillies' service with the RAMC ended on 8 October 1919, but he continued the treatment of patients at Sidcup and the same year was joined by two RAMC captains who were destined to become prominent figures in British surgery: Pomfret Kilner[†] and Ivor Magill.

Kilner had served with casualty clearing stations in France, and by 1918 was in charge of an orthopaedic unit at No 4 Base Hospital at Camiers. Having decided on a career in surgery, he was advised that an appointment might be available with Major Gillies at Sidcup in the new specialty of plastic surgery. Kilner knew no plastic surgery but was a fast learner and soon became second-in-command. By 1920 the treatment of facial injury cases was rapidly diminishing, and the committee arranged with the Ministry of Pensions for the admission of general medical and surgical cases. By 1925 the number of cases had been reduced to 70 and these were moved to Queen Mary's Hospital, Roehampton, where Gillies and Kilner continued to perform intermittent surgery until the work on these remaining patients was completed. The Queen's Hospital eventually closed in 1929. However, the following year it was sold

for £29,000 to the London County Council for use as a general hospital and renamed Queen Mary's Hospital, Sidcup. When Gillies set up in practice as the first plastic surgeon in the country, Kilner joined as his assistant – a relationship described by Richard Battle[†] as rather like an association between Oxbridge and redbrick. Although Gillies and Kilner had been working together for 10 years, they had no formal partnership agreement and eventually parted company under somewhat acrimonious circumstances.[36] The result was a rift that took many years to heal, and Kilner established his own practice on another floor of the London Clinic, much to Gillies' annoyance.

Ivor Magill, an Ulsterman who had served with the Irish Guards, and another ex-RAMC officer, Stanley Rowbotham,[37] who had also been posted to Sidcup, decided to focus their attention on the problem of administering general anaesthetics to patients with facial injuries; surprisingly, much of the maxillofacial surgery at Sidcup and elsewhere was performed under local anaesthesia. Together they are credited with laying the foundations of endotracheal anaesthesia – although Magill became the better-known public figure, helped no doubt by being the one to administer anaesthetics to members of the royal family, and by contributing a chapter to *The Principles and Art of Plastic Surgery* (1957), Gillies' second autobiographical work, co-authored with Ralph Millard Jr.

The Gillies Archive

The Gillies Archive at Queen Mary's Hospital, Sidcup, was a unique collection of over 2500 case files documenting the development of plastic and maxillofacial surgery at Sidcup between 1917 and 1925. At the end of the war each of the national units from Canada, Australia and New Zealand removed its wartime records. The Canadian records unfortunately have disappeared. The Australian records are located in the archives of the Royal Australasian College of Surgeons in Melbourne. Most of the New Zealand records resurfaced in Dunedin when they were rescued by AD (Sandy) Macalister, Professor of Oral Surgery at the Dental School, and were returned to Sidcup in 1989. They are known as the Macalister Archive and are discussed further in Chapter 6. Some of the medical notes from Rooksdown House where Gillies operated during the Second World War (see Chapter 11) were added in 2001, together with a number of cine films of Gillies operating in the 1930s and 1940s, plus colour prints and his personal collection of reprints and glass slides.[38]

In 2011, as the result of hospital reorganisation, the building housing the archive at QMH was decommissioned and the archives distributed to a number of other organisations. The First World War case notes from Aldershot and Sidcup, comprising the extant British and New Zealand Section notes, as well as the records from Rooksdown House, Basingstoke, up to 1960, have been transferred to the Royal College of Surgeons of England, Lincoln's Inn Fields. Plastic surgery instruments, material relating to Sir Harold Gillies and other ephemera have been moved to the archive of the British Association of Plastic, Reconstructive and Aesthetic Surgeons (BAPRAS) at the Royal College of Surgeons of England. However, the Gillies Archive website at www.gilliesarchives.org.uk will continue to be maintained by Dr Bamji for the foreseeable future.

CHAPTER 6

Pickerill joins the war effort and returns to England

Written in collaboration with Andrew N Bamji

BEFORE THE OUTBREAK OF the First World War, New Zealand was in a state of military semi-preparedness. Amid growing tension in Europe and concerns about the defence of Australia and New Zealand following the rapid growth of the German fleet, the New Zealand Defence Act of 1909 was introduced by the Liberal administration of Sir Joseph Ward. New Zealand did not have a standing army; the Act replaced the existing volunteer force with a Territorial Army and, at the same time, established the principle of universal service by means of compulsory military training. This applied to all males aged 14–21 years: senior cadets from 14 to 18, and territorials from 18 to 21, later extended to 25 years. Men were posted to the reserve until they were 30. This meant that by August 1914 when war was declared, New Zealand had a fairly well-trained defence force of 66,738 men out of a total population of 1.1 million.[1] Prime Minister William Massey was determined to provide full military assistance to Britain – or, as it was referred to at the time, the Mother Country. The first belligerent action of New Zealand troops, which took place at the request of the British government, was the unopposed occupation of German Samoa on 29 August 1914 by 55 officers and 1358 other ranks. Both the Samoan Expeditionary Force and the 360 officers and 8139 other ranks that volunteered

for the 1st New Zealand Expeditionary Force (1NZEF), which sailed for Egypt on 16 October 1914 under the command of Major-General Sir Alexander Godley, came from the Territorial Army. The NZEF was initially reinforced by volunteers at the rate of about 2000 per month, but the constant demand for manpower eventually led to the introduction of conscription on 1 August 1916. From the outbreak of war to the armistice, more than 100,000 men out of an eligible male population of fewer than 250,000 had served with the NZEF in France, Gallipoli and Egypt.[1]

New Zealand Dental Corps

New Zealand holds the proud position of being the first country to recognise the necessity of making arrangements for the systematic dental treatment of its expeditionary forces. Two dental officers attached to the NZMC accompanied the Samoan expedition, and a dental officer was detailed for duty on each of the 10 transports which carried the NZEF to Egypt.[2] Meanwhile, a large number of otherwise fit men were being rejected for military service during the first months of the war because of gross dental neglect. Recognising this as a waste of manpower, in June 1915 the New Zealand Dental Association offered to treat recruits free of charge, provided the government reimbursed members for the cost of materials. The proposal was accepted and following the arrival from England of Surgeon-General RSF Henderson RAMC, Director-General Medical Services, who approved the scheme, in November 1915 the New Zealand Dental Corps (NZDC) came into being. From the very beginning it was a separate organisation from the NZMC, controlled by a director, Lieutenant Colonel TA Hunter[†], and two assistant directors with the rank of major, JN Rishworth[†] and HP Pickerill.

No 2 New Zealand General Hospital, Walton-on-Thames

In 1916 Pickerill took leave of absence from the University of Otago to join the war effort, and on 30 December 1916 sailed from Wellington with the 20th Reinforcements NZEF on the troopship *Athenic*. Pickerill had been commissioned as a territorial captain in the NZMC in June 1915; and in November, with the formation of the NZDC, he was transferred to the new corps together with the other dental officers attached to the NZMC. However, after arriving in England in March 1917, Pickerill transferred back to the NZMC and was posted to No 2 New Zealand General Hospital at Walton-on-Thames in Surrey, the first of the New Zealand military hospitals to be established in the United Kingdom. His orders were to set up a unit for the treatment of facial and jaw injuries.

In June 1915 a large Italianate house called Mount Felix, at Walton-on-Thames in Surrey, had been requisitioned and converted into a 350-bed hospital exclusively for New Zealand wounded. The grounds were extensive, with pleasant walks, flowerbeds and green fields, and one side of the estate bordered the River Thames..The hospital opened on 1 August 1915 and accepted patients from the Gallipoli campaign within two days. It consisted of two parts: the main hospital on the banks of the Thames, which could accommodate up to 1900 patients; and Oatlands Park, an historic country-house hotel in nearby Weybridge. This had been acquired by the New Zealand Medical Board to relieve the pressure on Mount Felix after the Battle of the Somme, and it functioned as an auxiliary hospital with special rehabilitation facilities for the disabled and those with tuberculosis. Generally there were about 1000 patients undergoing treatment or convalescing at any one time, but after a 'push' the hospital was filled to overflowing.[3] From August 1915 to the end of the war, a total of 27,000 patients were cared for in the military hospitals at Mount Felix and Oatlands Park.[4] Mount Felix closed as a hospital in March 1920 and Oatlands Park a short time later. There is still a close association between Walton-on-Thames and New Zealand – an ANZAC Day service has been held in St Mary's Parish Church on 25 April every year since 1920.

Maxillofacial surgery at Mount Felix

By 1917 Pickerill had metamorphosed from being a university dean, teacher, administrator and dental caries researcher into a maxillofacial surgeon.[5] Although he was doubly qualified in medicine and dentistry, he had received no formal surgical training and did not have a surgical fellowship. Given that an FRCS was a sine qua non for specialist surgical practice throughout most of the dominions of the Empire, not having one was likely to have been a considerable irritant to Pickerill – and was probably the reason why his request for promotion to consultant status in June 1918 was turned down.

However, the removal of cysts and tumours of the mouth and jaws and the treatment of fractures and other forms of facial trauma would have been part of Pickerill's clinical responsibilities during his time in Dunedin; and in 1912 he felt confident enough in his ability to carry out a two-stage bilateral resection of the lower jaw in a patient with mandibular prognathism[6] – a particularly heroic operation at the time. He had also acquired some international recognition for his expertise in cleft palate surgery.[7] In the early years of the war, while still in New Zealand, he had discussed the challenges of managing facial trauma arising from gunshot wounds and new methods for treating fractures of the jaws.[8] It is not clear where the patients discussed in the article came from, but presumably they were returned servicemen from France or the Middle East.[5]

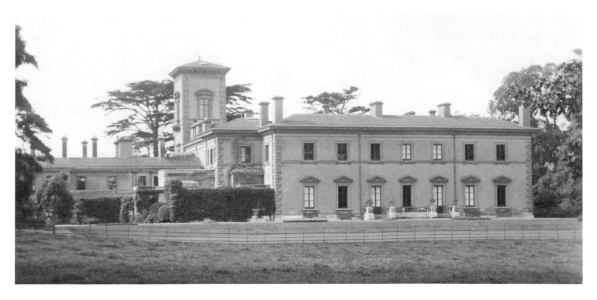

FIGURE 6.1. *Mount Felix, Walton-on-Thames, Surrey. The Italianate villa with a large, square, two-storey porte cochère entrance was designed for the fifth Earl of Tankerville in 1836 by Sir Charles Barry, best known for his role in the rebuilding of the Palace of Westminster. At the time it was requisitioned in 1915 for use as No 2 New Zealand General Hospital, the house was uninhabited and had been in decline for some years. After the war, Mount Felix entered another period of decline and was demolished in 1966 when severely damaged by fire.* (Photograph and narrative kindly provided by Matthew Beckett: www.lostheritage.org.uk: England's Lost Houses)

In a preliminary report of the work of the unit in the *New Zealand Dental Journal* published in 1917, Pickerill separated his cases into old ones which had been under treatment elsewhere, and fresh cases direct from the front.[3] The old cases he divided into three categories:

1. Adhesions along bullet wounds between the upper and lower jaws, treated by plastic operation within the mouth with the excision of facial scar tissue if necessary. Vulcanite shields were inserted immediately to prevent fresh adhesions forming and to keep the tissues stretched until healing was complete. However, until Pickerill adopted the Esser technique to line surgically created intraoral wounds with skin grafts (see Chapter 5), this approach was ultimately doomed to failure.

2. Un-united fractures of the mandible. Pickerill had a number of these, which were treated by opening up the fracture line from below and wiring the bone, followed by immobilisation of the jaws for a few weeks with splints.

3. Fractures with loss of substance. At the time of writing he had only once attempted reconstructing the mandible with bone from the tibia; it is not clear whether this was autogenous bone, but is likely to have been the case.

The American orthopaedic surgeon Fred Albee[†], who pioneered the use of tibial grafts of autogenous bone to fuse and immobilise the spine in patients with tubercular osteomyelitis, had published his acclaimed book *Bone Graft Surgery* in 1915,[9] and in the summer of 1916 was operating in Allied military hospitals in France. (Contrary to widespread opinion, including his own,[10] Albee was not the first surgeon to cure a patient with a bone graft. That honour goes to Sir William Macewen, Regius Professor of Surgery at the University of Glasgow, who restored the humerus of William Connell with tibial bone from three different donors in 1879, and 33 years later had the X-rays to prove it.)[11]

Fresh cases always arrived in a very septic condition, and usually with pieces of shrapnel or other foreign bodies embedded in the tissues. Patients were first cleaned up and X-rayed, and septic mouths treated with a pressure atomiser using peroxide or weak iodine solution 2–6 times a day depending on the level of infection (at Sidcup, Eusol replaced iodine for irrigating wounds). In patients with fractured jaws the usual operative procedure was to wire the bone ends together using a direct approach, while at the same time removing any foreign bodies such as shrapnel and tooth fragments – not an easy task, given their habit of moving around. The jaws were immobilised for at least a fortnight using cap splints or intermaxillary wiring, followed by a limited amount of mandibular movement to prevent adhesions developing in the temporomandibular (jaw) joint. This demonstrated

an understanding on the part of Pickerill of the importance of maintaining joint mobility during fracture healing that was ahead of orthopaedic practice at the time.

The move to Sidcup

Sir Fred Bowerbank, who was Director of the Medical Division at No 1 New Zealand General Hospital at Brockenhurst in Hampshire, gives an interesting insight in his autobiography into the circumstances surrounding Pickerill's move to Sidcup.[12] Queen Mary, who took a great interest in plastic surgery and visited Walton-on-Thames frequently, told Pickerill it would be better if his staff and patients were transferred to the newly opened Queen's Hospital for facial injuries at Sidcup. Neither Pickerill nor the patients were keen to move, and when Her Majesty visited the hospital

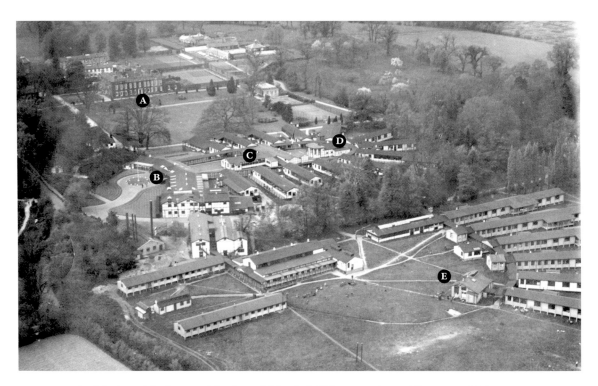

FIGURE 6.2. *Aerial view of the layout of the Queen's Hospital, Sidcup.* (A) *Frognal House.* (B) *Main entrance and administration block.* (C) *Dental workshop and surgeries.* (D) *Operating theatres.* (E) *New Zealand Section operating theatre. In 1930 it was sold to the London County Council for use as a general hospital and renamed Queen Mary's Hospital, Sidcup. The hospital buildings were demolished in 1975.* (Courtesy of the Gillies Archive, Queen Mary's Hospital, Sidcup)

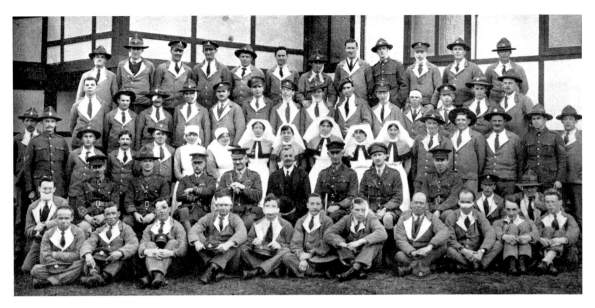

FIGURE 6.3. *New Zealand Section, the Queen's Hospital, Sidcup. Officers sitting in the front row (from left): Major BS Finn DSO, NZDC, Deputy Director Dental Services, NZEF; Major JN Rishworth NZDC; Lieutenant Colonel JR Colvin (Commandant); Brigadier-General GS Richardson CB (GOC Administration, NZEF); Colonel R Heaton Rhodes (Special Commissioner, NZ Red Cross); Colonel WH Parkes CMG (Director of Medical Services, NZEF); Major HP Pickerill NZMC; Lieutenant GC Birt RAMC, attached to the NZ Section. Photograph taken 21 March 1918 on the occasion of the visit of General Richardson and Colonels Heaton Rhodes and Parkes to the hospital.*

(Source: Otago Witness, *19 June 1918, courtesy of the Hocken Library, Uare Taoka o Hakena, University of Otago*)

some weeks later she expressed surprise that the jaw section was still there. One week later an instruction came from the War Office transferring Major Pickerill to Sidcup with immediate effect. (Pickerill has left a somewhat different version of events.)[5] In any event, on 9 January 1918 the Face and Jaw Unit, consisting of Pickerill, his dental mechanic (technician) and twenty-nine patients, arrived at Sidcup, where they were assigned three wards and at the same time inherited a number of British patients.

Extra officers were attached to the New Zealand Section: Major JN Rishworth NZDC[†] (Figure 6.3) was seconded to the unit as senior dental surgeon on the same day as Pickerill (he remained until 10 May, when he replaced BS Finn DSO, NZDC as Deputy Director of Dental Services, NZEF); followed by A McP Marshall NZMC[†] as specialist anaesthetist. (Marshall is incorrectly reported

in *History of the New Zealand Medical Service* as having been severely wounded just before the Battle of Messines;[13] the medical officer wounded on 2 June 1917 at Messines was Captain JA Marshall NZMC, and there is no record of an injury in A McP Marshall's New Zealand Defence Force record.) In August 1918 Captain SD Rhind MC, NZMC[†], who had twice been hospitalised following mustard gas attacks while serving in France, was appointed as a surgical assistant to Pickerill. New Zealand-born Rhind had been studying medicine in London when the war broke out, and he enlisted in the NZEF in 1916. In November 1917, while attached as an RMO to the Second Battalion of the Canterbury Regiment, he had been awarded the Military Cross 'for conspicuous gallantry and devotion to duty for three days and nights at his regimental aid post, repeatedly having to attend to men outside under heavy fire. He also organized parties of stretcher

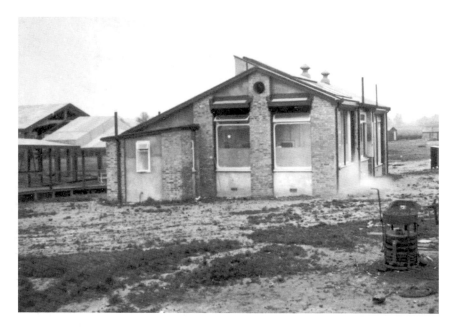

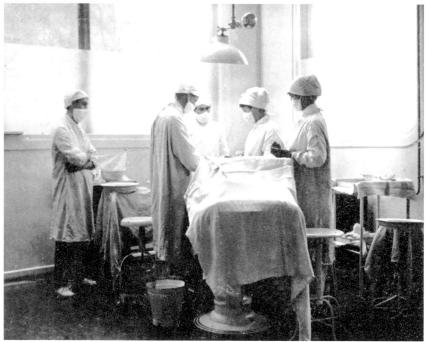

FIGURE 6.4. TOP: *New Zealand Section theatre block.* ABOVE: *Major Pickerill operating, assisted by Sisters Finlayson and McBeth; the orderly standing behind Pickerill is named as Gibbard. Captain Marshall is administering the anaesthetic at the head of the operating table – a triple extension dental chair with an easily adjustable head-rest.* (Photographs from Captain Rhind's memoir Plastic Facio-Maxillary Surgery, *and reproduced with the kind permission of Gillian Martin, Captain SD Rhind's daughter.*)

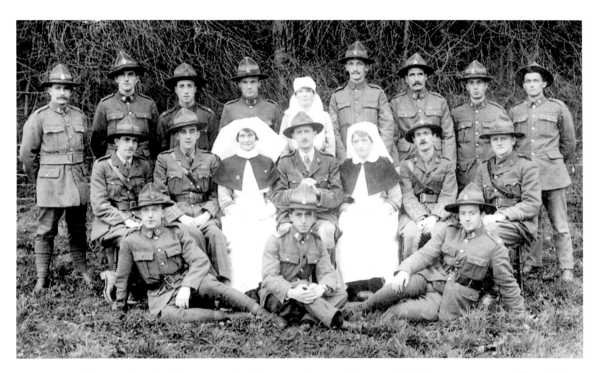

FIGURE 6.5. *Officers and staff of the New Zealand Section, the Queen's Hospital, Sidcup, 1918. Sitting, (from left): Captain JM Turner NZDC, Captain SD Rhind MC, NZMC, Sister McBeth, Major HP Pickerill NZMC, Sister Finlayson, Captain AMcP Marshall NZMC, Captain WS Seed NZDC.* (Photograph from Captain Rhind's memoir Plastic Facio-Maxillary Surgery *and reproduced with the kind permission of Gillian Martin, Captain SD Rhind's daughter)*

bearers for their removal'. (*London Gazette*, 17 December 1917). Two assistant dental surgeons, Captain JM Turner NZDC[†] and Lieutenant WS Seed NZDC[†], were posted to the unit on 23 March and 17 October 1918 respectively.

The generation gap between the three dental surgeons is instructive. Rishworth was an Auckland-based general dental practitioner, who had come to prominence nationally through the affairs of the NZDA, becoming its president in 1912. He lacked a formal dental qualification, having been brought up the hard way via the old apprenticeship system – one of the likely reasons why Pickerill and Rishworth never seemed to have the same respectful professional working relationship enjoyed by Gillies and Kelsey Fry. Nevertheless, Rishworth was a technically gifted clinician, who designed many of the internal and external appliances on which Pickerill's surgical procedures depended for

their success. Seed and Turner, on the other hand, were both members of the new breed of university-trained dental surgeons, former students of Pickerill in Dunedin who had graduated BDS (NZ) from the University of Otago Dental School in 1911 and 1912 respectively. Like Gillies and, later, McIndoe, they were schoolboy scholastic and sporting all-rounders – Seed had been in the Christchurch Boys' High School Rugby First XV and Turner in the Otago Boys' High School Football First XI. Although they lacked the professional experience of Rishworth, they were more highly educated, having had the benefit of a well-structured four-year academic and clinical training programme. One suspects that Pickerill carefully maintained the master–pupil relationship during their time at Sidcup.

As head of the New Zealand Section, Pickerill clearly benefited from the unique opportunities

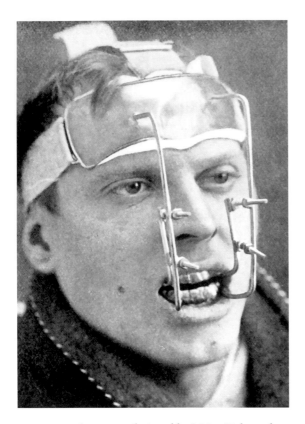

FIGURE 6.6. *Apparatus designed by Major Rishworth NZDC to produce forward displacement of the maxilla. It consisted of a headpiece attached by two vertical bars to a splint cemented to the teeth of the mandible, which was fixed in the slightly open opposition. A splint was also cemented to the teeth of the maxilla and the necessary forward traction produced by the paired screws attached to the short vertical bars. This represents an early form of distraction osteogenesis, widely used today in orthognathic surgery to advance the maxilla.* (Figure 363 in the chapter by W Kelsey Fry on prosthetic problems in Gillies (1920), Plastic Surgery of the Face)

the hospital had to offer to further his surgical expertise, probably more than he cared to admit, and during this period he established a considerable reputation as a plastic and reconstructive surgeon. He published papers on methods to control jaw fragments following gunshot wounds, the surgical reconstruction of the face and nose, the grafting of bone from the tibia and rib, pin fixation of the jaws, as well as the use of orthodontic external fixation to distract impactions of the middle third of the face.[14-17]

Facial Surgery

In 1924 Pickerill published *Facial Surgery*,[18] a small volume based on his wartime experiences but also containing some civilian cases, which he had submitted prior to publication to the University of Birmingham for the degree of Master of Surgery (MS). The preface provides an interesting insight into Pickerill's character. Whereas Gillies in the preface to *Plastic Surgery of the Face* manages to thank by name 39 individuals associated with Aldershot and Sidcup, practically down to the cleaning ladies, Pickerill acknowledges just three – Sir William Arbuthnot Lane, Lieutenant Colonel Colvin and a Mr Cathcart for preparing the index – and a rather inadequate one it is too. No mention of Gillies (undoubtedly a calculated snub) or any of the other section leaders, all of whom went on to distinguished careers in surgery; no mention of his dental and medical colleagues in the New Zealand Section who performed or assisted in many of the operations; no thanks to the nursing staff who looked after the patients, or the artists and photographers who documented the cases, or the technical staff who constructed the appliances that were essential to many a successful surgical outcome. With the exception of Marshall, who anaesthetised most of Pickerill's patients, none of the others is mentioned by name in the text. Even allowing for the fact that multiple or even joint authorship was unusual for the period, particularly among clinicians, where the surgeon-in-charge took most of the credit, Pickerill seems to have been pathologically incapable of acknowledging the work of others. He was also clearly envious of the reputation and position enjoyed by Gillies, and in discussing the tubed pedicle flap (p. 21) even reduces him to second billing: 'It was extensively used by Lieut-Col Newlands, Major Gillies, Major Waldron and myself.' To quote Fred Albee, a man in a position to know: 'When the Almighty passed out jealousy he gave most of it to the medical profession.'[19]

By this time Pickerill had learned that while losses involving the cavities of the mouth and maxillary antrum may be repaired locally, great care must be taken to restore the mucous membranes of the mouth with epithelial linings; this was particularly important for the later successful construction and wearing of artificial dentures. In February 1918 he had started restoring the mucous membrane lining the cheek directly in the mouth with intraoral skin grafts: pressure and the elimination of dead spaces were the essential factors for success. The question of precedence over who first used this adaptation of the Esser technique to skin-graft a defect in the mouth was another subject of disagreement between Pickerill and Gillies. In *Facial Surgery* Pickerill clearly states he was first to employ the method, and he makes a point of noting the date of the operation; whereas in the preface to *Plastic Surgery of the Face* Gillies had attributed it to Waldron, 'closely followed by Pickerill'.

The anonymous reviewer of *Facial Surgery* writing in the *British Journal of Surgery* (1926, Vol. 13, Issue 51, pp. 591–92) was not overly enthusiastic about such a small book and felt that given the advances in maxillofacial surgery since the war it would have been better if the author had confined himself to the treatment of one particular branch. The reviewer – and it is not difficult to guess who it might have been – then goes on to say, 'In a rapidly developing and comparatively new branch of surgery it is always difficult to decide to whom the credit of introducing some new procedure belongs: it is difficult to believe that the author was entirely responsible – working as he did in close association with the heads of the other sections of the hospital – for all he claims to.'

Three cases from the New Zealand Section

Nevertheless, the plastic and maxillofacial surgery carried out by Pickerill and the New Zealand Section at Sidcup was of the highest contemporary standards. Three cases from *Facial Surgery* serve as typical examples. The first demonstrates the sequence of operations required to reconstruct lost cheek tissue; the second, reconstruction of the soft tissues of the chin and lower lip followed by a bone graft to restore the continuity of the lower jaw; and the third, reconstruction of the upper and lower lips. Pickerill had found his métier – a discovery that was to profoundly change his professional and ultimately his personal life.

Private Mallon

In the first patient, Private Mallon, whose treatment was started at Sidcup and completed in Dunedin, the extensive loss of facial tissue extending into the antrum and floor of the orbit was repaired by grafting a large area of skin and fat from the chest (Figure 6.7). Nourishment and vitality were maintained by means of a tubed pedicle, which was subsequently divided and returned to the neck. Any raw exposed tissue at the donor site below the clavicle was covered by Thiersch split-skin grafts from the inner surface of the upper arm. All operations were carried out under local anaesthesia with Novocaine. After some months the bone of the lost zygoma (cheekbone) and the lower orbital margin were reconstructed with a rib cartilage graft, and the missing right eye was replaced with an orbital prosthesis.

Private Skurr

Private Skurr, whose treatment was also completed in Dunedin, suffered extensive loss of tissue involving destruction of the chin and lower lip, plus loss of two-thirds of the mandible from second molar to second molar (Figures 6.8, 6.9). As an emergency measure it was first necessary to do a high tracheotomy to prevent the patient from suffocating, as the swelling from the wound and loss of control of the tongue almost completely blocked the airway. Once this had healed, according to the case notes the surgical repair was undertaken as follows:

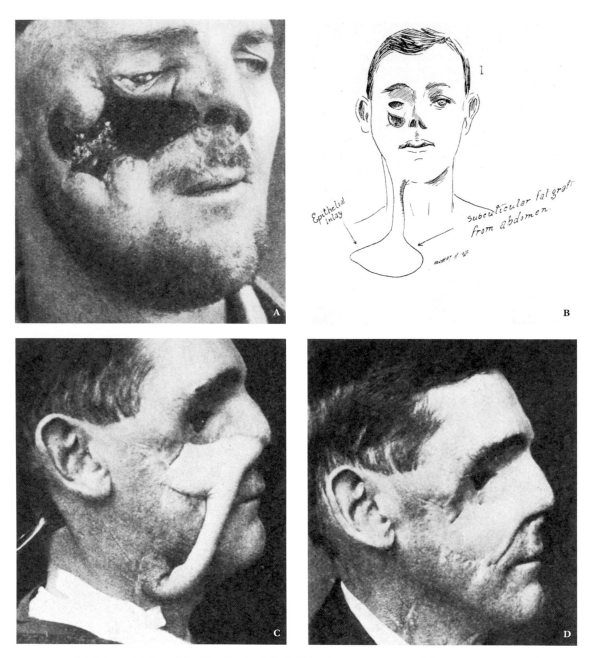

FIGURE 6.7. (A) *Private Mallon of the New Zealand Cycle Brigade on admission to Sidcup, 17.5.1918.* (B) *Planning diagram by Herbert Cole showing how this extensive loss of cheek tissue involving the antrum and floor of the orbit was reconstructed by grafting a large area of skin and fat from the chest by means of a tubed pedicle flap.* (C). *31.7.1920.* (D) *22.2.1921. The neck tube was subsequently divided and returned to the neck and the donor site below the clavicle covered by Thiersch split-skin grafts from the arm. All operations were carried out under local anaesthesia. After some months a rib cartilage graft was inserted and shaped to reconstruct the lost zygoma and orbital margin to accommodate an artificial eye.* (From Pickerill (1924), Facial Surgery)

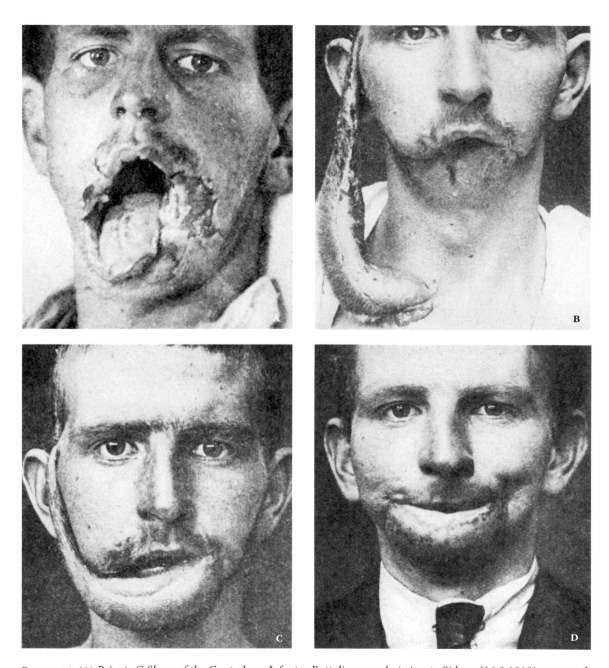

FIGURE 6.8. (A) *Private G Skurr of the Canterbury Infantry Battalion on admission to Sidcup (16.9.1918) presented with destruction of the chin and anterior part of mandible.* (B) *A double scalp-chest tubed pedicle flap was formed to restore the soft tissues of the chin.* (C) *The lower end of the double scalp-chest flap was detached and sutured below and to the left.* (D) *The tubed flap was then divided and returned. Graft sutured on the right side with hair-bearing skin on the outside with smooth hairless skin on the inside forming the vermilion of the lip. Photograph taken 5.12.1919.* (From Pickerill (1924), Facial Surgery)

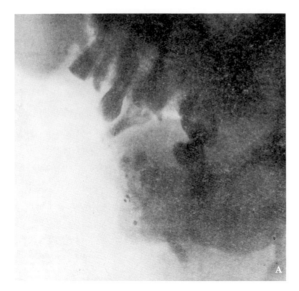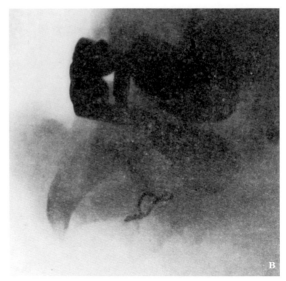

FIGURE 6.9. *Private G Skurr. Although the quality of the radiographs (skiagrams) is poor, they do show the extensive loss of bone pre-treatment.* (A) *The angle of the mandible is visible with a single molar tooth.* (B) *Dated 10.2.1924, showing how the missing anterior segment was reconstructed with a rib graft wired to the posterior segments; also visible is a cap splint that had been cemented to the upper teeth to immobilise the mandible.* (From Pickerill (1924), Facial Surgery)

Stage 1: *The amount and exact size of the tissue necessary for the repair of the chin and lip were determined from a reconstructed plaster cast. Pewter foil patterns were obtained and from these the following flaps were cut:*

(1) *A lining flap from the clavicle to the level of the fifth rib, detached at its lower end, tubed in its upper portion and thrown upwards to the neck, raw surface outwards.*

(2) *A scalp flap of similar dimensions cut from the zygoma to the vertex, tubed in its lower half, swung downwards and superimposed on the chest flap. The two flaps were sutured together and allowed to unite.*

Stage 2: *The chest flap was severed at its lower end and the double tubed flap was swung across and sutured into position, Nourishment of the flap was maintained by the posterior branch of the superficial temporal artery.*

Stage 3: *The tubed scalp flap was then divided and returned. The graft was sutured on the right side with hair-bearing skin on the outside, and smooth hairless skin on the inside forming the vermilion of the lip. Twelve months later the missing anterior segment of the mandible was successfully reconstructed by separating the flaps and inserting 5 inches of rib. Silver wire was used to maintain close approximation to the remains of the mandible on each side.*

Private Green

The case of Private P Green of the 2/12th Battalion, the London Regiment, was first reported by Pickerill in an article published in 1922 in the *British Journal of Surgery*.[20] Both the journal article and *Facial Surgery* discuss the case in some detail and include a photographic record of the sequence of operations. However, Private Green is of interest not only because of the severity of his wounds, but also because the watercolours painted by Herbert

Cole, which are held in the Gillies Archive and the Hocken Library, constitute the most complete set of portraits of any patient treated at Sidcup (Colour plate 11).

Private Green had been admitted on 21 August 1917 with severe gunshot wounds to the face. He was first seen by Captain Aymard, who removed a lachrymal sac and some fragments of dead bone. When Green was transferred to Pickerill, his condition was recorded as a total loss of the upper and lower lips as well as the premaxilla, with backward depression of the nose (Colour plate 11(A)). According to the case notes, the aim of Pickerill's first operation carried out on 11 June 1918 was to establish a lower labial sulcus; tissues adherent to the lower jaw were divided freely down to the mental process of the mandible and a large intraoral skin graft was inserted and secured by circumferential ligatures:

Operation 5.9.1918: *To obtain tissue for the formation of the lower lip and lining of the upper lip, a strip of skin and subcutaneous tissue was raised from the neck – the incision extended from the mandible to below the clavicle on the left side; the flap was tubed and left attached at both ends and the resulting raw area closed by undermining the skin on each side* (Colour plate 11(B)).

Operation 25.9.1918: *The remains of the lower lip were freshened and a bed prepared for the tube flap which was amputated at its lower end and then swung across and anchored into position by three rows of sutures* (Colour plate 11(C)).

Operation 17.10.1918: *The pedicle of the new lip was divided at the left angle, opened up and then converted into a free flap attached to the left angle of the jaw* (Colour plate 11(D)). *A long flap was next cut from the scalp extending diagonally backwards from the zygoma to the crown of the head. This was swung downwards keeping the hair surface outwards. The attached portion of the scalp flap was tubed and the lower free portion was united by catgut and horsehair sutures to the skin flap which had previously been used for the lip pedicle* (Colour plate 11(E)).

Operation 31.10.1918: *Under local anaesthesia the margin of the scalp flap was reduced and the skin flap brought further round to form the future lip margin* (Colour plate 11(F)).

Operation 23.11.1918: *A small piece of cartilage was inserted into columella to give stiffness prior to next operation.*

Dental operation 10.12.1918: *Captain Turner. Upper skeleton splint carrying vulcanite piece to mould upper lip cemented into position.*

Operation 11.12.1918: *Lip flap formed by junction of neck and scalp flaps swung across and inserted into prepared bed on the right side.*

Dental operation 21.12.1918: *Captain Seed. Nasal tubes with springs inserted (presumably to apply pressure to a skin graft).*

Operation 2.1.1919: *Scalp for new upper lip returned.*

No further entries are recorded in the notes.

Pickerill's return to Dunedin, 1919–21

The rehabilitation of the wounded did not end with the war. In March 1919 Pickerill, together with 59 patients, embarked from Plymouth on the SS *Tainui* and returned to New Zealand, where the long-term care of the patients continued in the Facial and Jaw Department at Dunedin Hospital. By June 1919 Pickerill had been promoted to lieutenant colonel and awarded an OBE 'for valuable services rendered in connection with the War'.[5] His staff at Dunedin Hospital consisted of Captains Marshall and Seed, three nursing sisters and four sergeants: an artist (Herbert Cole[†]), a photographer, a modeller and a dental mechanic.

Captain Turner stayed behind in England and was discharged from the army in September 1919. His next move was to Philadelphia and further study at the University of Pennsylvania Dental School (DDS, 1920). On his return to the United Kingdom, Turner went into practice in Torquay, Devon, where he remained until his death in 1975. Captain Seed worked in the Dunedin

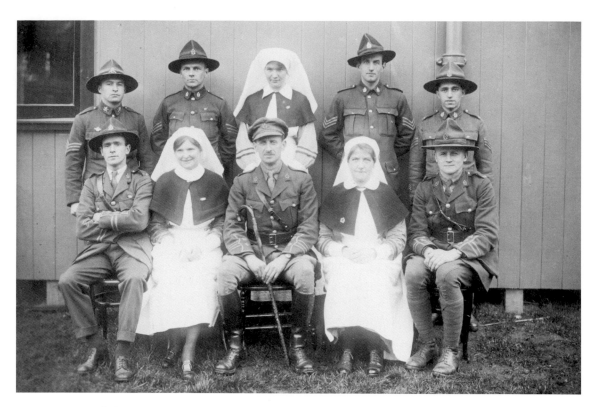

FIGURE 6.10. *Staff of the Facial and Jaw Unit outside the technical annex in the grounds of Dunedin Hospital. Back Row: Sergeant Ferguson, Sergeant Thomson, Sister Erwin, Sergeant Cole, Sergeant Meltzer. Front Row: Captain Marshall (anaesthetist), Sister Millar, Lieutenant Colonel Pickerill, Sister Finlayson, Captain Seed (dental officer).*
(Otago Witness, *1919*)

unit until discharged in January 1920, then he returned to dental practice in Christchurch until his retirement in 1952; he died two years later. Captain Rhind, whose health had been seriously compromised after two episodes of mustard gas poisoning, contracted pneumonia during the 1918 influenza pandemic and returned to New Zealand in March 1919 on the SS *Maheno*, a trans-Tasman passenger vessel that had been converted into a hospital ship. He was admitted to the Queen Mary Hospital at Hanmer Springs in North Canterbury in a much debilitated state. There, however, the alpine air and thermal pools restored his health, and he joined the staff and remained until May 1921, when he was discharged from the army (or in military parlance 'struck off the strength') and left for London to continue his surgical training at St George's Hospital in London. In 1924 he returned

with his FRCS (Eng) to surgical appointments in Wellington and Lower Hutt hospitals. He died in 1956 at the early age of 61.

To provide a convalescent home for the patients between operations, the Red Cross leased Woodside, a prominent Dunedin architectural landmark completed in 1876 for Judge Henry Chapman, Chancellor of the University of Otago 1876–79. The house was designed by the Dunedin architect FW Petrie, and at the time of its construction it was reputed to be the first concrete home in monolithic form to be built in the southern hemisphere.[21] It was renamed the Woodside Auxiliary Hospital for Facial Injuries (known locally as the 'Jaw Hospital') and re-equipped to accommodate 36 patients, with the overflow lodged at Montecillo, the Red Cross veterans home, and later at what became known as the Sidcup Ward in Dunedin

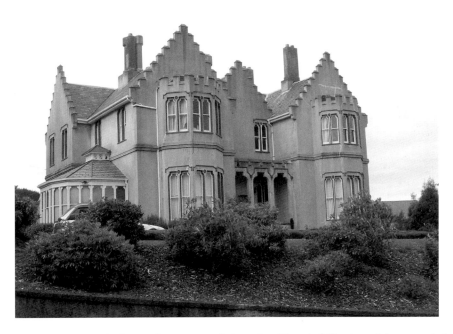

FIGURE 6.11. *Woodside Auxiliary Hospital, Dunedin. The rehabilitation of the wounded continued after the war and in 1919 the New Zealand Unit was transferred to Dunedin, where Pickerill continued the long-term care of injured servicemen. Sited at the corner of Dundas Street and Lovelock Avenue, the building was leased by the Red Cross to provide a convalescent home and was known locally as the Jaw Hospital. Originally called Castlemore, the building is now known as Lovelock House in memory of Jack Lovelock, former University of Otago medical student, Rhodes Scholar and winner of the gold medal for the 1500 metres at the 1936 Berlin Olympic Games.*

(Photograph (2007) courtesy of Harriet Meikle)

Hospital.[5] With a diminishing number of patients under his care, the unit closed in December 1921 and Pickerill was able to return full time to his position as Dean and Director of Dental Studies at the Dental School.

Captain Marshall's story does not have a happy ending. On returning from Sidcup, Marshall continued to anaesthetise Pickerill's patients in the Facial and Jaw Unit, and from 1921 he was Chief Anaesthetist at Dunedin Hospital. However, on 31 July 1927 he inexplicably took his own life with an overdose of hyoscine (scopolamine), leaving a wife and two children. He did not seem to have had a history of depression or any financial or family worries. Nevertheless, the statement made by his wife at the inquest is significant '… I think he had been worrying over his projected departure from Dunedin for Australia and was uncertain whether

he had taken the right step. This I think preyed on his mind. He told me he had taken a large dose.'[22]

In 1927 Pickerill had resigned from the University of Otago for personal reasons and to revive his career as a plastic surgeon in Australia. While there is no supporting documentary evidence, it is difficult to escape the conclusion, given their long-standing professional relationship, that Pickerill had managed to persuade Marshall to accompany him to Sydney as his anaesthetist. Marshall went so far as to resign his post at Dunedin Hospital, but must have had second thoughts, failing to attend the leaving function organised for him by his colleagues. Dr Marion Whyte, the anaesthetist who succeeded Marshall at Dunedin Hospital, when interviewed in 1969 expressed the opinion that Pickerill was a ruthless man in getting what he wanted and had persuaded Marshall against his better judgement to move to Australia.[23] Why he then took such an irrevocable step is difficult to understand. The Coroner, however, had no doubt: his verdict was that on the 31st day of July 1927, Angus McPhee Marshall died from the effects of hyoscine, a poison self-administered, while in a state of mental depression.[22]

The Macalister Archive

At the end of the war the New Zealand Section records returned to Dunedin with Pickerill and the Facial and Jaw Unit, and when the unit closed down they were transferred to the Dental School. Having survived two further moves to new Dental School buildings in 1927 and 1961, they were saved some years later from imminent destruction by the intervention of Professor AD Macalister, during one of those perennial clearouts of old patient notes (familiar to anyone who has ever worked in a clinical department) and were destined for the dump; for many years they were stored in Macalister's garage. In 1987 Macalister delivered the Menzies Campbell Lecture at the Royal College of Surgeons of England, entitled 'The Queen's Hospital, Sidcup: the Foundation of British Oral Surgery'.[24] After the lecture it was suggested the records could be given a permanent home at Queen Mary's Hospital, and arrived back in Sidcup via his son, Donald Macalister, 70 years after they had left.[25] The collection, known as the Macalister archive, consists of 282 sets of case notes containing typescript summaries, clinical photographs and radiographs, drawings, 77 watercolours and a life-size wax model of the head and upper torso (Colour plate 12). Many of the watercolours are unsigned, but most are almost certainly the work of Herbert R Cole, the artist attached to the New Zealand Section (not to be confused with Herbert Cole (1867–1930), a prolific illustrator of books and magazines in the Art Nouveau style). The collection also includes three watercolours by Daryl Lindsay, the artist attached to the Australian Section.

In addition to the 282 patient files returned to Sidcup from the Dental School in 1989, another 62 sets of case notes are in the Hocken Library at the University of Otago (Reference number: ARC-0187). These were given to Dr John Borrie by Pickerill's second wife, Dame Cecily Pickerill, and became part of the Medical Library Historical Collection in 1981. The records are named but in many cases are disappointingly incomplete, consisting mainly of photographs and the occasional watercolour. For some patients, particularly those with fractures or bone grafts of the jaws, X-rays are included, often with line diagrams drawn by Captain JM Turner to aid radiographic interpretation. The collection also includes an additional 19 watercolours of wounded servicemen undergoing treatment at Dunedin Hospital, painted by Cole, including the four used by Pickerill as the frontispiece to *Facial Surgery* (Colour plate 13).

Captain Rhind also put together an album of some of the cases treated by the New Zealand Section at Sidcup, entitled *Plastic Facio-Maxillary Surgery*. The collection consists of patient photographs and an occasional watercolour mounted on grey cardboard, each with a hand-written commentary. Following Captain Rhind's death in 1956, three copies were made and the original album was given by his daughter, Gillian Martin, into the care of Brigadier WH Blinman Bull, who in 1971 donated it to the Royal New Zealand Army Medical Corps Museum at Burnham Camp in Canterbury. One of the copies, with typed commentaries made by Mrs Martin, has been lodged with the Gillies Archive.

CHAPTER 7

McIndoe, Mowlem and the interwar years

GILLIES AND PICKERILL MADE their reputations in plastic and maxillofacial surgery in the First World War. McIndoe and Mowlem represent the next generation, who established their reputations during the Second. Both were born in New Zealand – McIndoe in Dunedin and Mowlem in Auckland – and they were contemporaries at the University of Otago, although McIndoe was senior by one year. The common factor in determining the future direction of their careers was the influence of Harold Gillies – or, as he had become in 1930, the year before McIndoe's arrival in London, Sir Harold Gillies. His knighthood was regarded by many at the time – including, it seems, Buckingham Palace – as an overdue and well-deserved honour.

The McIndoe family

The New Zealand McIndoes can trace their family roots back to Iain Dhu (Black Ian) Cameron who was born in Lochiel, Scotland, date unknown.[1] In 1746 he either fought in, or became a victim of, the Battle of Culloden – a brutal encounter in which the Jacobite army of mainly Highland clansmen led by the Young Pretender, Charles Edward Stuart (Bonnie Prince Charlie), and Lord George Murray was heavily defeated by the British redcoats under the command of the Duke of Cumberland, third son of the Hanoverian King George II, thereby bringing to a decisive end the final attempt to restore the

House of Stuart to the British throne. After the battle, indiscriminate killing by the government troops went on for several days; all men bearing arms were hanged on location, their women raped and their families forced from their burning homes and left to starve, earning for their commander the epithet 'Butcher' Cumberland. The bearing of arms and the wearing of all items of Highland dress, including the kilt, were banned.

To avoid the ongoing slaughter, Iain Dhu anglicised the Gaelic Mac Iain Dhu to McIndoe,[1] and fled with his wife Janet and son to Killearn on the Kintyre peninsula in Argyll. Ian Dhu's son, William (1746–1826), moved to Rothesay on the Isle of Bute around 1770 and progressed from being a pedlar and shopkeeper to being a successful merchant. His son Archibald (1791–1847), McIndoe's great-grandfather, followed his father into the family business and was an influential and respected member of the local community, succeeding the Earl of Bute as the first commoner to become the provost (mayor) of Rothesay.[1] However, as a result of the conflict and divisions within the Presbyterian Church, the next generation decided to leave Scotland and take advantage of the opportunities offered by a new life in New Zealand. In 1850 McIndoe's grandfather, James McIndoe (1824–1905), a Free Churchman and member of the Otago Association, married Elizabeth Gillies.

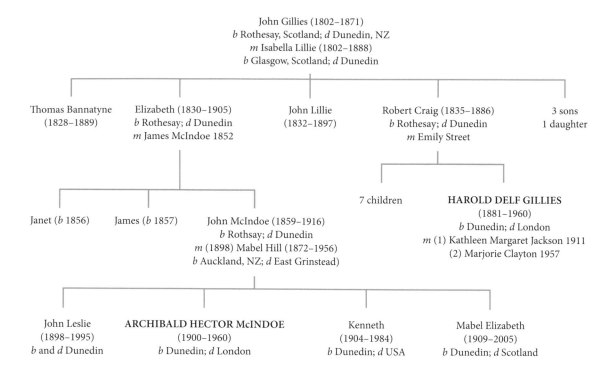

John Gillies (1802–1871)
b Rothesay, Scotland; *d* Dunedin, NZ
m Isabella Lillie (1802–1888)
b Glasgow, Scotland; *d* Dunedin

Thomas Bannatyne (1828–1889)

Elizabeth (1830–1905) *b* Rothesay; *d* Dunedin *m* James McIndoe 1852

John Lillie (1832–1897)

Robert Craig (1835–1886) *b* Rothesay; *d* Dunedin *m* Emily Street

3 sons 1 daughter

7 children

HAROLD DELF GILLIES (1881–1960) *b* Dunedin; *d* London *m* (1) Kathleen Margaret Jackson 1911 (2) Marjorie Clayton 1957

Janet (*b* 1856)

James (*b* 1857)

John McIndoe (1859–1916) *b* Rothsay; *d* Dunedin *m* (1898) Mabel Hill (1872–1956) *b* Auckland, NZ; *d* East Grinstead)

John Leslie (1898–1995) *b* and *d* Dunedin

ARCHIBALD HECTOR McINDOE (1900–1960) *b* Dunedin; *d* London

Kenneth (1904–1984) *b* Dunedin; *d* USA

Mabel Elizabeth (1909–2005) *b* Dunedin; *d* Scotland

FIGURE 7.1. *Gillies–McIndoe family tree.* *(Courtesy of John Hector McIndoe)*

Two years later Elizabeth's father, John Gillies, and the rest of her immediate family left for Otago (see Chapter 2), where they became well established in the commercial, professional and political affairs of the province. Archibald McIndoe's grandmother Elizabeth and Harold Gillies' father Robert were brother and sister – Gillies and McIndoe were therefore first cousins once removed.

James and Elizabeth McIndoe and their three surviving children, Janet (b 1856), James (b 1857) and John (b 1859), followed the Gillies to New Zealand on the *Alpine* (1100 tons), which sailed from Glasgow on 10 June 1859 with 460 passengers. It arrived at Port Chalmers, Dunedin, three months later on 12 September; there had been nine deaths on the voyage, all bar one under the age of three years, as well as four births.[2] The conditions for steerage passengers on a crowded sailing ship were a frequent cause for criticism, and the McIndoes' voyage proved to be no more pleasant than the Gillies' experience on the *Slains Castle*. On arrival at

Port Chalmers, the *Alpine* achieved some notoriety when, acting on complaints from the passengers, the immigration officer brought the captain before a bench of magistrates and fined him £500, with a special allowance made to each of the passengers claiming damages.[3]

James set up in business in Dunedin as a merchant, but following a successful gold-prospecting expedition with his brother-in-law, John L Gillies, relocated to Lawrence in 1861, where he opened the first general store at Gabriel's Gully in a calico tent – the usual building material on the early goldfields. When the miners moved on to fresh diggings, the family returned to Dunedin living at Hinemoa, a large stone farmhouse and its attendant farm, which occupied a large part of what is now South Dunedin. The farm had been bought for Elizabeth by her father, but because married women were not allowed to own property in their own right, it automatically became the property of her husband. Elizabeth was a strong-willed woman,

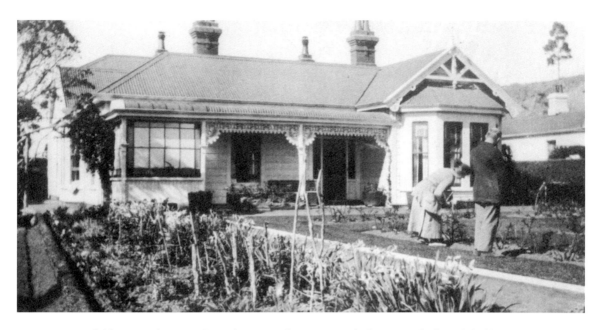

FIGURE 7.2. *Seafield, Macandrew Road, St Clair, Dunedin, ca 1912: the house in which Archibald McIndoe grew up. John McIndoe built this large villa in 1898 for his future wife, Mabel Hill, next to his parents' house, Hinemoa, at the corner of Forbury and Macandrew Roads – known locally as 'McIndoe Corner'. The house was compulsorily purchased in 1945 under the Public Works Act by the Education Department for no good reason, and in the 1960s was demolished and replaced by two ugly flats.* (Reproduced with the kind permission of John H McIndoe)

and she became an outspoken advocate for a change in this law.[1] (The Married Women's Property Act was eventually adopted in 1884.) James McIndoe took an active interest in local and national politics; he was elected to the Otago Provincial Council and, in 1870, briefly served as the member for Caversham in the House of Representatives at Wellington. A keen botanist and polemicist, he wrote articles for the *Otago Witness*, the *Otago Daily Times* and his old local newspaper *The Bute*, and two books on the early history of the settlement: *Early Days in Otago* and *A Sketch of Otago*.[4]

Archibald Hector McIndoe

Archibald Hector McIndoe was born on 4 May 1900, the second of four children of John McIndoe and his wife Mabel Hill, who was an accomplished and well-known New Zealand artist (Colour plates 14 and 15). The family lived at Seafield, a large wooden villa built by John in 1898 for his future wife in Macandrew Road, St Clair. John McIndoe

(1858–1916) had been educated at the local school in Caversham and at the age of 16 was apprenticed to Coulls and Culling, printers in Dunedin. He was an artistic and practical-minded young man, who earned praise for the quality of his typographical designs. After working as a compositor for some years, in 1893 he went into partnership with David Cherrie and in 1900 set up in business on his own as John McIndoe, Printer and Bookbinder. The business built a reputation for artistic and creative printing and proved very successful; in addition to Seafield, the family built a weekend crib (seaside cottage) at Brighton, on the coast south of Dunedin. Unfortunately, illness forced John to retire early, and he died at Seacliff near Dunedin on 4 April 1916.[5] On his death the business continued under the management of his oldest son, John Leslie McIndoe (the McIndoe and Gillies families had a weakness for calling their sons John), a personal sacrifice that enabled Archibald to study medicine at the University of Otago.

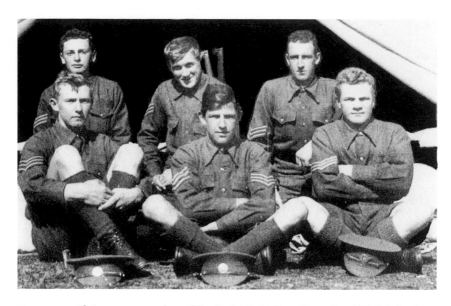

FIGURE 7.3. *Platoon commanders of the Cadet Battalion, Otago Boys' High School, summer camp, Tahuna Park, Dunedin, 1917. Back Row: DW Faigan, GA Holmes, PA Treahy. Front Row: D'AH Moir, AH McIndoe, GA Fairmaid. Absent: JM Twhigg, JD Hunter. Moir, McIndoe, Hunter, Treahy and Twhigg all went on to study medicine at the University of Otago. Holmes, dux in 1917, became an agricultural scientist; Faigan principal of a teachers' training college; and Fairmaid a mining engineer in Malaya.* (Photograph courtesy of the late David C Billing, OBHS Archives and Museum)

Archibald McIndoe, known as Archie to family and friends, was educated at Otago Boys' High School during the years of the First World War. Founded in 1863 by the provincial council, the school was an uncompromisingly academic institution with an ethos designed to produce future leaders in the professions and commerce – in an atmosphere of muscular Christianity, rugby and cricket were compulsory. For many boys the school was remarkably successful in achieving these aims. Of the eight platoon commanders of the Cadet Battalion in 1917, six of whom are shown in Figure 7.3, all went on to university (five to study medicine) and all became highly successful in their chosen careers. This environment clearly suited McIndoe's temperament and he had a notable academic and sporting career as a schoolboy. He was a prefect for two years, a member of the Gymnastics VIII for three, and in 1918 was captain of the Second Cricket XI, Cadet Battalion sergeant-major, school rifle champion in the Challenge Cup, and gained

a credit in the Scholarship exams. He was also an accomplished pianist – photographs of wartime and postwar Guinea Pig Club reunions show McIndoe at the piano surrounded by admiring current and former patients.

A career in medicine

In 1919 McIndoe matriculated at the University of Otago Medical School. He graduated MB ChB (NZ) in 1923, and went on to achieve the distinction of winning the Junior Clinical Medicine Prize in 1923 and the Senior Clinical Surgery Prize in 1924 – a notable double.[6] In his fifth and final year, he carried out 'A Survey of a Group of Slum Houses'[7] – a study of the environmental impact of housing and diet on health, particularly of children, in a rundown area of Dunedin. As Sir Arthur Porritt, who was a contemporary of McIndoe at Medical School, commented 40 years later, 'He was good-looking, had a good brain, a good physique and was a good mixer, but he also had ambition

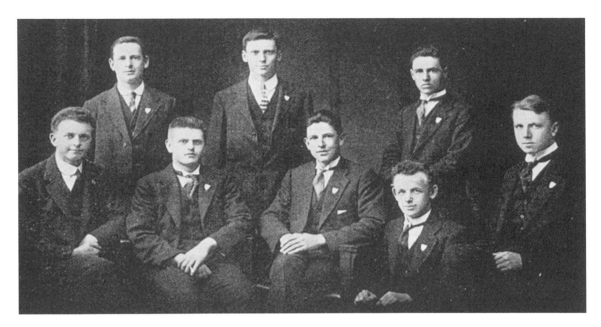

FIGURE 7.4. *Otago Boys' High School prefects, 1918. Back Row: WW Bridgman, HL Webb, JT Burton. Front Row: FM Campbell, RG Stokes, AH McIndoe, AL Sutherland, M Macbeth.* (Photograph courtesy of the late David C Billing, OBHS Archives and Museum, taken by Barry Cardno)

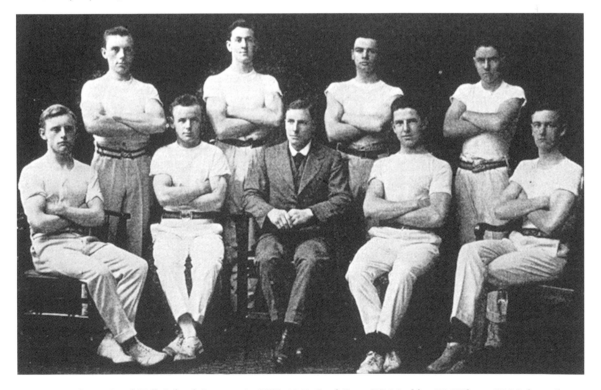

FIGURE 7.5. *Otago Boys' High School Gymnastics VIII, 1918. Back Row: RR Markby, BL Wilson, GM Salmond, JT Burton. Front Row: JHR Fulton, AL Sutherland, Mr L Phillips, AH McIndoe, HS Wilkinson.* (Photograph courtesy of the late David C Billing, OBHS Archives and Museum, taken by Barry Cardno)

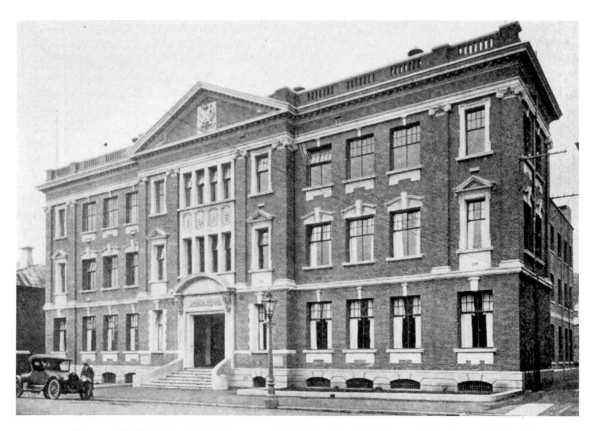

FIGURE 7.6. *The new Medical School building, opened in 1917, where McIndoe and Mowlem studied medicine. Built of brick in the textile factory style favoured by academic institutions at the time, it sits opposite Dunedin Hospital on Great King Street. Half the cost was raised by public subscription from the citizens of Dunedin, and this was matched by a government subsidy. It was named the Scott Building after JH Scott, Professor of Anatomy and Physiology and Dean of the Medical School 1890–1914.* (From GE Thompson (1919), A History of the University of Otago 1869–1919)

and vision and could not see in the small country where he was born, that either could be fulfilled.'[8] In this he was not alone: young New Zealanders have always travelled abroad to test themselves on a broader world stage, commonly referred to as OE (overseas experience), particularly to the United Kingdom with its family and cultural ties. Porritt was himself a good example: a man who left Dunedin for Oxford as a Rhodes Scholar in 1923, and returned in 1967 as New Zealand's first native-born governor-general.

After graduating, McIndoe worked as a house surgeon in Waikato Hospital at Hamilton in the North Island. In 1924 he secured the first fellowship granted to a New Zealander by the Mayo Clinic at Rochester, Minnesota (at the time arguably the outstanding centre for surgical and medical training in the world), to study pathological anatomy.[7] There was only one problem with this: the appointment required the fellow to be single and McIndoe had recently married Adonia Aitken.[9,10] To secure the fellowship they decided to keep the marriage a secret and he sailed for the United States without her. It could not be kept a secret indefinitely, however, and Adonia joined him 12 months later. He held the Mayo Fellowship until 1928, having obtained an MSc at the University of Minnesota in 1927. In 1929 he was appointed First Assistant in Surgery, and was awarded an MS (Master of Surgery) by the University of Minnesota. McIndoe made his mark at the Mayo Clinic, and published a number of papers on hepatic disease with DC Balfour, Chief Surgeon, and VS Counciller, including two on the importance of portal cirrhosis and the structure of the biliary canaliculi. At the same time he developed a name for himself as an expert abdominal surgeon, reputedly removing a 'metallic object' from the abdomen of a gentleman from Chicago with several large friends, who turned out to be Al Capone's brother.[10]

The turning point in his career came with a visit to the Mayo Clinic by Berkeley Moynihan, 1st Baron Moynihan of Leeds, who at the time was president of the Royal College of Surgeons of England. Moynihan recognised a good abdominal surgeon when he saw one, and apparently told McIndoe that with the planned expansion of the Royal Postgraduate Medical School at Hammersmith in London a professorship in surgery would be available and he would recommend him for the post.[9,10] Whatever transpired between the two men, it seems likely that life on the prairies had lost some of its charm, and McIndoe seized on their conversation as the opportunity to make a career move. On the strength of this encounter he resigned from the Mayo Clinic and sailed for England with Adonia and their daughter in the winter of 1931. Unfortunately, talk of the expansion of the medical school and the surgical professorship turned out to be premature and McIndoe found himself and his family in a basement flat in Maida Vale, West London, out of a job.

McIndoe was thrown a lifeline by Sir Harold Gillies, the cousin he had never met. Gillies took a liking to his country cousin and started to pull a few strings, arranging a post for him as a clinical assistant at St Bartholomew's Hospital and inviting him to join the plastic surgery practice he had established at the London Clinic (T Pomfret Kilner had left the partnership). After much criticism from Adonia, who regarded plastic surgery as nothing more than a cosmetic luxury, he accepted the offer. In 1932 McIndoe obtained a permanent appointment as lecturer and general surgeon at the Hospital for Tropical Diseases, where he continued his abdominal surgery, and later in

the same year was admitted FRCS (Eng). In the period leading up to the Second World War, like many of his contemporaries, he led a somewhat peripatetic existence with appointments at St Bartholomew's Hospital, the Chelsea Hospital for Women, St Andrew's Hospital Dollis Hill, St James' Balham, and the Children's Hospital Hampstead. He was also consulting plastic surgeon to the North Staffordshire Royal Infirmary and Croydon General Hospital.[11] In 1938 Gillies helped McIndoe again by relinquishing his appointment as consultant plastic surgeon to the RAF in his favour – a generous gesture that proved to be the foundation of McIndoe's subsequent international fame.

The Mowlem family

The Mowlems are descended from Durand de Moulham, who was given land at Moulham by William the Conqueror, for keeping the Great Tower of Corfe Castle on the Isle of Purbeck in Dorset in good working order. The Domesday Survey of 1087 records that Durand held Moleham *in capite* (directly from the Crown) and was commanded to undertake what is probably Britain's oldest recorded maintenance contract – he had to 'find a carpenter to work about the Great Tower of Corfe Castle when the King wishes to have it repaired'.[12] The residue of the land which constituted the De Moulham Estate, Swanage's biggest and oldest estate, was inherited by Rainsford Mowlem from his great-uncle John Ernest Mowlem (1868–1946), and on his death in 1986 it was gifted to the town of Swanage. A building gene was clearly embedded in the Mowlem family – John Ernest was the great-nephew of John Mowlem (1788–1868), who became a successful businessman by importing Purbeck limestone into London and who founded the Mowlem Construction Company.

Rainsford Mowlem's branch of the family came to New Zealand by way of Australia. His great-grandfather, Henry Hibbs Mowlem (1817–1874), had left England for Australia in 1851 with his wife Sarah Manwell and three children, and settled in Melbourne, Victoria. One of the sons, Fred (1846–1925), married Mary Emma Ward, and in 1872 Rainsford Mowlem's father Arthur was born.

In the second half of the nineteenth century New Zealand was firmly established as a sister colony to those in Australia. Indeed, New Zealand was involved in the protracted discussions between the six self-governing Australian colonies which led to the formation of the Commonwealth of Australia in 1901, but decided not to join (good news for the Bledisloe Cup). Many colonists thought nothing of moving from one country to the other – an itinerant workforce did it regularly, particularly during the days of the goldrush, and the journey from Dunedin to Melbourne was regarded as no more significant than from Dunedin to Auckland.[13] As part of this trans-Tasman migration, in 1874 the Mowlem family decided to try their luck in New Zealand, and settled in the small township of Wainuiomata, near Wellington. However, the isolated nature of the Wainuiomata valley with narrow hill routes being the only access presented a problem for early settlers in the area, with the local economy heavily dependent on timber milling. In 1877 the Mowlem family moved again, this time to Palmerston North.

Arthur Rainsford Mowlem

Arthur Rainsford Mowlem was born in Auckland on 1 December 1902, the son of Arthur Manwell Mowlem (1872–1936) and his wife Marion Beecroft. His father had trained as a solicitor and served as a stipendary magistrate (equivalent to a District Court judge) in Auckland, New Plymouth and Napier. At the time of his birth the family lived at 31 Shelly Beach Road, Herne Bay, in a house that has since been demolished. Rainsford Mowlem (he was always referred to as Rainsford, presumably to distinguish him from his father Arthur) was educated at Auckland Grammar School (Colour plate 16) – like Otago Boys', another uncompromisingly academic single-sex institution. The school had been founded and endowed by Governor Sir George Grey in 1850, but the good burghers of Auckland did not get around to opening it until 1869. This was not entirely the fault of the trustees, who had been slowly accumulating sufficient funds to make the school financially viable: secondary school education was not free at

the time. Auckland had none of the early wealth of Otago and Canterbury, and was preoccupied with the ongoing conflict between the Crown and Maori tribes in the Waikato. It was not until the endowments became the responsibility of the provincial council, and the passage of the Auckland Grammar Appropriation Act in 1868, that the school came into being.[14]

Mowlem was an academically able boy, and during his four years at the school (1916–19) was fed an unrelieved diet of English, Latin, French, mathematics and science. For the first three years he remained firmly anchored in the bottom half of the A-stream, but in the Lower Sixth he appears to have applied himself: with the exception of mathematics, he finished in the top six places in a class of 30 boys and left with the Higher Leaving and Medical Preliminary Certificates.[15] As he was not a prefect, was not in a top sports team and did not earn a University Scholarship, there are no photographs of him on record at the school.

Mowlem's obituary in *The Lancet* records that initially he trained for a legal career like his father, but soon changed to medicine.[16] However, it was not possible to obtain supporting documentary evidence for this statement (the University of Auckland declined to confirm it on the grounds that under the 1993 Privacy Act they were not permitted to release such information to a third party). Whatever the truth of the matter, in 1920 he enrolled as a student at Auckland University College and passed the intermediate medical examination (in biology, organic and inorganic chemistry, and physics), which enabled him to start the medical course proper in Dunedin. Up until the end of the war the number of medical graduates had averaged in the mid-twenties, but by the time McIndoe and Mowlem entered the Medical School, returned servicemen had swelled numbers in the postwar graduating classes to more than 60.

Having apparently tired of the student digs at the YMCA, where he spent his first year, Mowlem applied to join Knox College – a residential college and training establishment affiliated with the Presbyterian Church – and he lived there from 1922 to 1924. This proved to be a fortunate decision

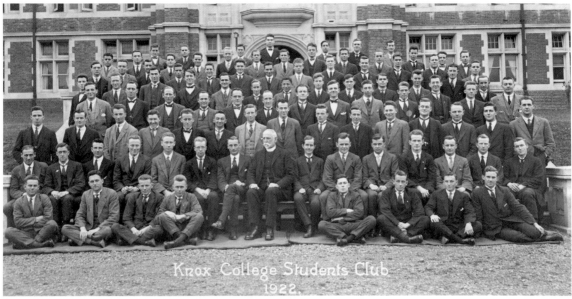

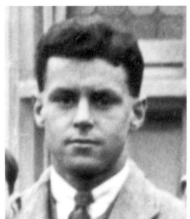

FIGURE 7.7. *Knox College students, 1922. Rainsford Mowlem is at the extreme left of the back row (detail left). The college was established in 1909 as residential accommodation for male students and the training of Presbyterian ministers. The bewhiskered gentleman in the middle of the front row is the master, the Reverend Professor William Hewitson.* (Photograph kindly provided by Donald Cochrane, Curator of Photographs, Archives Research Centre, Knox College, Presbyterian Church of Aotearoa New Zealand, and published with their permission)

for the photographic record; Mowlem seems to have been camera-shy, and the only images available anywhere of him as a young man are the annual Knox College student photographs. At the time McIndoe and Mowlem were in Dunedin the medical course was four years in duration (five years including the intermediate year), and Mowlem graduated MB ChB (NZ) in 1924. After spending two years as a house surgeon at Auckland Hospital and in general practice, he worked his passage to England around the Cape of Good Hope in that time-honoured manner as a ship's surgeon, with the intention of pursuing a surgical career.

Mowlem encounters Gillies

After six months in a general practice at Dorking in Surrey, Mowlem became a house surgeon, first at the Seamen's Hospital in Greenwich and then in Woolwich. To prepare for the Primary FRCS he enrolled on the refresher course at the Middlesex Hospital, which was then at the height of its fame, with Tim Yeates teaching anatomy and Samson Wright teaching physiology (his *Applied Physiology* was still in use 40 years and several editions later). Having 'satisfied the examiners', Mowlem became the Resident Surgical Officer (RSO) at Queen Mary's Hospital at Stratford in

East London, and after qualifying FRCS (Eng) in 1929 was appointed one of five RSOs at the Hammersmith Hospital.[17] Early in 1930 Mowlem was packed up to go home to Auckland with the intention of practising general surgery when he received a call to say that the Welsh medical officer in charge of the ward in which Gillies had four beds had become ill and would he stay on as a locum? (Gillies, in characteristic fashion, later claimed the Welsh doctor had died suddenly after eating too much Christmas pudding.[18]) Mowlem agreed and, although he was initially unsympathetic to the need for what he regarded as 'cosmetic surgery', began to assist Gillies. He became increasingly impressed with the potential of plastic operations and as a result changed his career plans. (Apparently he was won over by a patient with syphilis whose nose had been reconstructed by Gillies.) In 1933, when the Hammersmith changed from being a London County Council (LCC) hospital to a teaching hospital for the Postgraduate Medical School, Mowlem moved with Gillies to St James' Hospital in Balham. From 1933 to the outbreak of the war he was also the assistant medical officer in charge of the plastic unit at St Charles' Hospital, Ladbroke Grove.

The best description of Mowlem during this period comes from the autobiography of Sir Benjamin Rank. Not long after his arrival from Melbourne, Rank had been successful in gaining an RSO appointment at St James' Hospital, and in 1938–39 worked closely with Mowlem, learning the basic principles and techniques of plastic surgery. At the outbreak of war Rank was conscripted into the Emergency Medical Service (EMS) 'as an assistant plastic surgeon at the North London Centre attached to St Bartholomew's Hospital, to function at Hill End Hospital' at St Albans. According to Rank, in *Heads and Hands* (p. 23):

> *Mowlem's forte was good organisation, clear thinking and deft techniques. He introduced the use of spongy bone as living grafts – one of the few subjects on which he wrote. He was never prone to rush into print. Always direct and outspoken, his frankness often made him unpopular with the more conservative elements of the profession – he … was also allergic to bureaucracy. However, perhaps because we both appreciated a frontal approach, I was never put off by his lack of hesitation to call a spade a spade and accepted his lessons with gratitude, knowing that behind any superficial brusqueness lay genuine kindness. Rainsford Mowlem was a sprightly person with a sharp, decisive mind – often the mark of a man of slight build. Like Gillies and McIndoe, with whom he was so closely associated in hospital and private practice, he too was a New Zealander. Their relationship was a chain reaction. Each was attracted to something new or different from the general run of practice and each was exposed to plastic surgery by a chance encounter.[19]*

In 1936 Rainsford Mowlem became consulting plastic surgeon to the Middlesex Hospital in London, and in the same year became the junior partner in the partnership of Gillies, McIndoe and Mowlem that lasted until the outbreak of the Second World War.

Plastic surgery during the interwar years

In the years following the First World War, despite the lack of after-care facilities and the difficulties of operating in unfamiliar surroundings, Gillies and Pomfret Kilner (later joined by McIndoe and Mowlem) would go anywhere to advance the reputation of plastic surgery at unfashionable district general hospitals (many of which have since been demolished: St Andrew's, Dollis Hill; St James', Balham; Lord Mayor Treloar, Alton). With the drop in military patient numbers this mobility was necessary to keep the specialty alive as well as provide some sort of service for the rest of the country. Gillies eventually managed to get four beds at St Bartholomew's (1936) and Kilner four at St Thomas' soon after. An anonymous review of *Plastic Surgery of the Face*, published in *The Lancet* in 1920, sums up the ambivalent attitude of many in the medical profession towards this new branch of surgery – they couldn't see the need for it, and were uncomfortable with the idea of surgical operations that did not involve the curing of disease or the

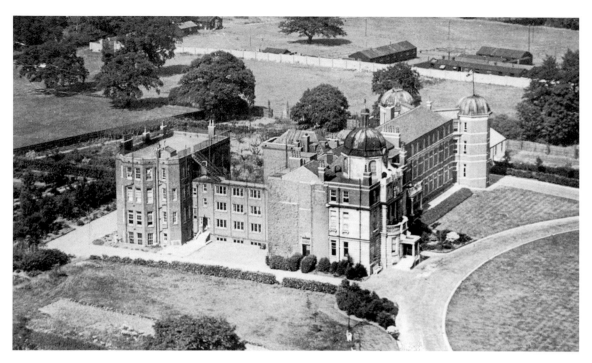

FIGURE 7.8. *St Andrew's Roman Catholic Hospital, Dollis Hill Lane, in the London borough of Willesden, viewed from the south, ca 1920 (Pritchard Photographic Co). The building of the hospital was financed by a wealthy Frenchwoman, Marguerite Amicie Piou (1847–1917), who wished to remain anonymous during her lifetime, and was administered by the Poor Servants of the Mother of God. It opened in 1913 with 100 beds and during the First World War became a military hospital.[31] Plastic surgery techniques were pioneered there by Gillies and McIndoe in the 1930s, but the hospital did not become part of the NHS. In 1972 it was sold to Brent Council; it was closed a year later and was subsequently demolished.* (Courtesy of the Gillies Archive, Queen Mary's Hospital, Sidcup)

removal of some offending organ. The reviewer praises the book, and the considerable progress made by Gillies and his colleagues in plastic surgery during the last war, but goes on to say (p. 169):

> *Mr Gillies in the preparation of his book has fully recognised the value of the graphic record in this branch of surgery … And this is well, for the general application of the same methods to the conditions met with in civil practice is of immediate importance, although the time may hardly be ripe for a department of plastic surgery in a general hospital. The defacements of heredity, disease, and accident are insignificant compared with the results of high explosives.*[20]

That may have been so, but the writer's ambiguous comment suggests he had yet to decide whether plastic operations were morally and ethically justifiable or simply cosmetic – a term loaded with somewhat pejorative overtones. The potential psychological benefits of plastic operations were misunderstood or simply ignored, which is hardly surprising given the temper of the times.

Much of Gillies' surgery was carried out at the Prince of Wales Hospital in Tottenham, where he had worked as an ENT surgeon before the war, and at St Andrew's Hospital in Dollis Hill. In 1923 the *British Medical Journal* announced that £23,000 was to be raised to provide a wing for housing a plastic surgery unit at St Andrew's.[21] The hospital was the first in London to provide free places for patients of the professional and middle classes who, while they did not qualify for free treatment in charitable institutions, were unable to meet the charges in private nursing homes or the fees for plastic surgery. It was while he was operating at Dollis Hill that McIndoe discovered John Hunter, the anaesthetist with whom he was to work closely both in private practice and at the Queen Victoria Hospital, East Grinstead for the next twenty-odd years.

Gillies and Kilner were also honorary consultants to the Lord Mayor Treloar Hospital at Alton in Hampshire. Originally built by public subscription in 1901 for sick and wounded soldiers returning from the Boer War, the hospital was taken over in 1907 by the Lord Mayor of London, Sir William Treloar, and converted into a children's hospital, particularly for those crippled by tuberculous disease of the bones and joints. In the early 1920s Sir Henry Gauvain, the hospital's medical superintendent, invited Gillies and Kilner to visit the hospital and carry out reconstructive work on cases of lupus, where the original disease and its treatment had produced disfigurement. The Lord Mayor Treloar Hospital thus holds the honour of being the first hospital in the country, outside London, to appoint a visiting plastic surgeon. As the incidence of lupus became less frequent, the hospital became an important centre for the treatment of cleft lip and palate, when Kilner transferred all his cleft patients to Alton from St Thomas' and the Princess Elizabeth of York Hospital for Children in East London.[22] Gillies was on the visiting staff of the North Staffordshire Royal Infirmary at Stoke-on-Trent, and carried out cosmetic and reconstructive surgery on private patients attending his Harley Street practice in order to earn a living. It must have taken considerable stamina to maintain such a punishing schedule.

Another hospital that played an important role in the development of plastic surgery when Gillies and Mowlem transferred their patients from the Hammersmith was St James' Hospital, Balham. Built by the Wandsworth Board of Guardians in 1910 as the St James' Infirmary, it was renamed in 1920 when the London City Council took over, and was enlarged into a hospital of nearly 900 beds, serving the local population, which included an abundance of poor, sick and undernourished people. No patient could be refused a bed, and with plenty of clinical material, St James' between the wars provided the blueprint for a modern accident and emergency service.[23] Sadly, as the result of yet another bureaucratic reorganisation of hospital services in Greater London, St James' Hospital was demolished in 1988 and its services transferred to the St James' Wing of St George's Hospital at Tooting, South London.

Gillies, Kilner, McIndoe and Mowlem all had sessions at St James'; between the four of them they conducted the only centralised plastic surgery clinic of any size in the country. Dental expertise was provided by Alex Fraser, who had worked with Gillies at Aldershot and Sidcup during the war (see Figure 5.4), plus two dental technicians. The unit had a total of 25 beds – 10 male, 10 female and five children's.[17] The volume and variety of plastic surgery carried out at St James' was extensive and varied, and between the wars the hospital became something of a Mecca for young surgeons from the world over.

Plastic surgery training in the United Kingdom and the United States

Wherever he went, Gillies was always accompanied by his 'foreign legion' – a group of four to eight surgical trainees, mostly from Europe, the dominions of the British Empire and the Middle East, who trailed him from one institution to another. Since there were no formal postgraduate training schemes at the time, the experience gained by aspiring surgeons was distinctly ad hoc. They had to plan their own careers, gaining an RSO appointment or arranging a clinical attachment at a hospital with the leading surgeons in their chosen field and, most importantly, gaining an FRCS from one of the four royal surgical colleges. Would-be surgeons from the United Kingdom were dissuaded from a career in plastic surgery by medical opinion and the surgical establishment; with the limited opportunities it offered for hospital and private practice most wisely chose general surgery. David Matthews and Richard Battle were the only two British surgeons from the next generation to have

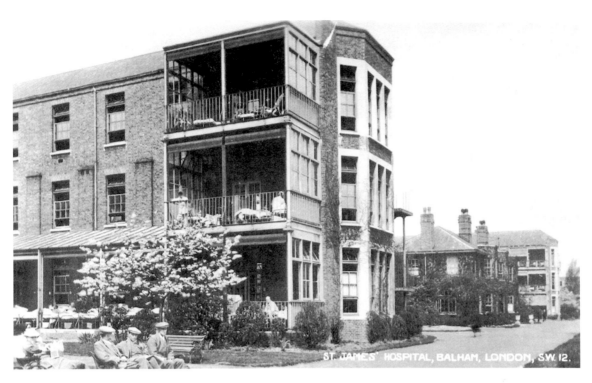

FIGURE 7.9. *St James' Hospital, Sarsfield Road, Balham. During the 1930s the hospital played a key role in the development of plastic surgery in the United Kingdom when Gillies and Mowlem transferred their patients from the Hammersmith Hospital. It was amalgamated with St George's Hospital and demolished in 1988.*

had any training in plastic operations during the late 1930s (at St Andrew's, Dollis Hill, and the Lord Mayor Treloar Hospital, Alton), and they subsequently became the vital link with the famous four.[21] It was not until the Second World War and the establishment of the EMS Maxillofacial Units at East Grinstead, Hill End, Roehampton and Rooksdown House that plastic surgeons began to be trained in significant numbers in the United Kingdom. This was markedly different from the United States, where around 60 plastic surgeons had been trained by 1940. Robert Ivy (p. 54) describes the catalyst for change:

> *The visit of Gillies to the United States in 1920 and the presentation of accounts of our treatment of war cases by men in this country, made the profession aware that there was room for specialisation in the field of plastic and maxillofacial surgery, which up until that time had been unorganised.*[24]

There is any number of reasons why plastic surgery flourished in the United States but not in Britain, including geography, population and economics, but the most significant was the way in which specialty training evolved in the two countries during the interwar years.[25,26] Fraser and Hultman,[25] writing from the American perspective, attribute this to two events. The first was the Flexner Report of 1910, restructuring medical education in North America.[27] This was unquestionably important in raising educational standards across the board in North American medical schools by bringing the curriculum and length of undergraduate training into line with universities in Europe. The commercial or 'proprietary' medical school – a distinctly American product – had resulted in an enormous overproduction of uneducated and ill-trained medical practitioners. The report forced privately owned medical schools to close or merge with existing universities. One consequence, intended or otherwise, was that medicine became much more expensive, and a profession made up largely of white middle-class males.

The second event, of much greater significance, was the establishment during the 1920s of training programmes in plastic surgery by Vilray Blair, Ferris Smith, Robert Ivy and others. Even so, most of the instruction in plastic surgery in both the United States and Canada was still by apprenticeship, that time-honoured model in which student surgeons acquired the knowledge, skills and professional values of their mentors in the course of caring for patients. In practice this meant that a good deal of the training was not comprehensive in scope and reflected the clinical practice of the preceptor: it was likely to be heavy, for example, in surgery of the head and neck, with limited exposure to the treatment of cancer and burns patients.[28] To deal with this deficiency, Blair was instrumental in creating a certifying board for the specialty. The American Board of Plastic Surgery, formed in 1937, required two years of general surgery and two years' plastic surgery training. The board also insisted that plastic surgery no longer applied to just maxillofacial procedures, but would fulfill Staige Davis' definition by extending from the top of the head to the soles of the feet.[28]

Furthermore – in keeping with the observations made by Alexis de Tocqueville during his travels throughout the United States about the fondness of Americans for forming clubs and other associations[29] – an American Association of Oral Surgeons had been created in 1921 by three MD, DDS surgeons representing the three dental schools in Chicago: Truman Brophy (Chicago College of Dental Surgery), Thomas Gilmer (Northwestern University) and Frederick Moorhead (University of Illinois). This made it the oldest plastic surgery society in existence, with a number of the surgeons who had been stationed at Sidcup as members.[24] Later that year it became the American Association of Oral and Plastic Surgeons (Oral was dropped from the title in 1942). One of the conditions of admission was that the candidate had to have dental as well as medical qualifications; this meant that until the rule was relaxed in 1923, Blair could

only be admitted as an associate member! In view of its exclusivity, a rival organisation devoted to the specialty – the American Society of Plastic and Reconstructive Surgery – was started in New York in 1931: so the United States now had two national societies. In contrast, the British Association of Plastic Surgeons was not established until 1947 and a formal examination in plastic surgery equivalent to American Board Certification did not come into existence in Britain for another 38 years.[26]

Brian Kingcome

Of the many patients treated by Gillies and McIndoe during the 1930s, only one has left an account of his experiences – Brian Kingcome in *A Willingness to Die*.[30] Charles Brian Fabris Kingcome (1917–1994) DSO, DFC & Bar[†], entered RAF Cranwell as an officer cadet in 1936. Soon after he began his pilot training he received serious facial injuries when he overturned his Clyno open two-seater on a foggy night in the fens of Lincolnshire. The bones of the middle third of his face – nose, cheeks and jaw – were crushed or broken. As Kingcome points out, in those days the armed services tended to provide a refuge for doctors and surgeons who were unable to earn a living in the outside world, and the surgeons of the RAF who attended him certainly lived up to this reputation. After six weeks he was unable to open his mouth, his nose was flattened and inoperative, but worst of all, his left eye had dropped down his face resulting in double vision – a fault that, if left uncorrected, would mean the end of his flying days. Since the RAF was not going to spend money bringing in outside specialists for a mere flight cadet hardly into his first term, his mother sprang into action (p. 30):

> She took me to see one of the most eminent surgeons of the day, a New Zealander by the name of Harold Gillies (later Sir Harold), doyen and pioneer of the new science of plastic surgery ... Mr Gillies studied me intently, then asked to speak to my sister Patricia, who was waiting outside. 'Was brother's face like sister's?' he asked. 'Good heavens no,' said Pat with an indignation that startled me. 'My brother's nose was straight!'

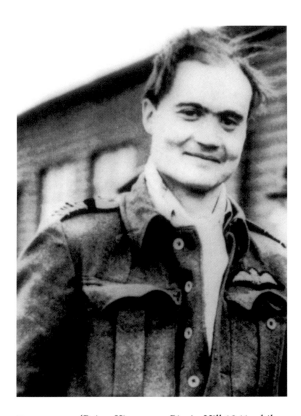

FIGURE 7.10. *'Brian Kingcome: Biggin Hill 1941 while CO of 92 Squadron'. Detail from a photograph on the back of the dust jacket of* A Willingness to Die: Life & memories from Fighter Command and beyond, *first published in 1999.* (Reproduced with the kind permission of Lesley Kingcome)

Peering again at the battered blob somewhere about the middle of my asymmetric features, Mr Gillies masked his incredulity, doubtless marvelling at the strength of sibling loyalty. Then he declared that he would accept the challenge, obviously glad to come across a guinea pig to help him extend his knowledge within this field of specialty. He was assisted in the operation by his cousin, a rising young surgeon called Archie McIndoe (later Sir Archibald), who would become the founder of the world-famous Guinea Pig Club at East Grinstead, where the formidable skills of his powerful, almost stubby square hands and the force and warmth of his personality made miracles a daily routine as he rebuilt the shattered bodies and minds of the burned casualties of the Second World War.

Judging by the photograph of Kingcome taken in 1941 at Biggin Hill, given the circumstances they made a good job, enabling him to resume his flying career, although his nose is flatter than photographs taken when he was at Bedford School. In any event, their intervention enabled Kingcome to complete his training at Cranwell and join the RAF in 1938 with a permanent commission, and he was posted to 65 Squadron at Hornchurch in Essex, which was equipped with Spitfires. Which brings us to the Second World War.

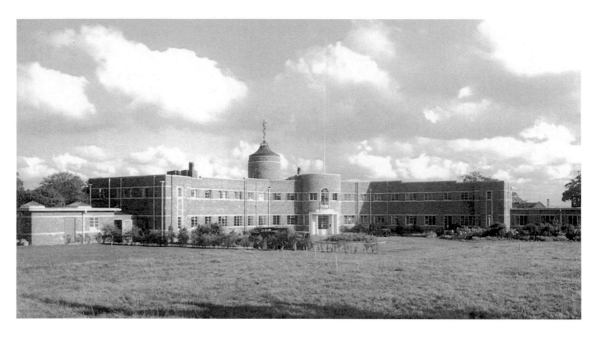

FIGURE 8.1. *The Queen Victoria Cottage Hospital, East Grinstead, 1936. The 36-bed hospital, completed at a cost of £25,000 raised largely by public subscription, was officially opened on 8 January 1936 by Princess Helena Victoria. QVH is a good example of how hospitals were built and maintained prior to their nationalisation and the introduction of the NHS. Within a few days of the opening of the hospital, however, the matron became ill and two patients died. Some of the more superstitious locals decided the Serpent and Staff of Aesculapius (the symbol of healing) on the top of the central dome was a bad omen and wanted it removed; the hospital management prevaricated, but eventually refused when they discovered it would cost £63 to do so.*[3] (*Courtesy of the Queen Victoria Hospital Archives, East Grinstead*)

CHAPTER 8

McIndoe and the Queen Victoria Hospital, East Grinstead

Written in collaboration with Robert (Bob) Marchant

In May 1932 an Army Advisory Standing Committee was appointed by the Army Council to investigate and report on facilities for the treatment of maxillofacial injuries in the event of war.[1] The members of the committee were Gillies, Kelsey Fry and W Warwick James, under the chairmanship of Colonel JP Helliwell, Assistant Director-General Army Medical Services (for Dental Services). In their report published in 1935 they recommended that special hospitals of 200 beds reserved solely for the treatment of maxillofacial injuries were preferable to special departments in general hospitals. Each special hospital should be capable of expansion to 500 beds and reserved for (a) the treatment of fractures requiring the attention of the dental surgeon, and (b) gross injuries to hard and/or soft tissues requiring treatment by plastic or other specialist surgeons and dental surgeons. Furthermore, based on the experience of treating maxillofacial injuries in the First World War, an auxiliary hospital or annex should be attached to each special hospital to provide accommodation for the convalescence of patients during the often protracted intervals between treatment.[1]

Early in 1939 and with war imminent, Gillies and Kelsey Fry were consulted by the Ministry of Health regarding the establishment of such specialist maxillofacial centres under the Emergency Medical Service. The EMS had been established in October the previous year to reorganise hospital services in response to the threat of bombing by the Luftwaffe. Specialist maxillofacial centres were also urgently required to train more plastic surgeons. After touring the country, Gillies and Kelsey Fry recommended that nine centres should be established. Four were set up near London, and the others at Birmingham, Leeds, Newcastle-upon-Tyne, Gloucester and Scotland. As civilian consultant to the Royal Air Force, McIndoe was appointed to the Queen Victoria Cottage Hospital at East Grinstead in West Sussex. Mowlem, by this time consultant plastic surgeon to the army and the Middlesex Hospital, was seconded to Hill End Hospital at St Albans in Hertfordshire, 22 miles north of central London. Kilner went to the Ministry of Pensions unit at Queen Mary's Hospital, Roehampton (because of its vulnerability, in 1941 the unit was transferred to Stoke Mandeville Hospital in Buckinghamshire). Gillies chose Rooksdown House at Basingstoke in Hampshire, 48 miles southwest of London, which, as luck would have it, was a 30-minute drive from the River Test, arguably the most famous fly-fishing river in the world. The Queen Victoria Cottage Hospital, located midway between London and the south coast, owed its inclusion to Kelsey Fry's choice of school for his son – Brambletye, a preparatory boarding school one mile south of

East Grinstead.[2] East Grinstead also happened to be on the way from London to Gillies' favourite golf course at Rye on the Sussex coast, where each January the Oxford and Cambridge Golfing Society played for the President's Putter – the winner in 1925 being a certain HD Gillies.

The origin of the Queen Victoria Hospital (QVH) can be traced back to 1863 when Green Hedges, a cottage hospital with seven beds, was opened by Dr John Henry Rogers, one of the local medical practitioners. Prior to this, admission to hospital had meant a difficult journey to London or Brighton by coach or train, and as a consequence many seriously ill people had to remain in their homes where they were largely dependent on charity.[3,4] Cottage hospitals thus arose from an urgent need to provide local treatment facilities for accidents and illnesses affecting the poor, and East Grinstead was the fourth of its kind in the country. Dr Rogers' experience of running Green Hedges was not altogether a happy one, however, and after 11 years, 'having experienced for some years the meanness of the wealthy, and too often the ingratitude of the poor', he closed the hospital.[3] Fourteen years elapsed before a second cottage hospital with five beds, Lansdowne House, was opened in 1888 by Mr and Mrs Oswald Smith at their own expense, with the three local medical practitioners, Drs Covey, Collins and Wallis, offering their services gratis.[3] By 1939 and after two further relocations, East Grinstead Cottage Hospital, which had been renamed the Queen Victoria Cottage Hospital in 1901 as the town's memorial to the late Queen, had developed into a modest 36-bed facility serving a local population of about 30,000. With the expansion of the hospital during the war, by 1943 the number of beds had increased to 230 and the word 'Cottage' was dropped from the title.

'Mr McIndoe has arrived to take over the Hospital'

In the minutes of a meeting of the board of management dated 4 September 1939, the day after war had been declared, is recorded what turned out to be arguably the most important event in the long history of the hospital: 'Mr McIndoe has arrived to take over the Hospital on behalf of the Ministry of Health as a Maxillo-facial Hospital, although he had no written instructions.'[3] If that sounds overly dramatic, the board had been informed earlier in the year by the ministry that the hospital was to be included in its emergency plans, and that something of the kind might happen. Indeed, in May 1939 the ministry had asked permission to erect huts at the rear of the hospital to accommodate 100 extra beds, and work on them had already begun. Three main wards were constructed: Ward I for male civilian dental and jaw injuries, Ward II for women and children, most of whom were air-raid casualties, and Ward III, the soon-to-be famous burns ward, its patients known as 'guinea pigs'. When McIndoe arrived at QVH he was 39. The board knew nothing of his character and outstanding qualities, and neither he nor the board could have foreseen how fruitful their association was to become.[3]

If the First World War had established Gillies' reputation as a plastic surgeon, the Second was about to make McIndoe a household name. He had been lucky. With the RAF in action from the outset of the war, and the Battle of Britain in the summer of 1940 being fought largely over the skies of southeast England, the bulk of the airmen requiring plastic surgery in the early days eventually arrived at East Grinstead. During the Battle of Britain the majority were Hurricane and Spitfire pilots, but later, as the bombing campaign against the industrial centres and cities of Germany intensified, 80 percent came from Bomber Command, many of them Canadians. By 1940 the Maxillo-facial Unit was firmly established and the staff listed as follows.[3]

Surgeons
Archibald H McIndoe, MSc, MS, FRCS, FACS, Surgeon-in-Charge
Nils L Eckhoff, MS, FRCS
David N Matthews, MCh, FRCS (Established Maxillo-facial Unit at RAF Halton in 1941)

RAF Registrar
Squadron Leader George H Morley, FRCS (Established Maxillo-facial Unit at RAF Ely in 1941)

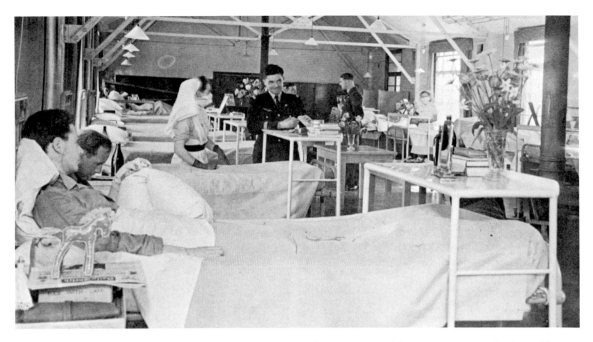

FIGURE 8.2. *Ward III: otherwise known as The Sty. 'Ward III housing some of the worst cases stands about fifty yards away from the main hospital. It was a long, low hut, with a door at one end and twenty beds down each side … Windows were let into the walls at regular intervals on each side: they were never open. Down the middle there was a table with a wireless on it, a stove, and a piano. On either side of the entrance passage were four lavatories and two bathrooms. Immediately on the left of the entrance was the saline bath, a complicated arrangement of pipes that maintained a constant flow of saline around the bathed patient at a regular temperature.' – Richard Hillary,* The Last Enemy. *(Courtesy of the Queen Victoria Hospital Archives, East Grinstead)*

Resident Medical Officer

Percy H Jayes, MB, BS

Dental Surgeons

W Kelsey Fry, MC, MRCS, LRCP, LDSRCS,
    Consultant, Ministry of Health
D Greer Walker, MA, MB, BChir, MDS
    (Transferred to Stoke Mandeville in 1941)
Alan C McLeod, BSc (Toronto), DDS (Penn),
    LDSRCS (Eng)
P Rae Shepherd, LDSRCS (Eng)
AH Clarkson

Anaesthetists

J Truscott Hunter, MRCS, LRCP, DA
Russell M Davies, MRCS, LRCP, DA

Consulting Ophthalmologist

Frederick Ridley, MB, BS, FRCS

Photographer

Miss Lehmann

Challenging the system

Apart from his skill as a surgeon, McIndoe's strengths were his refusal to accept a commission in the RAF despite pressure from the Air Ministry (which offered him the relatively lowly rank of wing commander), and a well-developed irreverence for rank and officialdom inherited from his Celtic ancestors – further fine-tuned, it must be said, by his Antipodean upbringing. This was to be expected since attitudes to hierarchy and respect for authority are culturally determined – what the Dutch psychologist Geert Hofstede has referred to in his influential book *Cultures Consequences* as the power distance index (PDI), the basic issue of which is how different societies handle inequality, usually formalised in boss–subordinate relationships. Although one's inclination is not to take the findings of research by questionnaire too seriously, there seems little doubt Hofstede's basic thesis is correct. Cultures with low PDI scores are not afraid to challenge the status quo or express disagreement with management, and Hofstede rated New Zealand a particularly low PDI country, even lower than Australia, somewhat surprisingly.[5] Remaining a civilian enabled McIndoe (like Gillies and Mowlem) to avoid the conventions of military custom and protocol such as importance based on rank; or having to go through formal or official channels, characterised as they are by interminable delays: if he wanted something done he could go straight to the Secretary of State for Air. It has been said that McIndoe's greatest quality was his courage and his belief there was a proper course of action for treating the injured. To achieve this he was prepared to challenge authority using any means he thought necessary.[6]

A good deal has been written about McIndoe's decision to allow commissioned and non-commissioned ranks at East Grinstead to occupy the same wards – an arrangement that was contrary to common practice at the time. Whether this arose from a heavy demand for beds, thereby making a virtue out of a necessity, is not entirely clear, but it had been observed that the recovery of officers was slower if they were isolated in side cubicles; when transferred to the rough and tumble of the ward they picked up and made a normal recovery. The democracy of Ward III may therefore have stemmed more from the urgent needs of accommodation than from any carefully crafted psychological plan on the part of McIndoe.[7]

At the same time, such a break with military tradition was undoubtedly helped by the more relaxed service discipline of the RAF compared with the army and navy. The technical nature of the service meant the RAF had to look outside the traditional recruiting grounds for officers and men, which meant the service was more socially mixed and meritocratic.[8] And as Lord Moran observed, the RAF was a ruthless service where seniority counted

for little – successful pilots had proved themselves capable in the air of quicker and tougher thinking than the rest.[9]

The unconventional arrangement was also helped by the presence of airmen of several nationalities from the dominions, including Australians, Canadians, New Zealanders and South Africans, with their more egalitarian attitude to social class. Moreover, many of the pilots in Fighter Command were non-commissioned sergeant-pilots from the RAF Volunteer Reserve, while the aircraft of Bomber Command were crewed by young officers and NCOs who formed a unique, tight-knit partnership; the pilot was the captain of the aircraft regardless of his rank. In these circumstances the distinction between officers and other ranks was difficult if not impossible to maintain. As a result there was no respect for rank or privilege in Ward III.

Communal wards also highlighted another inequality that existed between officers and other ranks. While officers were allowed to wear their service uniform, non-commissioned ranks were required by *King's Regulations* to wear a hospital uniform consisting of a particularly ill-fitting and unattractive blue suit, white shirt and red tie. McIndoe's answer to this degrading and divisive practice was quite simple – he ordered the stock of uniforms to be taken out and burnt, and had the men issued with their service uniform.[6] A different approach, however, was required for two of his major challenges: first, persuading the War Wounds Committee to abandon tannic acid or any form of coagulation treatment for burns; and second, battling the Admiralty and Air Ministry over the 90-day rule, which stated that a man who did not return to active duty after three months was invalided out of the service.

The airman's burn

Surgical teams in the First World War had been confronted with the issue of how to reconstruct lost tissue. In the Second they were faced by an additional problem: the treatment of severe burns. Although there had been an ever-present risk of fire in the aircraft of the First World War, constructed as they were from a highly combustible combination of wood, canvas and glue. Allied pilots were not issued with parachutes, based on the tortured logic that they would leap to safety rather than engage the enemy, and few airmen who sustained major burns during aerial combat survived. In the event of an aircraft catching fire, the inevitable consequence was a crash and almost certain death. Indeed, parachutes did not become standard equipment in the RAF until 1928. Improvements in parachute technology between the wars saved the lives of a trickle of airmen whose aircraft had caught fire, but by 1939 no substantial series of cases had been published, and none in which a rational plan of repair had been proposed.[10]

Sidney Camm and Reginald Mitchell had designed two beautiful fighting machines – the Hurricane and the Spitfire. Unfortunately for the pilots, economy of space meant the Spitfire had two fuel tanks situated immediately in front of the cockpit behind the instrument panel: the top one held 48 gallons and the bottom 37 gallons of performance-enhancing 100-octane gasoline. The Hurricane was not much better: it had two 33-gallon tanks in the wings, which were self-sealing; and a reserve or header tank behind the instrument panel holding 27 gallons, which was not. If either plane caught fire, flames swept into the cockpit and the pilot had little chance unless he could get clear of the aircraft in a matter of seconds. It is estimated that approximately 4500 airmen were recovered from crashed planes or parachuted to safety in flames, and 80 percent of these men had burns to the face and hands[10,11] – referred to by McIndoe as the 'airman's burn' (Colour plates 17 and 18). This was largely caused by the pilots' habit of removing their gloves, goggles and masks – many found that gloves interfered with their manual dexterity, while the helmet, oxygen mask and goggles were liable to induce feelings of claustrophobia. From the various RAF Burns Units scattered around England (at Cosford, Rauncey, Ely and Halton) and eventually in the Middle East, 600 of the more severe facial burns were selected by McIndoe making his rounds and transferred to East Grinstead. 'Of this number, 200 were regarded as being of major severity or as

total facial burns. They were in and out of hospital for an average of three years and sustained between them approximately 3000 operations, ranging between 10 and 50 each.'[10]

In 1939 the method approved by the Medical Research Council (MRC) War Wounds Committee for the treatment of burns was coagulation therapy with tannic acid gel, which had become the method of choice for the localised treatment of burns shortly after its introduction by Davidson in 1925.[12,13] Because tannic acid lacked any bactericidal action, gentian violet and, later, the triple dye solution were favoured by some surgeons. Given that tanning is the process of making leather from the skins of animals using tannins (astringent plant polyphenols), in retrospect the use of tannic acid seems to have been a strange choice, but for first-degree domestic burns or scalds involving the surface layer of the skin with minimal tissue damage it was often very effective, and it had its firm adherents. Tubes of tannic acid gel (tannic acid with 0.5 percent phenol in a water-soluble base, marketed as Tannafax by Burroughs Wellcome) were included in every first-aid kit and could be applied to affected areas as a frontline treatment by anyone with minimal training. Problems arose when principles based on civilian injuries were applied to the type of severe burns caused by war, and it soon became apparent that coagulation treatment with tannic acid had serious disadvantages and was frequently disastrous – particularly when applied to second-degree (partial skin loss) and third-degree (destruction of full thickness of the skin) burns of the face and hands[14, 15] – in other words, the degree of injuries suffered by the majority of air crew who survived.

Tannic acid applied to the hands formed a hard, inelastic glove or eschar, which could lead to compression of the circulation, necrosis of the fingers and deformities of the hands. Mowlem also had first-hand experience of the dangers of tannic acid – on the eighth or tenth day a little pus would seep out of the various cracks in the armour, and the coagulum eventually separated off piece by piece to expose the hands covered by thin scar tissue, without a great deal of the subcutaneous tissue of the fingers remaining, and probably without one or more terminal phalanges (ends of the fingers).[15] Tannic acid also stiffened eyelids, endangering sight, and it could destroy intact epithelium, thereby inflicting further damage by converting second- into third-degree burns. The tanning of burns was also characterised by a high incidence of secondary infection, septicaemia and death. An additional problem was that general surgeons, who were responsible for the initial care of most of these men, were ill-equipped either by training or temperament to undertake the surgery necessary to prevent scarring of the affected areas. They knew burns were to be covered with tannic acid gel, but not what to do next. Primary skin grafting of the raw surface at a much earlier stage in a patient's clinical history would have prevented the development of many of the more gross deformities.[16] McIndoe knew more about these problems than any other surgeon – most of the airmen he collected and transferred to Ward III at East Grinstead from other hospitals around the country provided unwelcome examples of the devastating effects of coagulation treatment. It was obvious that something had to be done.

At a special meeting requested by McIndoe at the Royal Society of Medicine on 6 November 1940 to discuss the treatment of burns, he showed a series of photographs of cases treated with tannic acid, illustrating such points as deformities of the hands with necrosis and loss of fingertips from gangrene, and contractures of the eyelids leading to corneal ulceration.[14] One of McIndoe's first innovations had been to abandon coagulation treatment and introduce two-percent saline baths at 105°F for half an hour or more (Figure 8.3). Saline baths had been revived by Vilray Blair and Barrett Brown in St Louis during the 1930s, but it had also been noted during the evacuation from Dunkirk that burn patients immersed in sea water suffered less infection than expected. The patient could be completely submerged, and this usually gave some relief from pain. After the patient had been carefully lifted out of the bath, the burned areas were cleansed, dusted with sulphonamides and covered with tulle gras dressings (an open mesh material impregnated with Vaseline containing 1 percent Balsam of Peru, an

antiseptic). In those burns involving extensive skin loss where regeneration occurred only from the margins, early surgical intervention was directed towards the epithelialisation of raw surfaces with pinch or Thiersch split-skin grafts,[16,17] using a technique that had been developed at Sidcup during the First World War. These were designed to prevent the development of ectropic deformities of the eyelids and mouth, thereby preserving sight and protecting the teeth.[6] The RAF medical chiefs, convinced by the evidence, immediately banned the use of tannic acid on third-degree burns. The members of the MRC Burns Subcommittee, however, although unable to bring themselves to completely abandon coagulation therapy, had by April 1941 recommended the regime developed at QVH for managing burns to the face, hands and feet, and McIndoe was recognised as the leading expert on the treatment and reconstruction of burn injuries. (For those tempted to read about this further, Emily Mayhew has trawled the Public Records Office and written a detailed account of the controversy and the search for alternatives in *The Reconstruction of Warriors*.)[18]

The 90-day rule

Changing *King's Regulations* was a much more formidable challenge. Under the 90-day rule an injured serviceman was given three months to return to active duty. If he was still unfit after that time he was invalided out of the service as being of no further use, and passed on to civilian hospitals for additional treatment. If the convalescence was a long one, this system absolutely guaranteed the man would arrive back in civilian life without hope, broken in spirit, bitter and disillusioned. He could also be in debt, for his service pay ceased and his eventual pension would not be settled for a long time.[19] McIndoe had a large number of men under his long-term care who would suffer the same fate. He concluded the only way to overturn what he regarded as an unjust and bureaucratic regulation was to create a precedent with a cast-iron case.

The case he selected for the task was that of a Fleet Air Arm pilot by the name of Colin Hodgkinson†. McIndoe first met Hodgkinson in

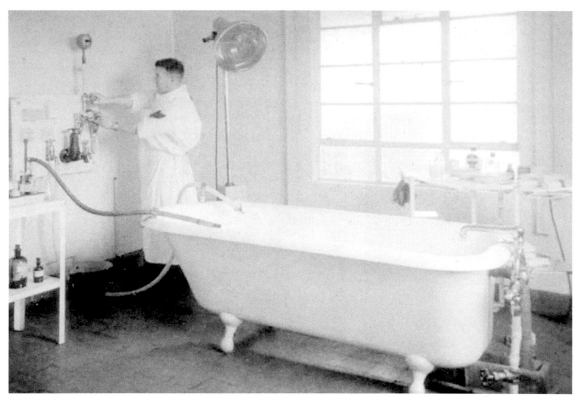

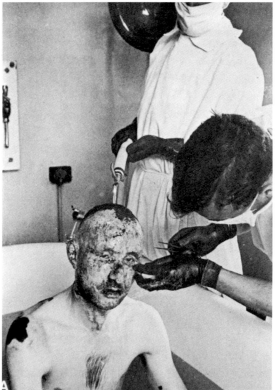

FIGURE 8.3. *At the beginning of the war the standard first aid treatment for burns was coagulation therapy with tannic acid gel; this formed a hard crust that immobilised fingers and toes, stiffened eyelids and made skin grafting difficult. One of McIndoe's first innovations was to abandon tannic acid and introduce saline baths. After the patient was lifted out of the bath the burned areas were cleansed, dusted with sulphonamide powder and covered with tulle gras dressings before skin grafting. Staff Sergeant Salmon oversees the saline bath, 1942.* (Courtesy of the Queen Victoria Hospital Archives, East Grinstead)

September 1940, while making the rounds of his patients at Dutton Homestall – a spacious house two miles from QVH that had been loaned to the Red Cross as a convalescent home by Kathleen Dewar and her husband John, a member of the whisky distilling family; they retained one small wing for their own use. Hodgkinson, who was precariously balanced on two artificial legs, asked McIndoe if he could get him back into active service in the navy. As McIndoe wrote in the foreword to Hodgkinson's autobiography, *Best Foot Forward*:[20]

> *In 1939 Colin Hodgkinson was 6 feet 1 inch tall and weighed 189 pounds of solid and well-trained bone and muscle … In 1940 following a near fatal air crash, he was 5 feet 10 inches tall, and, minus two legs, weighed 168 pounds. He was 'on the beach,' having been invalided out of the Navy with a pension of £3 per week.*[19]

McIndoe, who was not bound by the etiquette of rank, together with Kathleen Dewar (a friend of Hodgkinson's mother when they were both on the stage in South Africa), made a formidable negotiating team. One of Kathleen's friends was Sir Victor Warrender (later Lord Bruntisfield), Parliamentary Secretary to the Navy; another friend, Charles Hughesden, helped Hodgkinson to regain his confidence by allowing him to fly a light aircraft to which he had access. Meanwhile, McIndoe had been lobbying vigorously behind the scenes. Three months later it all paid off when Hodgkinson, after being summoned by Sir Victor to the Admiralty for a medical, was told by McIndoe, 'The penny is about to drop.' A few days later Hodgkinson was informed by their lordships that he could rejoin the Fleet Air Arm as an Acting Sub-Lieutenant RNVR, thereby opening up the way for an alteration in *King's Regulations*. Admittedly it was only as an air watch officer at St Merryn in Cornwall, a non-flying appointment, but it was a start. How Hodgkinson eventually got back into the air and spent the rest of the war is described in Chapter 9.

Group therapy

The pilots and air crew who arrived in Ward III in 1940 were, with a few exceptions, young men in their early twenties. Apart from the injuries to their face and hands they were otherwise fit and healthy, exuberant and above all intelligent – this was absolutely essential for being accepted and trained by the RAF in the first place. They may have been wounded, but they were not sick. In addition to the surgical side of his work, McIndoe developed a deep humanitarian interest in the welfare of his patients. As he observed:

> *The impact of disfiguring injuries upon the young adult is usually severe. The majority have been strong and healthy, and have given no consideration to illness or injury, or to its possible future effects. They are usually unprepared mentally for the blow, so for a period they may be psychically lost, depressed, morose, pessimistic, and thoroughly out of tune with their surroundings.*[21]

McIndoe's answer was to brighten up the barrack-room appearance of the ward, changing its colour from institutional brown and cream to pastel green and pink; discarding the iron beds and replacing them with modern wooden ones; and, most revolutionary of all, allowing a plentiful supply of beer in the ward. Rules were conspicuous by their absence and the atmosphere can best be described as boarding-school rowdyism – noisy, irreverent and sometimes out of hand. The language was rough and sometimes offensive – essentially an extension of behaviour in the mess. It was not for the faint-hearted, particularly among the nursing staff.

After a difficult start – some of the patients, with their disfiguring injuries, were not very pretty to look at – the townspeople of East Grinstead played an important role in their welfare and rehabilitation, accepting them into the community, befriending, entertaining and taking care of them. It was not unusual to see men in the pub, or playing football or cricket, sporting tubed pedicles or other paraphernalia of plastic or maxillofacial surgery. The favourite watering-hole of the 'Guinea Pigs', as they were called, was the Whitehall – a pub-cum-restaurant-cum-cinema complex managed by the genial Bill Gardner in the High Street.[22] McIndoe also enlisted the help of the local press to disseminate news of the work of the hospital, which began to receive national publicity.[6] The involvement of the local community in the welfare and rehabilitation of the patients was as integral to their treatment as was surgery. There were no psychiatrists at QVH – there was no need for them. Although they didn't know it at the time the medical staff, patients of Ward III and the people of East Grinstead were pioneering what is now referred to in social theory as a 'therapeutic community' – a term that now seems to have become restricted to the field of mental health.

The Canadian Wing

In 1942 a Canadian Plastic Surgery and Jaw Injuries Unit under the command of Squadron Leader Ross Tilley[†], a plastic surgeon in the Royal Canadian Air Force (RCAF), together with an anaesthetist and three nursing sisters, had been attached to the hospital for training.[3] With the RCAF playing an increasingly active role in the air war, particularly the bombing campaign over Germany, there was a growing number of Canadian casualties at East Grinstead. In June 1943 the Canadian government granted £20,000 towards the cost of building a 50-bed Canadian Wing on land that had been bought for the hospital by the Peanut Club.[23] It was to be staffed by Canadians for the treatment of Canadians, and after the war it was to be handed over to the hospital as a living memorial to those Canadians who had lost their lives. Nine patients were admitted on 12 July 1944 and by early August all 50 beds were occupied.[4] Over the next 14 months the wing would accommodate 26 RCAF patients, 32 from the RAF and 80 from other Allied services, comprising five nationalities.[24] The Canadian Wing, a single-storey, T-shaped structure, is still in use today and holds the honours board listing the names of 642 Guinea Pigs (See Appendix III).

Surgery at East Grinstead

A wide variety of plastic and maxillofacial surgery was practised at East Grinstead during the war. There was a large Dental Department with four dental surgeons and five technicians, who treated a large number of patients with facial fractures. The concentration of cases involving maxillofacial trauma resulted in the 1942 publication *Dental*

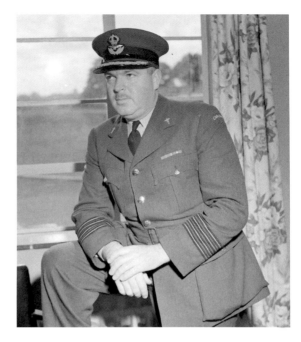

FIGURE 8.4. *Group Captain A Ross Tilley OBE, RCAF. In 1943, with Ward III filled to overflowing with casualties from the bombing campaign against Germany, Tilley played an influential role in persuading the Canadian government to fund construction of a separate Canadian wing at QVH. It was an all-Canadian operation: built by Canadian army engineers, staffed by Tilley, Dr Norman Park, his anaesthetist, and other Canadian surgeons, doctors, nurses and orderlies, but not confined to Canadian patients.[24]* (By kind permission of Library and Archives Canada/Bibliothèque et Archives Canada, Copy negative PA-205336)

Treatment of Maxillo-Facial Injuries by William Kelsey Fry, Rae Shepherd, Alan McLeod and Gilbert Parfitt,[25] a practical guide based on lectures and demonstrations given to members of the armed forces and which became a standard text for many years. It is interesting to note that by the end of 1941 the Ministry of Health had requested the Maxillo-facial Unit change its name to the Plastic and Jaw Injuries Centre, on account of the diversity of cases now passing through the unit. According to the QVH annual report for that year, only 547 of the last 1000 cases had been facial; the other 453 had been injuries to other parts of the body, requiring collaboration between general surgical, orthopaedic and neurological colleagues.[3]

The following examples from East Grinstead are typical of the sequence of operations required to rehabilitate a burnt airman. The first two are Hurricane pilots shot down over southeast England during the Battle of Britain, who later wrote about their experiences (see Chapter 9). The third was a crew member of a Hampden bomber shot down by a Junkers Ju 88 intruder as it was landing in East Anglia. It's all very well recording that patients went through 10 or 15 or so operations, but what does that mean, in reality? The following narrative is included for those who wish to know exactly what was involved in the reconstruction of a total facial burn and, in the cases of Geoffrey Page and Jack Allaway, the rather more difficult task of restoring the function of the burnt hand. Unlike conventional surgery, the reconstruction of a burns patient was a series of small engagements over several years, in which form and function were gradually restored. It required great patience and attention to detail on the part of the surgeon and, above all, skilful nursing, understanding and continuity of care.

Squadron Leader Tom Gleave

Squadron Leader Tom Gleave[†] of 253 Squadron (Colour plate 19), for many years the chief Guinea Pig, was one of the first Battle of Britain fighter pilots to arrive at East Grinstead. On 31 August 1940, while he was attacking a formation of Junkers Ju 88 bombers, a cannon shell from a Messerschmitt Bf 109[26] ignited the starboard wing gasoline tank. With his clothes on fire, Gleave managed to parachute to safety, but his hands, face and legs had been badly burned. He was picked up from Mace Farm near Biggin Hill in Kent and admitted to Orpington Hospital the same day in a state of shock, with extensive second-degree burns to his legs, both hands and forearms, and his face in the region of the eyes, forehead and nose. Tannic acid was applied to the hands and legs, and his face treated with 10 percent silver nitrate over 5 percent tannic acid. On 29 October 1940 he was transferred to East Grinstead, where daily saline baths were

immediately started and tulle gras and saline dressings were applied to the legs and wrist. Three weeks later McIndoe began the series of operations to give him four new eyelids and a new nose, while Percy Jayes re-epithelialised his legs. (McIndoe is referred to by Gleave in *I Had a Row with a German* (1941) as 'The Maestro' and 'The Doc'.)

Operation 20.11.1940: *McIndoe/Jayes/Hunter. At the first of Gleave's operations McIndoe applied Thiersch grafts from the inner side of the arm to both upper eyelids on Stent moulds. At the same time, Percy Jayes applied pinch grafts to granulating areas on the legs; these were sprayed with sulphanilamide powder and fixed with tulle gras, paraffin flavine wool, and crepe bandaging. Both the eyelid and pinch grafts had a 100% take.*

Operation 4.12.1940: *McIndoe/Hunter. Thiersch grafts on Stent moulds were applied to both the lower eyelids. After 8 days' leave, Gleave was readmitted on 29.12.1940 when it was noted that contraction of scar tissue across the bridge of the nose was pulling both inner canthi away from the eyes.*

Operation 2.1.1941: *McIndoe/Hunter. To correct this McIndoe excised the scar tissue from the nose extending the incision over the tip into the beginning of columella and a rhinoplastic forehead flap was raised and sutured to the nose. A Thiersch graft from the left thigh was applied to cover the forehead donor site.*

Operation 18.1.1941: *McIndoe/Beaver. The flap was divided and suturing around the nose completed, followed by the return of the forehead flap – any raw surfaces were dusted with sulphanilamide powder and Eusol dressings applied. Healing occurred after a slight infection and Gleave was discharged for 28 days.*

Operation 3.4.1941: *McIndoe/Morley. The left side of the nose flap was raised and a considerable amount of scar tissue excised from underneath; the flap was then replaced allowing the alar margin to come down satisfactorily. The right lower lid was freed from adhesions above the previous contracted graft and a second Thiersch graft set in the usual*

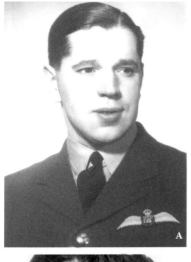
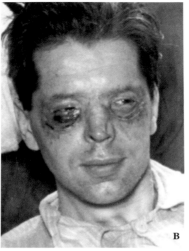
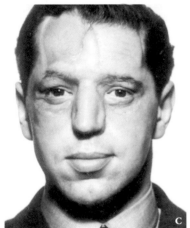
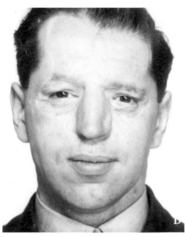

FIGURE 8.5 (A) *Prewar photograph of Squadron Leader Tom Gleave.*
(Kindly provided by Angela Lodge, Tom Gleave's daughter)

Thiersch grafts on Stent moulds were used to reconstruct the upper and lower eyelids and pinch grafts to re-epithelialise his legs. However, contraction of the scar tissue across the bridge of the nose was pulling both inner canthi away from the eyes. To correct this, scar tissue was excised from the nose and a rhinoplasty performed using a rotational forehead flap. (B) *13.12.1940, nine days after Thiersch grafts had been applied to his lower eyelids.* (C) *1.8.1941 following a forehead rhinoplasty.* (D) *Follow-up photograph taken 10.3.1943* (Photographs reproduced with the kind permission of Angela Lodge, Tom Gleave's daughter, and the Queen Victoria Hospital, East Grinstead)

manner with a Stent mould, paraffin flavine wool and a pressure bandage. The take was satisfactory and on 10.4.1941 Gleave was given 21 days' leave.

Operation 7.5.1941: *McIndoe/Hunter. The right side of the nose flap was lifted and shortened to raise the tip and a considerable amount of scar tissue excised. It was noted that the right anterior angle of the flap was a little shaky. The junction of the upper and lower right eyelid graft was excised and resutured; the left inner canthal defect was lifted and a small Thiersch graft on a button Stent set into place. A week later Gleave was seen by GH Morley who noted that he was healing well. He was given 28 days' leave, and on readmission was likely to require some trimming of the grafts.*

Operation 10.7.1941: *McIndoe. Some scars were excised from the forehead and excess tissue removed from the left lower eyelid.*

The date of Gleave's discharge and return to duty was recorded as 21 July 1941, when he was seen by DC Bodenham, who declared his condition to be satisfactory, recommending 14 days' sick leave and then a CME (Central Medical Establishment) Board at RAF Halton. From the time of his admission to QVH to his discharge nine months later, Gleave had undergone a total of seven operative procedures. He was seen again at QVH by McIndoe on 23 January 1942 and the decision was made to postpone any further treatment for two years. In fact, he was not seen again until

July 1945, when minor trimming operations were performed on his eyelids. In January 1950 and July 1953 McIndoe made two further adjustments to the upper eyelids with Thiersch grafts. Gleave was discharged on 28 July 1953 and no further entries were recorded.

Pilot Officer Geoffrey Page

Pilot Officer Geoffrey Page[†] of 56 Squadron, also equipped with Hurricanes, was shot down on 12 August 1940 while attacking a formation of 30 Dornier Do 215 bombers. The gasoline tank behind the engine blew up and the cockpit quickly became an inferno. Severely burned and in agonising pain, he managed to escape the aircraft and parachuted into the Channel; his abiding memory of the descent was the smell of burning flesh. He was rescued by the Margate lifeboat; his face and particularly his hands were badly burnt. Page spent three months at the Royal Masonic Hospital, London, and RAF Halton (graphically described in *Tale of a Guinea Pig* (1981)), before being transferred to East Grinstead from the RAF convalescent hospital in Torquay. This is his often quoted description of what it was like to have been on the receiving end of coagulation treatment, and the reaction of a Voluntary Aid Detachment (VAD) Red Cross nurse who was unable to hide her horror at the sight of his scorched flesh (p. 105):

> Following her hypnotised stare, I looked down watery eyed at my arms. From the elbows to the wrists the bare forearms were one seething mass of pus-filled boils … Then for the first time I noticed the hands themselves. From the wrist joints to the finger tips they were blacker than any Negro's hand, but smaller in size than I had remembered them to be. I shared the VAD's expression of horror until Skipper [the name of his nurse] intervened. 'That black stuff's only tannic acid. It's not the colour of your skin.'

Geoffrey Page was one of McIndoe's favourite patients and his case illustrates just how many operations many of the Guinea Pigs went through, as well as the surgical adjustments that continued for several years after the war had ended. It is clear from the photographs taken on admission to QVH that Page's hands were in a bad state (Figure 8.7), an unhappy reminder of the consequences of applying coagulants such as tannic acid and/or silver nitrate to third-degree burns and then failing to re-epithelialise the raw surfaces with skin grafts. Healing had been followed by the formation of keloids – thick scar tissue – resulting in skin contractures, typically causing loss of flexion or hyperextension of the metacarpo-phalangeal joints and flexion of the finger joints, the result being a so-called frozen or claw hand.

In Page's Queen Victoria Hospital notes the first operation carried out by McIndoe is recorded as taking place on 10 July 1941 – a puzzling gap of eight months after his admission in December 1940 – and there is no mention of it in Page's autobiography. However, considering the later entries and the priority given to preventing corneal ulceration, it is likely that during this period his eyelids had been reconstructed with Thiersch grafts, and since Page famously shot down one German for every one of his 15 wartime operations, four must have been performed before work began on reconstructing his hands.

> Operation 10.7.1941: *McIndoe/Davies. Scar tissue was excised from the front of the thumb, half the dorsum and the entire thenar eminence (the fleshy pad at the base of the thumb) of the left hand. This exposed the index finger and thumb and it was found that all the joints moved well. An intermediate skin graft was cut from the inner surface of the left thigh, sewn into place and sulfanilamide injected beneath the graft. By 20.7.1941 the graft had taken well, apart from a small area on the dorsal surface at the base of the index finger.*

> Operation 6.8.1941: *McIndoe/Hunter. Scar tissue over the face and neck excised by direct incision and repaired by the transfer of flaps forward from behind the ears. 21.8.1941. Neck now soundly healed – no sign of keloid.*

> Operation 17.9.1941: *McIndoe/Hunter. After 14 days' sick leave, Page was readmitted and the scar*

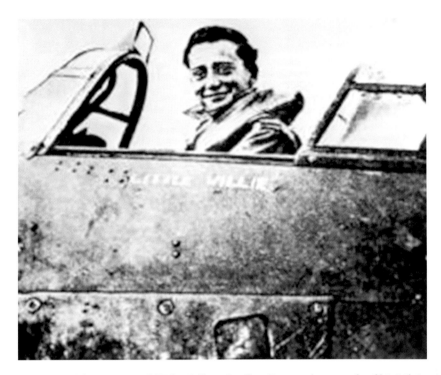

FIGURE 8.6. *Twenty-year-old Pilot Officer Geoffrey Page at the controls of his Mk I Hawker Hurricane US-X 'Little Willie', stationed at RAF North Weald with 56 Squadron during the Battle of Britain. There are 2½ swastika kill markings on the fuselage – the half was for a shared Junkers Ju 88. The squadron insignia, approved by King Edward VIII in July 1936, is a phoenix rising from the flames, which in Page's case unfortunately proved to be prescient.* (Photograph: Chaz Bowyer (1984). Fighter Pilots of the RAF, 1939–1945. William Kimber & Co)

on the right hand at the ulna border excised and the webs of tissue between three fingers including the index finger freed; the complete adhesion of the extensor tendons with no free movement in extension or flexion was noted – a large amount of scar tissue was dissected from the tendon sheaths and interosseous spaces including the metacarpophalangeal joints. Split skin grafts were sewn into place and pressure applied.

Operation 1.10.1941: *McIndoe/Davies. Excision of redundant skin on left eyelid and removal of web contracture on the inner canthus (there was some question whether the right eyelid should have a further graft). An internal canthoplasty was done together with the removal of keloid scar tissue and redundant skin of the lower lid.*

Operation 30.10.1941: *McIndoe/Davies. Remaining scars on the ulna side of the dorsum of the right hand removed including webs of the ring and little finger. Thiersch grafts were inserted with the usual technique and with sulphanilamide cover. Following a Medical Board, Page was then transferred to the RAF convalescent home in Torquay for 6 weeks.*

Operation 4.12.1941: *McIndoe/Hunter. Right thumb separated from index finger and flap brought round to line the medial surface. A further defect was filled with an intermediate graft on a Stent mould. The terminal phalanx of the index finger was straightened by arthrodesis (ankylosis) of the terminal joint and fixed in 15° of flexion. The proximal interphalangeal joint was straightened*

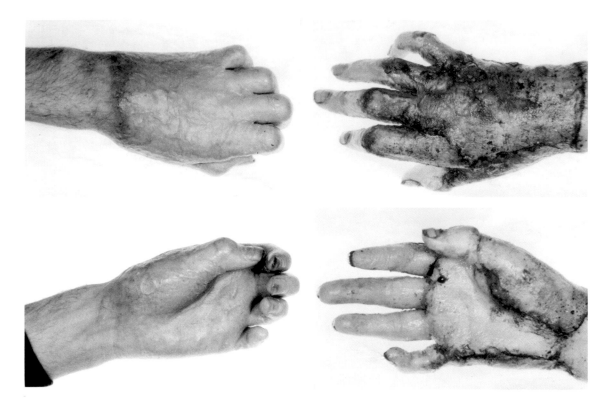

FIGURE 8.7. *The hands of Pilot Officer Geoffrey Page – photographs taken on 13 December 1940 a few days after his admission to East Grinstead. They are a graphic reminder of the consequences of treating second- and third-degree burns with coagulants and then failing to re-epithelialise the raw surfaces; healing has been by keloid scar tissue which has contracted the fingers of the left hand. Such a hand is functionally useless.* (Courtesy of the Queen Victoria Hospital, East Grinstead)

by division of the scar tissue band anteriorly and a graft inserted. The little finger was treated in a similar fashion. In January 1942 Page was discharged for light duties and return for further treatment in three months.

Figure 8.8 shows the condition of his hands on readmission.

Operation 3.4.1942: *McIndoe/Hunter. The middle and ring fingers were straightened after excision of anterior scar leaving an anterior gap on each finger of 2 x ¾ inches. A Wolfe graft from the outer side of the right thigh was over sewn into position and a pressure bandage applied.*

Operation 12.4.1942: *McIndoe/Hunter. Excision of scar from the right upper lid with insertion of a*

large Thiersch graft cut from the inner side of right arm on a Stent mould.

Operation 29.4.1942: *McIndoe/Hunter. Wolfe grafts applied to index and anterior surfaces of the middle finger. 2.5.1942: Owing to pain in the index finger grafts were taken down and found to have failed with evidence of pus underneath the graft. 4.5.1942: The little finger was taken down on 7th day and found to be a 75% take. Fingers were well-splinted and provided the position can be maintained will not be too bad.*

Operation 15.8.1942: *McIndoe/Davies. The graft on the thenar eminence and palm of the left hand spread to take a Wolfe graft measuring 3½ x 1½ inches from the abdomen, resulting in considerable*

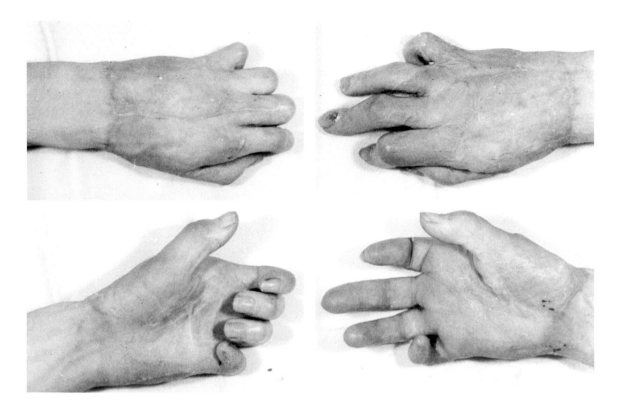

FIGURE 8.8. *The hands of Geoffrey Page photographed on 3 April 1942 following a series of operations performed over the previous 10 months to excise scar tissue and re-epithelialise the raw surfaces with skin grafts. Subsequent to these photographs he had further adjustments to straighten the fingers and a Wolfe graft applied to the thenar eminence and palm of the left hand, and was cleared to return to active flying duty in September 1942. By that time he had undergone 15 operations on his hands and face.* (Courtesy of the Queen Victoria Hospital, East Grinstead)

widening of the hand and separation of the thumb from the index finger.

Operation 29.8.1942: McIndoe/Hunter. Right eyebrow inserted from the left temporal region as a free graft. Keloid scar on the right side of the face excised. On 14.9.1942 Page was discharged for 3 days' sick leave with instructions to attend a CME Medical Board on 17.9.1942 and cleared to return to flying duties.

Page's operational flying days came to an abrupt end while he was providing ground support during the Battle of Arnhem in September 1944, when the ailerons on his Spitfire were hit by anti-aircraft fire and he crashed on landing, breaking a steel plate supporting the gunsight with his left cheek

and injuring his back. After being admitted to the nearest CCS in a Dutch convent, he was readmitted to QVH on 7 October 1944 with a fractured left malar (cheekbone). However, the bone was not displaced and no surgery was performed. He had a small piece of cannon shell removed from his left leg below the knee by Wing Commander Ross Tilley in April 1945 (the legacy of a shell from an Bf 109 that exploded in the cockpit over Normandy), and a tonsillectomy by Mr Scott-Brown in May of the same year. No further operations were performed by McIndoe on Page until 1947.

Operation 14.5.1947: McIndoe/Hunter. Incisions were made on each side of the 2nd, 3rd, 4th and 5th metacarpo-phalangeal joints of the left hand, and mobilisation of grossly adherent structures carried out. The extensor tendons were also mobilised subcutaneously up to the wrist. All wounds were sutured after obtaining marked improvement in the index and middle and some improvement in the ring and fifth fingers. On 17.5.1947 the dressings were taken down. The condition of the hand was satisfactory and in spite of some bruising Page was starting active movements. Penicillin (530,000 units) discontinued. He was then discharged to his unit on 21.5.1947.

Operation 7.4.1948: *McIndoe/Hunter. Vertical incisions were made dorsally in the interdigital spaces on either side of the ring finger of the right hand; through these incisions a large amount of solid scar tissue was removed. The metacarpo-phalangeal (MP) joints of the ring and little finger were exposed, and the collateral ligaments of the MP joint of the little finger and the radial collateral ligament of the MP joint of the little finger excised. The extensor tendon of the ring finger was mobilised back to the wrist; the extensor tendon of the little finger was degenerate. It was possible to produce a slightly increased range of flexion of the middle and ring fingers, but not as much as had been hoped – this seemed to be partly a shortage of skin on the dorsum of the hand. A Z-plasty was then carried out on the web between the index and middle finger and considerable release obtained. 12.4.1948. All incisions healed satisfactorily and fit for discharge.*

Operation 8.8.1948: *McIndoe/Hunter. A rotation flap was raised from the right side of the nose eliminating scar below right inner canthus. Scar excision and re-suturing of right upper eyelid. Arthrodesis of the first inter-phalangeal joint, little finger, left hand.*

Operation 15.6.1954: *McIndoe. Page returned to QVH complaining of retraction of the skin of the nail bed of the right middle finger, and hyperextension of the distal inter-phalangeal joint. This was corrected under local anaesthetic with a Thiersch graft taken from the flexor surface of the right forearm.*

The last entry in the QVH notes, dated 28 June 1963 at 149 Harley Street, is as follows: 'There is a band of rather tight scar tissue extending from the thumb into the palm but this does not cause any serious interference with function. This could be released by a small full thickness skin graft and if the patient decides to have this done later he will get in touch.' The identity of the examiner is not recorded.

Flight Sergeant Jack Allaway

The case of Flight Sergeant Jack Allaway[†] is a good example of the reconstruction of a total facial burn. Allaway was a wireless operator/air-gunner in a Handley Page Hampden bomber of 521 Squadron returning from a shipping strike in the Skagerrak on 10 October 1943, when it was shot down by a Junkers Ju 88 intruder as it was about to land in Norfolk. It was Allaway's twenty-seventh operational flight;[27] he was not wearing goggles or gloves. He managed to extricate himself from the aircraft and, after first-aid treatment, was transferred to the RAF Hospital at Ely near Cambridge. Routine burns treatment was carried out and grafts were applied to the upper and lower eyelids and both hands, including the fingers, by Wing Commander George Morley (Figure 8.9).

On 8 May 1944 he was moved to Marchwood Park, a rehabilitation unit near Southampton (see Chapter 9), and on 15 July 1944 he was transferred to East Grinstead as a walking case. His general physical condition was good and his local condition was described as follows:

> *Face: Healed second and third degree burns of the mask area. Eyes: Upper and lower lids completed, but requiring excision of redundant skin. Nose: Loss of right lower lateral ala cartilage – partial loss of left. Right ear: Loss of rim and upper third of cartilage with scar tissue extending down to right cheek.*

The operations carried out on Allaway at East Grinstead are as follows. It is interesting to note that while McIndoe is frequently reported as having been particularly pleased with the outcome of Allaway's surgery, most of the operations were carried out by George Morley at RAF Ely and by Ross Tilley.

22.7.1944: *McIndoe/Davies. Z-plasty performed between the thumb and index finger to deepen the web. Split skin grafts on moulds applied to the 2nd and 4th interosseus spaces.*

Operation 16.8.1944: *McIndoe/Hunter. Scar tissue excised from both lower lids and left upper lid. Scar tissue excised from upper lip and insertion of dermatome graft, oversewn on Stent mould using sino-glue technique and pressure.*

Operation 11.10.1944: *McIndoe/Hunter. Scar excised from palm of left hand, including separation of thumb – insertion of a large dermatome graft into the palm with Stent mould pressure. The take was good and patient discharged to Marchwood Park Rehabilitation Unit.*

Operation 31.1.1945: *W/C Tilley/SLdr Park. Trimming of lower eyelid grafts; web between middle and ring fingers opened and Thiersch graft inserted.*

Operation 8.3.1945: *W/C Tilley/SLdr Park. Acromio-thoracic pedicle 9 inches in length raised on right side of chest. Donor site closed with interrupted sutures and after sulphanilamide powder had been insufflated, dressings applied. 15.3.1945: sutures removed condition of pedicle very satisfactory and donor site well healed.*

Operation 30.3.1945: *W/C Tilley/SLdr Park. Distal end of acromio-thoracic pedicle freed from chest and defect closed with interrupted sutures. Scar keloid tissue excised from nose and lining flaps turned down. The distal end of the pedicle split, thinned and sewn into position on nose. Elastoplast dressings applied.*

Operation 20.4.1945: *W/C Tilley/SLdr Park. Acromio-thoracic pedicle detached near its nasal extremity and flap used to form nose. The remaining portion of pedicle returned to shoulder after excision of scars (Figure 8.10(C)). 30.4.1945: flap to nose is now well healed. Patient to continue wearing moulds in both nostrils, donor site now healed.*

Operation 7.6.1945: *W/C Tilley/SLdr Peart. Webs between index and middle finger, middle and ring*

finger of left hand opened up and Thiersch grafts from right thigh applied. 15.6.1945: incisions have healed and grafts settled in very well. Patient discharged to Marchwood Park.

Operation 9.2.1946: *SLdr Moore/Davies. Excision of scar tissue between the thumb and index finger; dermatome graft (4 x 1½ inches) from thigh sutured to raw area, and dressings applied under pressure. 19.2.1946: graft perfect – all stitches removed.*

Operation 6.3.1946: *McIndoe/De Zwaan. Nose thinned by lateral vertical incisions in the ala groove with undermining of the lateral sides of the nose beneath the ala skin. Flaps pinned down with Stent mould pressure to control.*

Operation 29.5.1946: *SLdr Szlazak/Major Shepherd. Scar tissue excised between the ring and middle finger, and thumb and index finger of the right hand. Both defects covered with dermatome grafts from the left thigh under pressure. 17.6.1946: discharged to Marchwood Park.*

Operation 21.10.1946: *McIndoe/Sherwood. Insertion of eyebrow graft from left temporal region, reversing the graft on the right side to suit the run of the hairs. Grafts sewn directly into place and pressure applied. 6.11.1946: discharged to Marchwood Park.*

Operation 14.2.1947: *SLdr Moore/Davies. Excision of scar and previous graft from dorsum of right hand from wrist to mid-phalanges and covered with a dermatome graft.*

Operation 25.3.1947: *SLdr Moore/Davies. Reconstruction of the right ear – a local flap was raised from posterior surface of ear based on free margin of helix. The role was held by mattress sutures tied over rubber wicks and raw area covered with a dermatome graft. 1.4.1947: shape of ear good with a 100% take.*

Allaway's last injury was a sporting one. On 11 April 1947 he injured his knee while playing football, resulting in an effusion into the lateral compartment and probable derangement of the lateral cartilage. After another stay at Marchwood Park for a period of recuperation he was discharged

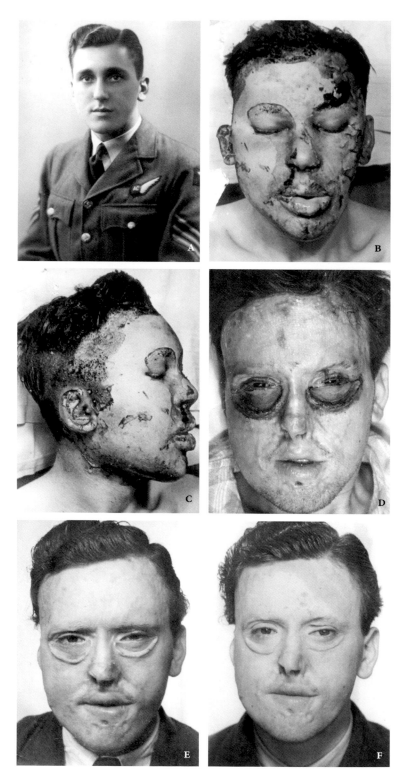

FIGURE 8.9 *Flight Sergeant Jack Allaway was an air gunner on a Hampden bomber that crashed on 10.10.1943 and he spent the next six months at RAF Ely. While there routine burns treatment was carried out and the upper and lower eyelids reconstructed with Thiersch grafts by Wing Commander George Morley.* (A) *Pre-treatment (undated).* (B, C) *His condition on 3.11.1943 when first photographed.* (D) *6.2.1944 following grafts to the lower eyelids.* (E) *26.4.1944.* (F) *17.7.1944 at time of admission to East Grinstead.* (Photographs reproduced with permission of the late Jack Allaway and the Queen Victoria Hospital, East Grinstead)

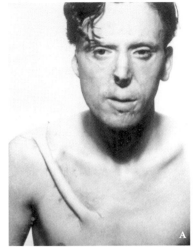
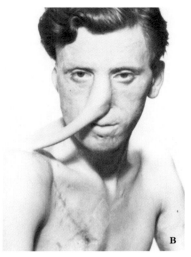
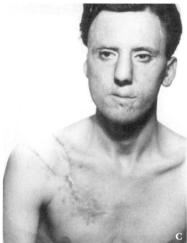

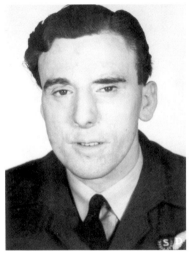

FIGURE 8.10 *Flight Sergeant Jack Allaway.* (A) *On 8.3.1945 an acromio-thoracic tubed pedicle 9 inches in length was raised on right side of chest. Photograph dated 29.3.1945.* (B) *Distal end freed on 30.3.1945 and sewn into position on nose. Photograph taken 18.4.1945.* (C) *On 20.4.1945 the pedicle was detached near its nasal extremity and used to form nose and the remaining portion returned to the shoulder. Photograph dated 23.5.1945. All three operative procedures were carried out by Wing Commander Ross Tilley, RCAF.* (D) *Appearance 19.2.1947.* (Photographs reproduced with permission of the late Jack Allaway and the Queen Victoria Hospital, East Grinstead)

from the hospital on 5 August 1947. The time from the date of injury on 10 November 1943 to the last operation on 25 March 1947 was over three years, and during that period he had been on the receiving end of a total of 14 operations at East Grinstead, plus those carried out earlier at RAF Ely.

Queen Victoria Hospital Archives

Up until 2008 artefacts from the hospital's history collected over many years, carefully cared for and curated by Bob Marchant, were available to view in the museum based at the hospital. In 2009 this collection, comprising several thousand objects, including equipment, surgical instruments and prostheses, photographs, paintings and other memorabilia, was transferred to the East Grinstead Museum in Cantalupe Road, West Sussex. The archives include handwritten papers by Sir Archibald McIndoe and medical records from Guinea Pig Club patients. At the time of writing, the records are in the process of being catalogued and housed in a new wing at the museum to make them more accessible to historians and students of medical history.

CHAPTER 9

The Guinea Pig Club

Written in collaboration with Robert (Bob) Marchant

GIVEN THE NUMBER OF BOOKS and documentaries that have appeared over the years about that extraordinary band of brothers, the Guinea Pig Club, one may well ask why yet another is necessary. The answer, for generations who have not had to test their courage in war, is simply to remind us of first, the price these men paid to preserve our freedom; and second, the capacity of the human spirit to triumph over adversity. It was also through the Guinea Pig Club that the public became aware of the rehabilitation of burned airmen in an otherwise obscure cottage hospital in Sussex, and the surviving Guinea Pigs remain the source of McIndoe's enduring fame.

In 1941, RAF Fighter Command and the Air Ministry, with its talent for publicity, had issued a bestselling booklet entitled *The Battle of Britain, August–October 1940*, an account of the first great air battle in history; this was followed up by a longer, more technical version in 1943.[1] The narrative opens under the heading 'The Scene is Set', with that famous quotation from Churchill's speech to the House of Commons at 3.52 pm on Tuesday 20 August 1940: 'Never in the field of human conflict was so much owed by so many to so few' – and just in case the reader had missed the significance of the defeat of the German Luftwaffe after 84 days of continuous attack, it ends with the single line: 'Such was the Battle of Britain in 1940. Future historians

may compare it with Marathon, Trafalgar, and the Marne.'

The young men of the RAF (average age twenty-four) had captured the imagination of the nation with their skill, great courage and devotion to duty. The majority of McIndoe's early patients were Hurricane and Spitfire pilots who had been injured in the Battle of Britain, and the conspicuous combination of the disfigured and heroic airman created an irresistibly powerful image in the mind of the public. Considering the amount of media exposure the hospital consequently attracted, it is easy to conclude that McIndoe was an extrovert publicity seeker, and no doubt some of the more conservative elements within the medical establishment saw it that way. An energetic and extrovert personality he certainly was, but any publicity McIndoe attracted was for the benefit of his patients, for whom he fought tirelessly up until his sudden and premature death at the age of 59. McIndoe and the maxillofacial unit at East Grinstead had a simple philosophy: once a patient, always a patient.

The Maxillonian Club

The social network that eventually became known as the Guinea Pig Club originated on the morning of Sunday 20 July 1941 in the surgeons' mess, where most of the inmates of Ward III were recovering

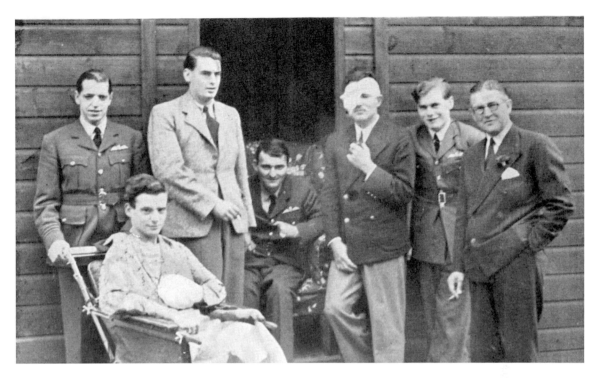

FIGURE 9.1. *An exclusive club: the Guinea Pig Club's first committee. From left to right: Tom Gleave (chief Guinea Pig), Geoffrey Page, Russell Davies, Peter Weeks (treasurer), Bill Towers-Perkins (secretary), Michael Coote, Archibald McIndoe (president).* (From RAF Casualty (1941), I Had a Row with a German)

from hangovers from the previous evening. When their mood had been revived with a bottle of sherry – perhaps not everyone's idea of the perfect restorative – it was decided to form a drinking society to be known as the Maxillonian Club (at the time QVH was a maxillofacial unit), whose members would be called Guinea Pigs,[2] a name adopted for obvious reasons, given the experimental nature of much of the surgery. Squadron Leader Tom Gleave, the senior officer present, became Chief Guinea Pig, and Pilot Officer Geoffrey Page took the minutes. With typical gallows humour, Flying Officer Bill Towers-Perkins was appointed secretary because he couldn't write, and Pilot Officer Peter Weeks was the club treasurer, a choice based on the equally sound reasoning that his badly injured legs prevented him from running off with the cash tin. McIndoe was elected president. (On his death he was succeeded by HRH Prince Philip, Duke of Edinburgh.) The Maxillonians, soon to be

known as the Guinea Pig Club, was composed of three classes of membership, all with equal rights:

1. The guinea pigs – serving airmen who had gone through at least one surgical procedure.
2. The medical staff at the Queen Victoria Hospital, East Grinstead.
3. The Royal Society for the Prevention of Cruelty to Guinea Pigs – friends and benefactors who, by their interest in the hospital and patients, made the life of the guinea pig a happy one.[2]

Although it started out as something of a joke and an excuse to hold an annual reunion, the Guinea Pig Club soon acquired a serious purpose.

Liaison with the Air Ministry: Smith-Barry and Philippi

The name of Smith-Barry may be found among the founder members of the Guinea Pig Club, a man who by the time he arrived in Ward III had led an extraordinary career as an aviator. Robert Smith-

---

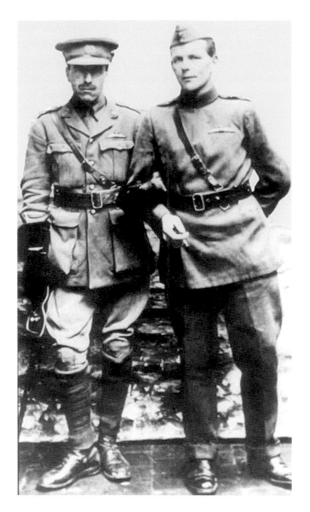

FIGURE 9.2. *Robert Smith-Barry (right) with his commanding officer FF Waldron: photograph taken at Gosport in April 1916 when they formed 60 Squadron RFC. Waldron was killed over the Somme in July and Smith-Barry took over command of the squadron, which claimed 320 aerial victories during the First World War – its aces included the VC winners Albert Ball and WA 'Billy' Bishop.* (Picture scanned by Ian Dunster from 'Not THE Smith Barry', an article in the July 1984 issue of Aeroplane Monthly posted on Wikipedia)

Barry AFC was an old Etonian from an Anglo-Irish landowning family, blessed with an Irishman's charm. He had learned to fly in 1911, and on the outbreak of the First World War joined the Royal Flying Corps (RFC). According to the history of 60 Squadron, during the retreat from Mons, Smith-Barry had crashed near Amiens, breaking both his legs leaving him permanently lame, and although beloved by the squadron, was often found to be a little trying by his superiors.[3]

Smith-Barry became one of the RFC's most skilful and daring pilots and was appalled by the standard of flying instruction in the RFC, which could only be charitably described as 'the blind leading the blind'. At the time, pilots were being sent to France with very limited training and no experience whatsoever of the aerobatics necessary to survive aerial combat – they were more likely to be killed during training than on active service. In August 1917, with the approval of Lord Trenchard, Smith-Barry put his ideas for improvement into practice at Gosport near Portsmouth.[4] Seen by his peers as an eccentric and colourful personality, he was the moving spirit behind the 'School of Special Flying' at Fort Grange Aerodrome, writing the RFC's first flying training manual, which revolutionised the way in which pilots in the RFC and its successor the RAF were trained. Lord Trenchard regarded Smith-Barry as 'the man who taught the air forces of the world how to fly'. In 1940 Smith-Barry shaved off his grey beard to appear more youthful, and at the age of 53 joined the volunteer reserve, dropping several ranks in the process, although he was still addressed as 'the Colonel' by his colleagues. He served as a ferry pilot and ground instructor until he crashed a Bristol Blenheim, fracturing his jaw, and, hearing good things about East Grinstead, managed to talk his way into Ward III.

McIndoe was ambivalent about his admission, but decided to take advantage of Smith-Barry's reputation and contacts in the RAF and asked him whether he would act as a liaison officer between the Air Ministry and East Grinstead. Smith-Barry declined, saying he was no good at that sort of thing (an accurate self-assessment, as it happens –

in 1916 when commanding officer of 60 Squadron he once dealt with a massive accumulation of official paperwork by burning down the squadron office), and suggested his equally venerable friend Lieutenant Colonel George Philippi[†], another 60 Squadron veteran of the First World War (Colour plate 21). In due course Philippi, freshly commissioned as a pilot officer in the RAF, arrived at East Grinstead. He was just the man for the job. Philippi knew everyone in senior RAF circles and had extensive business connections. He was on first-name terms with the Chief of Air Staff and the members of the Air Council, and the fact that his lowly rank was so obviously ridiculous (further highlighted by his MC and war service ribbons), served as a useful advertisement for his activities.[5] After a short period at East Grinstead studying the problem, Philippi departed for Adastral House in Kingsway, home of the Air Ministry, where he looked after the welfare of Guinea Pigs at a department called P5 (Rehabilitation), established specifically for the purpose.

A social and welfare organisation

To handle the day-to-day details at East Grinstead, Philippi recruited Flight Sergeant Edward Black-sell[†], an assistant schoolmaster from Barnstable in North Devon. At the outbreak of war, hoping to join the Royal Navy, Blacksell was rejected on medical grounds, but had been made a physical training (PT) instructor by the RAF (work that one out). Affectionately known as 'Blackie' by the Guinea Pigs, Blacksell found himself posted to East Grinstead and Ward III with his PT kit. It was an inspired choice – not that he was to do much PT. As Tom Gleave wrote in Blacksell's obituary, 'The grim side of this hilarious situation in which a physical training instructor was posted to the QVH, was the immobility of its patients with their cross-leg flaps, pedicles, amputations, blindness and so on.'[6] Blacksell's job was unofficially to act as welfare officer whose role, with the help of Philippi, was to look after the Guinea Pigs at work and play, arrange work, games and outings and otherwise prepare them for a return to life in the outside world. Visits and outings and other forms of entertainment

were all very well, but what was required was some regular, meaningful activity. Conventional occupational therapy soon proved a failure; burnt airmen in their early twenties were not interested in basket weaving, carpentry and embroidery, no matter how delightful the occupational therapist. What they wanted to do was something useful that would help the war effort.

To achieve these aims McIndoe sought the help of George Reid, a former RFC pilot who had helped establish an instrument-manufacturing company in Leicester, called Reid and Sigrist, which specialised in aviation instruments. A small satellite factory was set up in the hospital grounds, staffed by five of the company's employees; their function was to train and supervise the work done by the patients, who were paid a small hourly rate. It was the first real factory to be established in a hospital, and it helped to revolutionise rehabilitation.

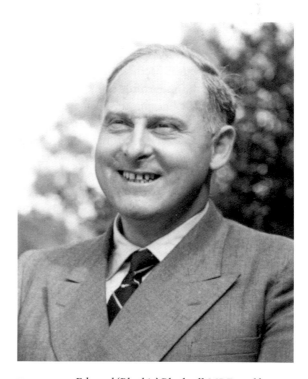

FIGURE 9.3. *Edward 'Blackie' Blacksell MBE, welfare officer to the Guinea Pigs, a role he fulfilled in one way or another for the rest of his life.* (Reproduced with permission of the East Grinstead Museum)

Jagdgeschwader 27. However, as described in Chapter 8, the next day while attacking a formation of Junkers Ju 88 bombers, an incendiary shell hit the starboard wing tank, which burst into flames. He was forced to abandon the aircraft, parachuting into a field near Biggin Hill, and was taken to Orpington Hospital. His hands, forearms and legs encased in dried tannic acid and with a face that felt like the proverbial melon, when told his wife had arrived Gleave was naturally anxious about her likely reaction. As he peered through slits in the mask, 'I heard footsteps approaching the bed and then saw my wife standing gazing at me. She flushed a little and said, "What on earth have you been doing with yourself, darling?" I found it hard to answer. "Had a row with a German," I replied.' (p. 80).

Richard Hillary, *The Last Enemy*

The most famous of the Guinea Pig books is *The Last Enemy* by Richard Hillary[†], another of the founder members of the Guinea Pig Club (Colour plate 22). Recognised as one of the classics of the Second World War literature, it was published in July 1942 to instant acclaim; by 1950 the English edition had sold 135,000 copies, the American edition 15,000 and the French 35,000.[11] It had been translated into every European language and was admired even in postwar Germany.[12] In 1941 Hillary had been given permission by the Air Ministry to travel to the United States on a speaking tour to win support for the war. However, when he arrived in Washington, the British Embassy took one look at him and concluded his face was too scarred for public appearances and restricted him to radio broadcasts. It was during this period in New York, at a time when RAF casualties were mounting and he was becoming increasingly frustrated, that Hillary wrote about his life and experiences. Before returning to England, he signed a contract with the New York publisher Reynal and Hitchcock, and the book first appeared in the United States as *Falling Through Space*,[13] a title he apparently disliked. It seems it was the fiancée of Peter Pease (a member of Hillary's squadron who had been killed in action in 1940), who is referred to only as Denise in the book, who came across that marvellous title *The Last Enemy* in Saint Paul's first Epistle to the Corinthians – 'The last enemy that shall be destroyed is death' – while thumbing through Hillary's Bible.[14]

At the outbreak of war Hillary enlisted in the RAF, and in July 1940 he was posted to 603 (City of Edinburgh) Squadron flying Spitfires at RAF Dyce in Aberdeenshire. In August the squadron was ordered south to RAF Hornchurch in Essex. During the Battle of Britain Hillary was credited with five enemy aircraft (therefore qualifying him as an Ace), before he was shot down over the North Sea on 3 September 1940 by Hauptmann Helmut Bode of Jagdgeschwader 26 in a Messerschmitt Bf 109. He was rescued by the Margate lifeboat, but his face and particularly his hands had been badly burnt. He was admitted to Margate Hospital and then spent three months at the Royal Masonic Hospital in London before being transferred to East Grinstead, where his bright red pyjamas, long cigarette-holder, intellectual superiority and cutting wit did not endear him to some of the members of Ward III.

Hillary's experiences while his face and hands were being rebuilt by McIndoe are described in two celebrated chapters of *The Last Enemy*, 'The Beauty Shop' and 'The Last of the Long-haired Boys' – the latter refers to those members of the Oxford and Cambridge University air squadrons who joined the RAF with Hillary in 1939, and who had all been killed in action apart from himself.

In January 1943 Hillary returned to operational flying, against the express wishes of McIndoe, and while on a night flying exercise crashed a Bristol Blenheim – a difficult aircraft to control with his deformed hands – killing both himself and his radio operator, William Fison. Much has been written about the short and tormented life of Richard Hillary by many distinguished writers, including Arthur Koestler, Eric Linklater and Sebastian Faulks[15] – not all of it accurate. Whether or not Dunedin is a dead-end town is debatable, but other comments by Faulks regarding McIndoe's early professional life are not correct. McIndoe did not train as a doctor at the University of

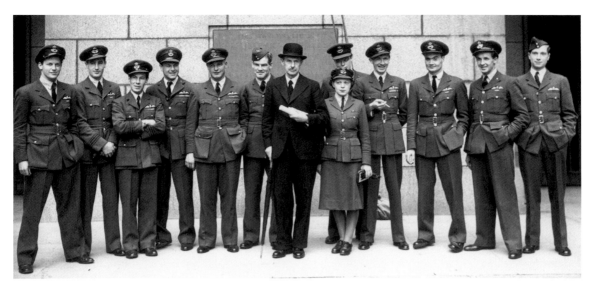

FIGURE 9.6. *Some of 'The Few'. Photograph of Air Chief Marshall Sir Hugh Dowding and aide with several Battle of Britain fighter pilots outside the Air Ministry on 14 September 1942. From left: S/Ldr AC Bartley DFC; W/Cdr DFB Sheen DFC and Bar (Australia); W/Cdr IR Gleed DSO, DFC; W/Cdr JWM Aitken DSO, DFC; W/Cdr AG Malan DSO, DFC (South Africa); S/Ldr AC Deere DFC and Bar (New Zealand); Air Chief Marshall Sir Hugh Dowding (later Lord Dowding) GCB, GCVO, CMG; F/O EC Henderson MM (WAAF); F/Lt RH Hillary; W/Cdr JA Kent DFC, AFC (Canada); W/Cdr CBF Kingcome DSO, DFC and Bar; S/Ldr DH Watkins DFC; WO RH Gretton. At the time the photograph was taken, Hillary had become something of an international celebrity after publication of* The Last Enemy. *Nevertheless, in the several photos taken that day he continued to hover in the background, giving the impression of not being quite sure whether he should be in such distinguished company.* (Photograph courtesy of Hulton Archive Getty Images)

Minnesota, and did not go to England to work with his cousin Sir Harold Gillies in 1929. (Gillies was not knighted until 1930.) When McIndoe turned up unannounced on Gillies' doorstep in 1931 looking for a job, they hardly knew each other. The most recent Hillary biography by David Ross includes a detailed account of his flying career and rehabilitation at East Grinstead.[16]

William Simpson, *One of Our Pilots Is Safe*

On 2 September 1939 – the day before the outbreak of the war – 12 Squadron, equipped with obsolete single-engined Fairey Battle bombers, was sent to an airfield at Amifontaine between Rheims and Laon as part of the RAF's somewhat optimistically designated Advanced Air Striking Force – a force of 160 aircraft accompanied by two fighter squadrons

(numbers 1 and 73) with orders to attack ground targets. These were difficult to hit and were usually heavily defended, and the Fairey Battle, which was painfully slow (top speed 241 mph), lightly armoured and ill-armed (a single forward-firing 0.303 gun operated by the pilot, and one Vickers rear-firing machine gun operated by the air gunner), was vulnerable to ground fire.

On 10 May 1940 the Germans launched their Blitzkrieg against the Low Countries, and two Fairey Battles, led by Flight Lieutenant William Simpson†, were ordered to attack enemy troops and convoys advancing on the road between Luxembourg and Junglinster. Both aircraft were hit by flak. Simpson managed to belly-land his aircraft (PH-V: L4949) in a field northwest of Virton in Belgium, but before he had time to unstrap his harness and exit the aircraft, the cockpit became enveloped in flames. His two-man crew, Sergeant Edward Nelson Odell and Corporal Robert Tod Tomlinson, braved the inferno and pulled him clear, but Simpson suffered severe burns, particularly to his face and hands. Tomlinson was also burned, although less badly. Both Simpson and Tomlinson were eventually treated at an emergency hospital near Verdun before being moved to a hospital in Bar-le-Duc, where they were separated. Simpson was later awarded the DFC and both Odell and Tomlinson the DFM.

Simpson wrote three critically acclaimed books about his subsequent experiences.[17] *One of Our Pilots Is Safe* (1943) describes the series of night-mare journeys and hospitalisations experienced in the face of the German advance. After five weeks he reached the relative safety of Vichy, France, where he was admitted to a military hospital at Roanne in the Loire; 13 months later he was transferred to the Michel Lévy Military Hospital in Marseilles. The treatment at both hospitals amounted to little more than palliative care and the application of mercurochrome to his burns, and in Marseilles the hospital director and medical staff proved to be anything but helpful. In due course he appeared before an international medical board, and in October 1941 was repatriated via Spain and Portugal to England, where he was admitted to Ward III. His eyelids had been burned off, along

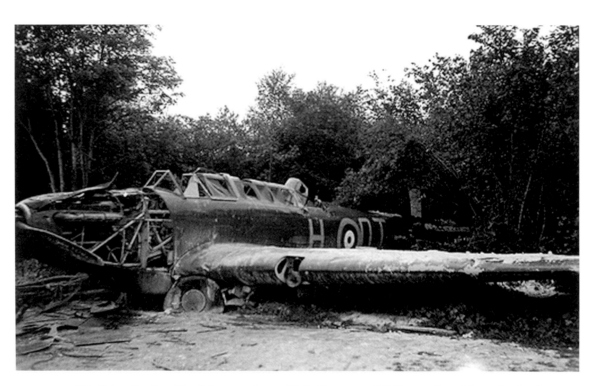

FIGURE 9.7. *This Fairey Battle suffered the same fate as Flight Lieutenant Bill Simpson's – of the 32 Battles that were ordered to attack German convoys advancing through Luxembourg on 10 May 1940, 13 were lost, including Simpson's, and the remainder were damaged. Two days later 12 Squadron led by Flying Officer Garland was ordered to destroy a vital bridge over the Albert Canal; of the six crews who volunteered for the raid, one had to turn back early due to technical problems and the remaining five were all shot down by ground fire. Garland and his observer Sergeant Gray were posthumously awarded the Victoria Cross, the first RAF personnel in the Second World War to receive such an honour. The third member of the crew, Leading Aircraftman LR Reynolds, a wireless operator/air gunner, received no award of any kind. (Image from www.tangmerepilots.co.uk)*

with part of his nose; and his mouth, cheeks and forehead were ribbed with keloid scars. But worst of all were his hands: most of his fingers had been destroyed – they had become gangrenous and had been torn off during dressings. None remained on his left hand, and only the proximal phalanges remained on his right hand.

It was during his time at East Grinstead that Simpson was encouraged by Katherine Dewar to record his experiences, using a dictaphone held between his wrists. His second volume, *The Way of Recovery* (1944), is concerned with the long process of rehabilitation, both physical and mental. Simpson had an excellent memory, an acute sense of observation and a gift for describing what he saw. This is his first meeting with McIndoe (pp. 20–21):

It was not long before Mr MacIndoe [sic] examined me. My hands had already been dressed and almost every part of my body had been photographed. I was waiting for lunch when he came into the ward. I saw that he was a man of medium height and solid build, with a bronzed complexion. His hair had begun to grey, and was parted in the middle. He wore horn-rimmed spectacles and behind them his eyes betrayed a keen sense of humour. His jaw was firm and he radiated confidence. His hands were powerful, and the ends of his fingers squared … In a few minutes of quiet observation he had examined me, decided what he was going to do, and explained to me his plan in simple detail. He had none of the hesitation of many other doctors I had known.

These few sentences tell us why McIndoe was able to exert such a powerful influence and induce lasting affection from his patients – he treated them with respect, communicating in detail exactly what surgical procedures were required and how long it would take; he answered their questions and encouraged them to attend operations so they knew in advance exactly what they would have to go through. Theirs was a meeting of equals, with none of the hierarchical attitudes, conscious or otherwise, normally associated with doctor–patient relationships.

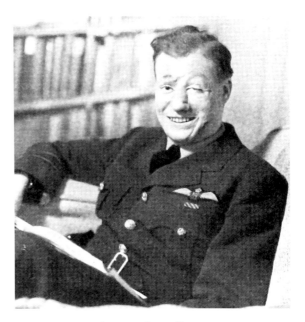

FIGURE 9.8. *Squadron Leader William Simpson DFC after reconstructive surgery to his face and hands at East Grinstead. Regrettably, it is the only illustration in his three books, and the grainy image reflects the standard of wartime publishing. The photograph was taken by Howard Coster and used as the frontispiece in* The Way of Recovery *(1944).*

I Burned My Fingers (1955), which appeared 10 years after the war, inevitably covers some of the same ground as Simpson's earlier books and chronicles his gradual return to civilian life. It also contains the best descriptions of the social and welfare role of the Guinea Pig Club and the people involved in their rehabilitation discussed earlier in the chapter. Simpson was not altogether happy to be back on English soil again having developed an affectionate regard for the French people, and his mind had been troubled by a premonition that his marriage would collapse on his return – and so it proved: his appearance was a profound and terrible shock to his wife Hope, and on seeing him she broke down and wept. As he admits, it was bitterly ironic that her instinctive compassion hardened him against her, and from that moment onwards, no matter how hard she tried, there was no way back into his heart. It had turned to stone (p. 53).

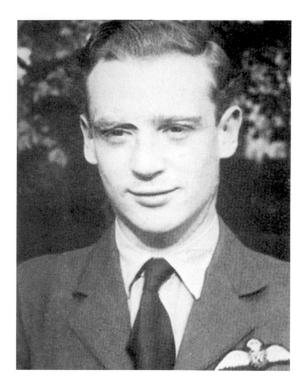

FIGURE 9.9. *Flight Lieutenant Geoffrey Page in 1943, shortly after being awarded the DFC for his part in the celebrated sortie to attack Luftwaffe night-fighter airfields south of Paris with Squadron Leader James MacLachlan DSO, DFC. They accounted for six enemy aircraft: three by MacLachlan, two by Page with one shared.* (Courtesy of Queen Victoria Hospital Archives, East Grinstead)

Geoffrey Page, *Tale of a Guinea Pig*

In *Tale of a Guinea Pig* (1981) Geoffrey Page[†] gives a rather droll account of his rescue by two merchant seamen and being welcomed at the quayside by the Mayor of Margate in mayoral regalia and a top hat, followed by his admission to Margate Hospital.[18] After a few days he was transferred to London in an ambulance driven by two members of the Women's Transport Service who hadn't the faintest idea where they were going (Hillary's experience had been similar). Eventually they arrived at their destination, the Royal Masonic Hospital at Hammersmith, where he suffered the first of a series of setbacks – and here the narrative takes on a more serious tone.

As the bombing of London by the Luftwaffe intensified, Page was evacuated to Princess Mary's Hospital at RAF Halton in Buckinghamshire, an institution in which service discipline and red tape were the order of the day and the Ward Sister made sure his stay there was not a happy one. The consultant RAF surgeon-in-charge, Wing Commander Stanford Cade (a Polish-Russian émigré originally named Kadinsky, later Sir Stanford Cade), who visited him each day, eventually decided to remove the tannic acid that had been applied to his hands. However, failure to re-epithelialise the raw surfaces with skin grafts following this procedure meant healing by keloid scar tissue, and the condition of his hands continued to deteriorate. The tendons contracted day by day until the tips contacted the palms, and the skin became toughened by degrees until it reached the texture of rhinoceros hide.

As noted earlier, a good deal of the suffering and surgical rehabilitation of burn victims during the early months of the war could have been avoided if the prescient advice of Pomfret Kilner in 1934 had been followed – namely, that any general surgeon should have a working knowledge of plastic surgical procedures, and should be prepared to cover any raw surface with a skin graft to prevent the extreme contractures that plastic surgeons frequently encountered.[19] (Although to be fair to Cade, he did become a strong advocate of Kilner's recommendations later in the war.)[20] Fortunately for Page, his luck was about to change for the first time in more than three months. Cade finally decided to refer him to McIndoe at East Grinstead. The protracted series of operations to reconstruct Page's face and hands, performed by McIndoe over a period of two years, are described in detail in Chapter 8.

Page was determined to get back into the air, and made a bitter vow that on his return to active service he would destroy one enemy aircraft for every operation he had endured (p. 140). Cleared to return to flying duties in September 1942, after serving with an anti-aircraft cooperation unit in Cardiff, early in 1943 he was posted to a Spitfire squadron based at RAF Martlesham Heath in

Suffolk, and then, hoping to see more action, he volunteered for North Africa. Unfortunately the heat of the sun on the newly grafted skin of his face proved too uncomfortable and he asked to be reassigned. Back in England he was posted to the Air Fighting Development Unit stationed at RAF Wittering in Cambridgeshire, which had been formed to assess types of fighter aircraft. There he teamed up with Squadron Leader James MacLachlan DSO, DFC, otherwise known as 'One-armed Mac' – a fighter ace who had lost his left arm during combat over Malta. In a famous 'rhubarb' (a low-level sortie by pairs of aircraft operating at low level over occupied territory) carried out on 29 June 1943, MacLachlan and Page flew two American P-51 Mustangs across France to attack the Luftwaffe night-fighter airfields south of Paris. As Page was to write later, 'Fine bloody pair we are, I thought. Going off to tackle the enemy with only one good hand between the two of us' (p. 160). In the course of the operation they accounted for six enemy aircraft – three by MacLachlan, two by Page and one shared. MacLachlan was given a second bar to his DFC, and Page was awarded the DFC. Their second attempt on 15 July was to end in tragedy, however, when MacLachlan's Mustang was hit by ground fire soon after crossing the French coast and he crash-landed into a field – MacLachlan survived, but died two weeks later in hospital at Pont-l'Évêque.[21] Page's own wartime flying service ended in September 1944 following his crash-landing during the Battle of Arnhem (see Chapter 8), but by that time he had achieved his ambition and destroyed at least 17 aircraft.

Richard Pape, *Boldness Be My Friend*

Richard Pape[†], a red-haired Yorkshireman, was the navigator on a Short Stirling bomber shot down on 7 September 1941 while returning from a night raid on Berlin; the target had been Göring's headquarters. The aircraft crashed near the Dutch border, and although he was helped by the Resistance, Pape was captured by the Germans and sent to Stalag VIIIB near Lamsdorf in Silesia on the East German border. His first book, *Boldness Be My Friend*,[22] which came out in

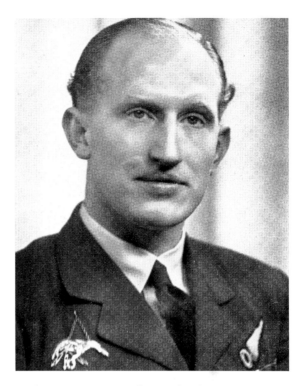

FIGURE 9.10. *Warrant Officer Richard Pape MM, RAFVR. The Military Medal could be awarded to RAF personnel for gallant service on the ground – in Pape's case for his exploits as a POW and dispatching coded messages of German troop movements and Allied bomb damage back to England. Over the left pocket is the Observer/Navigator brevet, abolished in April 1942 when it was split into the categories of Navigator and Air Bomber. Over the right pocket is the Polish Air Force Eagle. (From Richard Pape (1953),* Boldness Be My Friend)

1952 and eventually sold 160,000 copies, describes the three years he spent as a POW. Soon after his arrival he persuaded a New Zealand POW called Private Winston Yeatman to swap identities, and Pape managed to escape with a Polish airman referred to simply as Mietek C——. After a series of extraordinary adventures he was recaptured by the Gestapo and returned to Stalag VIIIB, where he suffered meningitis and temporary blindness. Eleven months passed before he returned to the main barracks. When his subterfuge with Yeatman was discovered, as an airman he was moved to Stalag Luft VI in southern Lithuania. The man in the next bunk was suffering from acute nephritis and had been cleared for repatriation. Pape closely observed his symptoms, and with swollen ankles (from constant flicking with a damp towel), a jaundiced complexion (from swallowing soap) and a sample of nephritis-laden urine from his bunk mate contained in an artificial penis, he managed to convince the medical commission he was seriously ill. He arrived in Sweden on 7 September 1944, three years to the day after he had been shot down.

However, Fate was not yet finished with Pape. Shortly after his return to England he returned to flying duties and, after a second crash on the Isle of Man, spent two years at East Grinstead. His book does not include a description of his time at QVH, but is dedicated to the Guinea Pig Club and its great benefactor, Sir Archibald McIndoe. Pape seems to have been something of a tortured soul; in the epilogue he recounts how at East Grinstead he met the finest bunch of RAF men he had ever encountered, the greatest body of men he was ever likely to know or live among. But perhaps East Grinstead's greatest gift to Pape was that while he was there (p. 309):

> I found that sanity of happiness and calmness that I had imagined would forever elude me. It was there that I experienced such humane, constructive decency that, in three months, it offset all the inhuman and destructive indecency I saw and experienced during my three years in German Occupied Europe.

Colin Hodgkinson, *Best Foot Forward*

Colin Hodgkinson was the legless pilot chosen by McIndoe to successfully challenge the 90-day rule described in Chapter 8; much of the narrative there is drawn from Hodgkinson's autobiography *Best Foot Forward*.[23] He rejoined the Fleet Air Arm as a ground officer, and was determined to return to flying. Sir Victor Warrender again came to the rescue and he was accepted for flying duties at the Royal Naval Air Station, Lee-on-Solent. However, his ambition was to fly Spitfires, which necessitated yet another begging letter to the long-suffering Sir Victor, who duly obliged, and in September

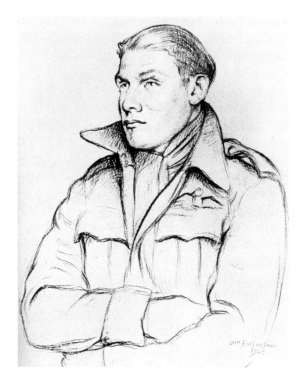

FIGURE 9.11. *Flight Lieutenant Colin Hodgkinson, 1943. Pencil portrait by Sir William Rothenstein.*[24]

(*From Colin Hodgkinson (1957),* Best Foot Forward)

1942 Hodgkinson was posted to the RAF as a pilot officer. He was successively with 610 and 510 Squadrons flying Spitfires on bomber escorts and in March 1943 was promoted flying officer and joined 611 Squadron, first at Biggin Hill and later at Coltishall in Norfolk. However, while he was on high-altitude weather reconnaissance his oxygen failed and he crashed in France. He became a POW, first at Dulag Luft (the Luftwaffe interrogation centre) minus one of his tin legs. Eventually he was transferred to Stalag Luft III in Silesia, and after 10 months Hodgkinson was repatriated to Britain. He had further surgery at East Grinstead, and ended the war flying with a ferry unit at Filton near Bristol. Hodgkinson was one of only two men in the Second World War to return to operational flying after losing both legs. The other was Douglas Bader.

Four Czech Guinea Pigs

Four Czech Guinea Pigs who went to extraordinary lengths to escape German-occupied Europe and join the RAF – Frankie Truhlar, Josef Koukal, Josef Capka and Alois Siska – were featured in *The Stories of Brave Guinea Pigs* by Vítek Formánek.[25] Two wrote autobiographies. The first, *Red Sky at Night* by Joseph Capka[†], appeared in 1958.[26] Capka was a pilot officer in the Czech air force when the Germans invaded Czechoslovakia in March 1939. He joined the Underground Movement, and when they blew up the Gestapo headquarters in his home town of Olomouc near Brno he fled to Poland. However, the Poles refused to let the Czechs fly in the Polish air force: Capka and his fellow pilots found the only way to fight for the Allies was to join the French Foreign Legion. He suffered the life and discipline of a Legionnaire at Sidi Bel Abbès in Algeria for several months, and when France entered into the war he became a caporal-chef in the French Armée de l'Air, flying hopeless missions against Panzer divisions in antiquated aircraft. After the fall of France in June 1940 he reached England in a boat out of Bordeaux with other Czechs and Poles, and was assigned to the RAF's all-Czech 311 (Bomber) Squadron: Capka flew Wellingtons on a total of 56 bombing missions, was awarded the DFM and was commissioned as a pilot officer in 1941.

He then converted to night-fighters, flying Bristol Beaufighters and then de Havilland Mosquitoes with 68 Squadron at Coltishall in Norfolk. His luck continued to hold until June 1944. While flying a daylight patrol over the Channel he noticed a badly shot-up USAAF Liberator flying on three engines, and as they drew up alongside to offer help, the rear turret traversed to follow them and fired. Capka was blinded in his left eye and covered in blood. After persuading his observer to bale out, he managed by holding his right eyelid open to crash-land in a wood. He was admitted to Colchester Military Hospital and then RAF Ely, where he was seen by McIndoe on his rounds. He was then transferred to East Grinstead, where his left orbit was reconstructed to accommodate an artificial eye.

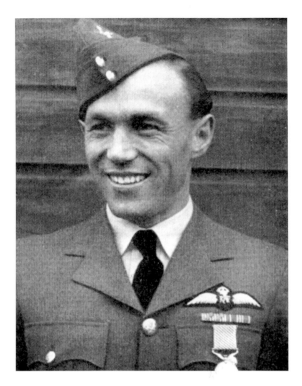

FIGURE 9.12. *Josef Capka after being awarded the DFM in 1941, 'In recognition of gallantry and devotion to duty in execution of air operations.'* (From Jo Capka (1958), Red Sky at Night)

While at East Grinstead he was visited by an officer from RAF Intelligence who explained that the Liberator was a rogue aircraft that had gone missing over Germany, been patched up by the Germans and sent on 'pirate' missions – not that Capka was ever completely convinced it wasn't a 'friendly-fire' incident. After the war, Capka the war hero and his English wife Rhoda returned to Czechoslovakia, where he ran a flying school. But in the Kafkaesque nightmare that followed the communist coup in 1948 he was charged with high treason and sentenced to 10 years in prison. Released after seven years, he was finally given permission to leave Czechoslovakia in May 1957, and was able to rejoin his wife in Essex and return to his original profession as an electrical engineer.

The second autobiography was by Alois Siska[†]. After the German occupation of Czechoslovakia,

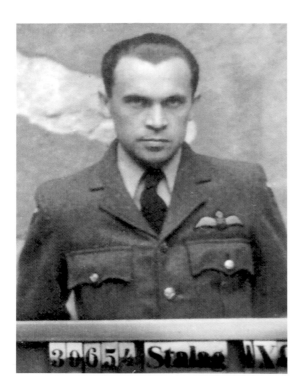

FIGURE 9.13. *Gestapo photograph of Alois Siska striking a suitably belligerent pose: Number 39654; Stalag IXC Obermansfeld, a POW camp near Frankfurt in Germany.* (From Alois Siska (2008) Flying for Freedom)

Siska fled to Hungary, where he was imprisoned but managed to escape. He too joined the Foreign Legion, and when they discovered he was a pilot they sent him to a Czech unit in France. After the French capitulated he escaped to England and also joined the RAF's all-Czech 311 Squadron, flying Wellingtons. While returning from bombing the Wilhelmshaven docks, the aircraft he was piloting caught fire and ditched in the North Sea. After several days in a dinghy, the surviving members of the crew were washed up on the Dutch coast. Siska's legs were severely frostbitten and gangrene had set in. He was moved to Germany and spent time in several POW camps, eventually ending up in Colditz Castle. In 1945 he was repatriated to East Grinstead. After two years at QVH recovering the use of his legs, in 1947 he returned to Czechoslovakia and, although he was regarded

with suspicion because he had served with the RAF, rejoined the Czech air force. After the communist takeover he refused to join the Communist Party. By the tortured logic of the Stalinist regime Siska was regarded as an enemy of the people, dismissed from the armed forces and banished from Prague to poor housing and menial jobs – a fate shared by many of his Czech and Polish contemporaries. However, with the collapse of communism in 1989, Siska was reinstated in the Czech air force and promoted to the rank of major-general. His autobiography, *Flying for Freedom*, was published posthumously by his daughter, Dagmar Johnson-Siskova, in 2008.[27]

John Harding, The Dancin' Navigator

In *The Dancin' Navigator* (1988),[28] Flight-Lieutenant John Harding[†] from Windsor, Ontario, described his wartime career as a navigator with Bomber Command in the Lancasters of 103 and 550 Squadrons stationed in Lincolnshire. Having survived two whole operational tours over Germany against almost impossible odds, in January 1945 he had the misfortune to be in a DC-3 (Dakota) carrying mail, which crashed in poor visibility while taking off from Biggin Hill. The port inner fuel tank burst inside the fuselage and ignited, producing a blowtorch effect and Harding, who was not wearing gloves or helmet, was severely burned. All the survivors had suffered burns and other injuries to varying degrees and were taken by ambulance to a civilian hospital in nearby Orpington. Harding was operated on to close a facial gash, and the medical staff began to treat his hands with the discredited gentian violet method. Fortunately, after a few days and before too much harm could be done, Ross Tilley visited the hospital and immediately transferred the crew to the Canadian Wing at East Grinstead.

Canadian Guinea Pigs have been particularly fortunate in having Rita Donovan undertake the mammoth task of tracking down and recording many of the personal stories – both during and after the war – of the members of the Guinea Pig Club who were Canadians. Her book, *As for the*

Canadians, which appeared in 2000,[29] is a valuable written and photographic record of the exploits of brave men and the surgeons and nurses who returned them to civilian life.

Postscript

The Guinea Pig Club was originally founded to maintain the bonds of comradeship, but developed into a society devoted to helping its weakest members. The names of 642 of the Guinea Pigs are recorded on the honours board that hangs in the Canadian Wing at Queen Victoria Hospital, East Grinstead (see Appendix III). It reads: 'The above are members of the Guinea Pig Club, founded in 1941 for Allied Serving Airforce Men who were treated at the Queen Victoria Hospital during the Second World War.' The majority of the names are British, with the next largest contingent coming from Canada; other nationalities included are Australia, New Zealand, South Africa and several other countries, notably those who had escaped the German occupation of Europe to join the RAF. After the second annual reunion dinner of January 1943, Simpson in *The Way of Recovery* ended a chapter on the Guinea Pig Club as follows (p. 143):

> *When eventually we broke up and returned to hospital or to the houses where we were guests for the week-end, there must have been few of us who did not feel, as I did, that this inspiring assembly was one man's triumph. Without the inspiration, skill and devotion of MacIndoe [sic], such a meeting could never have been possible.*

CHAPTER 10

Mowlem and Hill End Hospital, St Albans

Written in collaboration with Brian Morgan

HILL END HOSPITAL AT ST ALBANS in Hertfordshire was founded in 1899 as the Hertfordshire County Mental Hospital. In 1939 it was taken over by the Emergency Medical Service and in anticipation of an influx of casualties from the bombing of London, most of St Bartholomew's Hospital was evacuated to St Albans. Britain was thought to be defenceless against air attack, the thinking of the day being that the bombers would always get through. Extrapolating from the experience of the bombing raids carried out by the Luftwaffe Condor Legion on Guernica and Barcelona during the Spanish Civil War, it was estimated that a German air assault would result in half a million casualties. The hospital in Smithfield continued to provide medical services for the civilian population and also acted as a receiving and emergency clearing station for the wounded, but from 1939 to 1947 most surgical operations were carried out at Hill End.

The EMS Maxillofacial Unit at the hospital was established early in September 1939 by Rainsford Mowlem and JL Dudley Buxton[†]. Other key members of the professional staff during the war included John Barron[†], Alexander MacGregor[†] and Benjamin Fickling. The nursing and theatre staff at the unit were provided by Bart's, with 18 nurses and a sister to each ward. The unit was housed in two wards that had been vacated by the mental

patients, each with 33 beds, although at busy times the beds were moved closer together to accommodate up to 80 patients. The downstairs ward had an operating theatre and photographic department in continuity, and there was also an outpatient room, an office and a dental laboratory. Like most plastic and maxillofacial units attached to district general hospitals, it had a makeshift atmosphere about it. The unit remained in operation until 1953, when it was transferred to Mount Vernon Hospital at Northwood in North London, and Hill End was restored to its original function as a mental hospital.[1]

Mowlem did not have the high public profile of Gillies or McIndoe outside the surgical community – for a clinician to develop a reputation it helps to have famous patients. He had once joined the Prince of Wales for a quick cigarette while his mother inspected Queen Mary's Hospital in East London,[1] and had attended Sir Winston Churchill who had exploded a box of matches with a cigar and burnt his hand,[2] but the patients admitted to Hill End had none of the glamour of the RAF; for the most part they were ordinary men and women, soldiers who had been wounded in combat (during the evacuation of Dunkirk, May–June 1940, Hill End received 600 military casualties in one week) and civilians injured during the Blitz.

Mowlem was a quiet, unassuming man who did not socialise easily and to some contemporaries

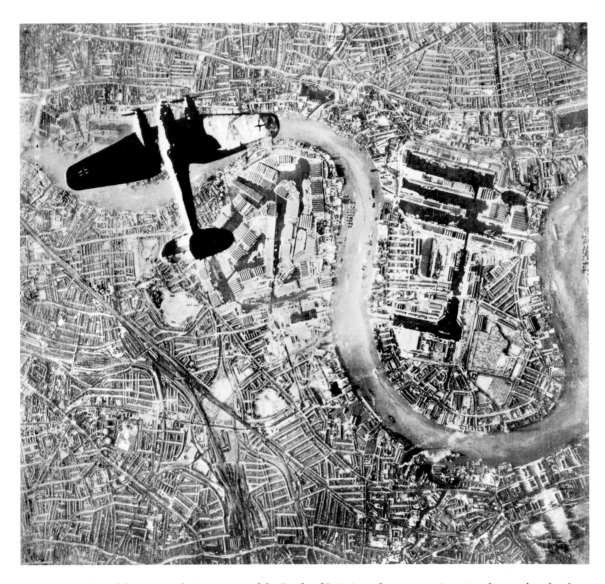

FIGURE 10.1. *One of the most enduring images of the Battle of Britain and an appropriate visual metaphor for the Blitz, which provided Hill End with many of its early patients. A Heinkel He III bomber is flying over Wapping and the Isle of Dogs in London's East End at the start of the Luftwaffe's evening raids of 7 September 1940 – the objective was the destruction of London's docklands.* (Copy negative of part of an aerial photograph taken from a German aircraft at 6.48 pm German time. By kind permission of the Imperial War Museum, London, IWM catalogue number C 5422)

appeared somewhat aloof – often a sign of shyness. Apart from the contributions of Benjamin Rank[3] and RLG Dawson, there is comparatively little written about his career and he published sparingly. Nevertheless, Mowlem together with his colleagues at Hill End made important contributions to surgical practice in several key areas, including: (1) pin fixation to stabilise fractures and bone grafts of the mandible; (2) the use of cancellous (spongy) bone chip grafts from the iliac crest (hip) to repair bone defects of the jaws and long bones; and (3) the early clinical trials of penicillin. Mowlem was also a skilful and well-regarded hand surgeon: when McIndoe required surgery to correct his Dupuytren's contracture, the surgeon he chose to perform the operation was Mowlem.

Early trials with sulphonamides

Before the arrival of war casualties, the early months of 1940 were spent working on the best method to control surface infection with the sulphanilamide group of drugs. Before Prontosil (para-aminobenzenesulphonamide) – the first synthetic drug used to treat bacterial infections – became commercially available in the mid-1930s, the failure rate of skin grafts from haemolytic streptococci was high. This was potentially a serious problem in patients with extensive burns or other war wounds. Building on the research of Leonard Colebrook and colleagues at Queen Charlotte's Hospital, London, which had shown the lifesaving power of sulphonamides in cases of puerperal fever, the Hill End team made an important advance with the demonstration that sulphonamides applied daily to a cleansed wound before grafting, followed by postoperative oral administration for 36 hours, minimised or prevented infection. At a meeting held at the Royal Society of Medicine in February 1941 to discuss the chemotherapy of wound infection, Mowlem reported that out of almost 40 patients treated by this method, there had been only one failure, where sulphonamides by mouth had unfortunately been omitted – none of the other patients had less than a 75 percent take. In the face of such compelling

evidence the technique was soon adopted at other EMS units for general use.[4]

The problem of flying glass

The advent of the Blitz and the night bombing of civilian targets in September 1940 brought a new problem: flying glass causing serious facial injuries (Figure 10.2). This presented new difficulties, because the complete removal of all glass splinters might take several hours – something that was often impracticable because of the patient's poor condition. Nevertheless, with adequate chemotherapy, residual glass fragments were seldom the cause of troublesome infection. Many such cases were also referred to EMS plastic units from other hospitals some weeks after healing had occurred – the result of marked disfigurement due to bluish-black scars scattered all over the face. Good results were usually achieved, however, by multiple scar excision and secondary repair, but loss of eyes from perforating wounds meant that reconstruction of the eyelids and the bony socket were usually required before artificial eyes could be fitted.[4]

Fixation of the jaws

At the beginning of the war several methods of fixation were available to immobilise the jaws. The choice depended on the site and the degree of fracture and also whether the surgeon or dental surgeon was working in the field, in a general hospital or in an EMS maxillofacial unit. The 1935 *Report to the Army Council of the Advisory Standing Committee on Maxillo-Facial Injuries* by Kelsey Fry, Gillies and Warwick James, mentioned in Chapter 8, discusses the methods of fixation for fractures of the jaws, and it is clear there were two distinct schools of thought for controlling the fragments. Warwick James strongly favoured interdental wiring whenever possible, while Kelsey Fry (supported by Gillies) just as strongly advocated cap splints.[5] Indeed, unable to reconcile their differences, Warwick James and Kelsey Fry battled it out in an Appendix to the Report: 'Mechanical Methods of Immobilisation of the Mandible and Maxillae', with separate memoranda extolling the virtues of their preferred method.

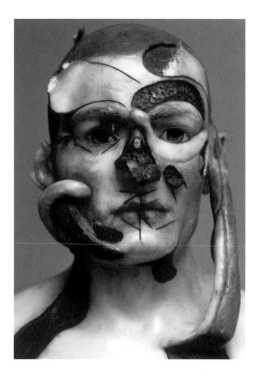

PLATE 12. *Life-size wax model of the head and upper torso constructed for teaching purposes by Sergeant Kelsey, illustrating surgical techniques including forehead and tubed pedical flaps. Part of the New Zealand records returned to Sidcup in 1989 and subsequently restored at Madame Tussaud's.* (Courtesy of the Gillies Archive, Queen Mary's Hospital, Sidcup)

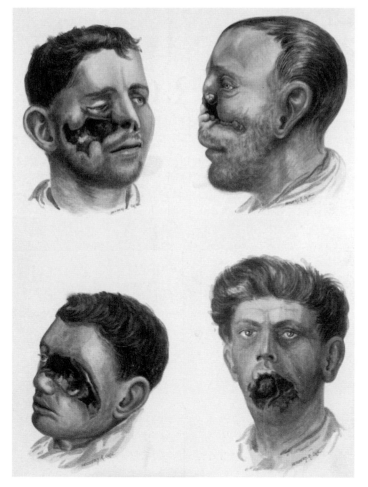

PLATE 13. *Four of the watercolours painted by Herbert R Cole and used by Pickerill as the frontispiece in* Facial Surgery (1924). *The soldiers are (clockwise from top left): Private Mallon, New Zealand Cycle Brigade; Private Wisely, Gordon Highlanders; Private G Skurr, Canterbury Infantry Battalion; Private A Grieve, Black Watch.* (The originals are in the Hocken Library, Uare Taoka o Hakena, University of Otago, Pickerill papers, Reference number MS-1620/013).

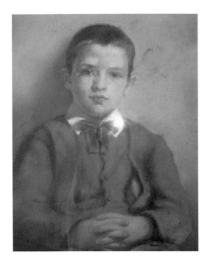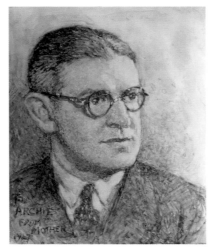

PLATE 14. LEFT: *Archibald McIndoe, 'Archie', aged eight. Pastel by his mother,*
Mabel Hill. Exhibited at the Otago Arts Society Annual Exhibition, Dunedin, in 1908.
Sale price: 5 guineas (16 cm x 48 cm). (www.mabelhill.net/catalogue)
PLATE 15. RIGHT: *'To Archie from Mother, 1947'. Miniature by Mabel Hill,*
watercolour and ink on paper (8 cm x 7 cm). Painted in London. (www.mabelhill.net/catalogue)

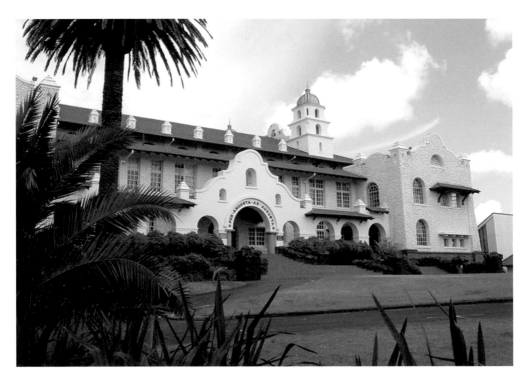

PLATE 16. *Auckland Grammar School, completed in 1916. This was the winning design in a competition by the*
Auckland architects Arnold and Abbott, who had returned from southern California much impressed by the
Spanish Mission style of architecture. It is listed as a Category I historic building by the New Zealand Historic
Places Trust. Rainsford Mowlem was a pupil at the school 1916–19. (Image from Wikimedia)

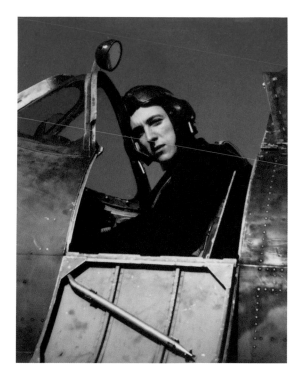
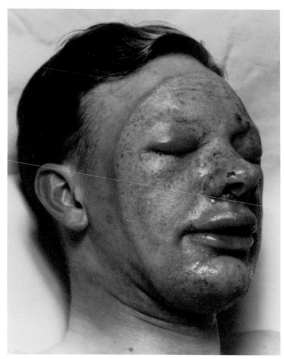

PLATE 17. *Pilot with a facial burn showing the area typically affected by not wearing goggles and oxygen mask. There is a moderate degree of edema with trumpeting of the lips even at this early stage of the burn – approximately 8 hours after the injury. On the left side of the face there is a third-degree burn, while the rest is approximately second degree. Both photographs were taken by Percy Hennell of the Metal Box Company.* (Courtesy of Brian Morgan and the Antony Wallace Archive, BAPRAS, Royal College of Surgeons of England)

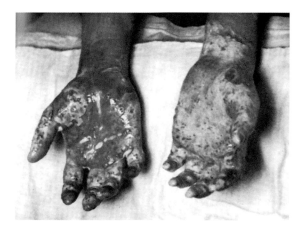
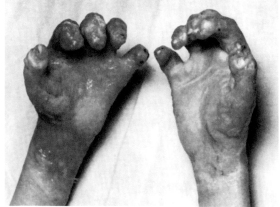

PLATE 18. *Burns of an airman's hands resulting from not wearing gloves. Photographs taken by Percy Hennell of the Metal Box Company.* (From History of the Second World War: Surgery (1953), ed. Sir Zachary Cope)

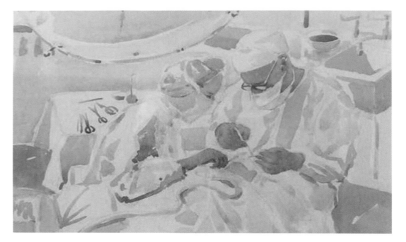

PLATE 19. *McIndoe operating, assisted by his theatre sister, Jill Mullins. Watercolour by his elder brother John McIndoe painted in 1945 soon after his release from a POW camp in Germany. The original hangs in the entrance hall of the Archibald McIndoe Building at Otago Boys' High School, Dunedin.* (With acknowledgements to OBHS: photograph taken by Barry Cardno)

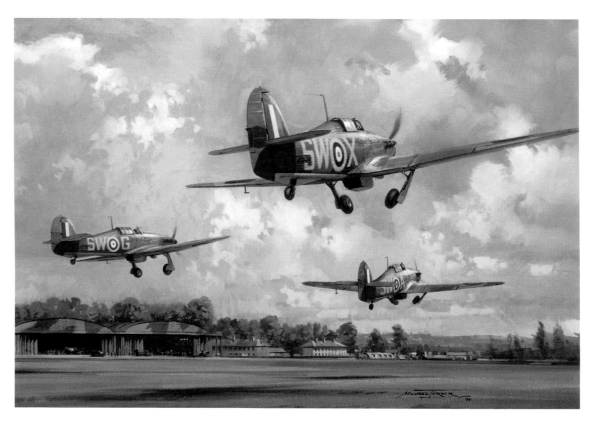

PLATE 20. Hurricanes from Kenley *by Michael Turner. A flight of Hawker Hurricanes from 253 Squadron taking off from RAF Kenley in August 1940, led by Squadron Leader Tom Gleave in SW-A. The other aircraft are piloted by Sergeant SF Cooper in SW-X and Flight Lieutenant GA Brown in SW-G. 253 Squadron took part in the Battle of Britain from the end of August 1940 and remained in southern England until January 1941. Gleave shared command of the squadron with Squadron Leader HM Starr until 31 August, the day he was shot down over Kent in Hurricane SW-K: serial number P3115.* (By kind permission of the artist, Michael Turner, Studio 88, Aylesbury, Buckinghamshire)

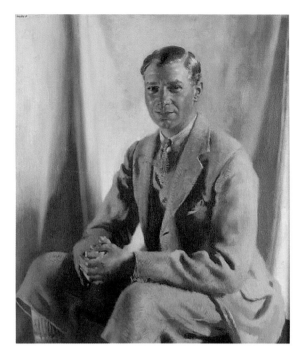

PLATE 21. *Lieutenant Colonel George Philippi by Sir William Orpen, father of Diana 'Dickie' Orpen who recorded the work of Rainsford Mowlem and his colleagues at Hill End Hospital, St Albans (Chapter 10). Portrait painted in 1926 and exhibited at the Royal Academy of Arts, Summer Exhibition 1927. Oil on canvas: 102.5 cm x 87 cm.* (Private collection: image from www.bonhams.com)

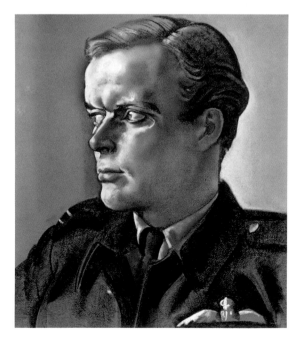

PLATE 22. *Flight Lieutenant Richard Hope Hillary, 1942, pastel portrait by Eric Henri Kennington. The original is in the National Portrait Gallery, London. Kennington (1888–1960) was an official war artist in both world wars.* Drawing the RAF: A book of portraits *is a collection of fifty-two pastel portraits (four in colour) of fighter and bomber pilots plus biographical notes commissioned by the Ministry of Information for the Air Ministry. As Lord Portal observed in the foreword to the book, 'the trouble about a Kennington portrait is that it gives one too much to live up to'.* (Reproduced with permission from the National Portrait Gallery, London, NPG 5167)

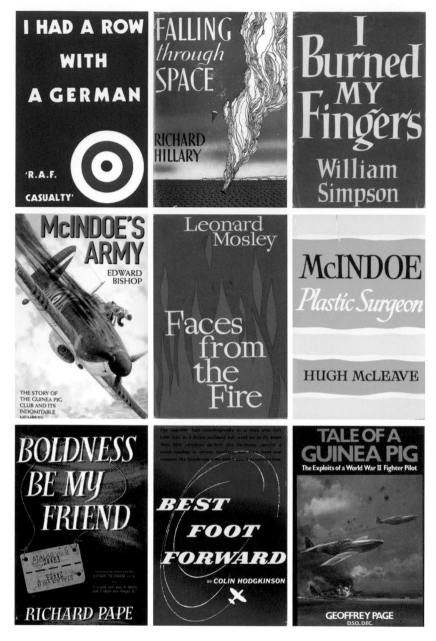

PLATE 23. *Some of the numerous books written about McIndoe, East Grinstead and the Guinea Pig Club, described by McIndoe as the most exclusive in the world.* I Had a Row with a German *by Squadron Leader Tom Gleave appeared in December 1941 under the nom de plume of 'RAF Casualty.'* Falling Through Space *(1942) was the American edition of* The Last Enemy. I Burned My Fingers *(1955) by William Simpson is the final book in a trilogy recounting his experiences after being shot down over Belgium.* McIndoe's Army *(2001) by Edward Bishop is a rewritten version of the* Guinea Pig Club *first published in 1963 – the cover illustration by Barry Weekley depicts Squadron Leader Tom Gleave exiting his burning Hurricane SW-K during the Battle of Britain.* Faces from the Fire *(1962) and* McIndoe: Plastic Surgeon *(1961) are McIndoe biographies.* Boldness Be My Friend *(1953) is the autobiography of Richard Pape.* Best Foot Forward *(1957) is the autobiography of Colin Hodgkinson, the pilot chosen by McIndoe to challenge the 90-day rule.* Tale of a Guinea Pig *(1981) is the autobiography of Geoffrey Page – the cover illustration is from a painting by Frank Wootton of Page and Squadron Leader James MacLachlan attacking an airfield in two P-51 Mustangs during their famous 'Rhubarb' on the 29th of June 1943.*

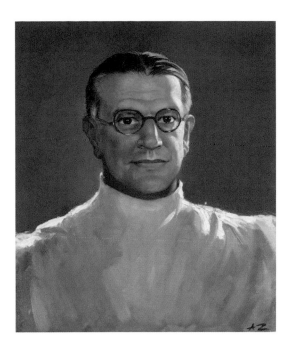

PLATE 24. *Sir Archibald Hector McIndoe (he was knighted in 1947). Portrait by Anna Katrina Zinkeisen (Mrs Heseltine), oil on canvas, painted ca 1944.* (By kind permission of the National Portrait Gallery, London, NPG 5927)

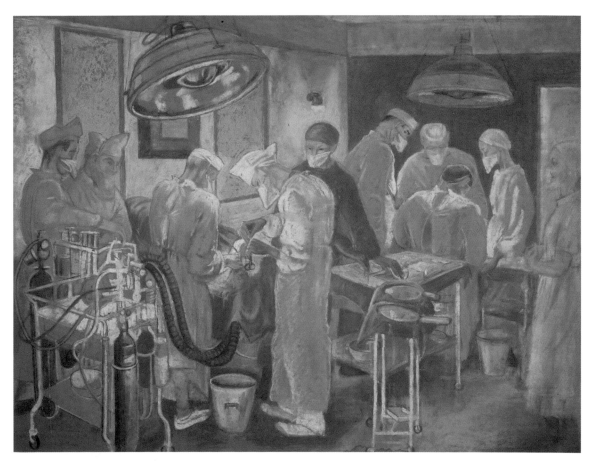

PLATE 25. The operating theatre, Hill End Hospital, St Albans. *Pastel by Diana Orpen, 1945. The surgeon at the head of the operating table in the middle foreground is Rainsford Mowlem; seated in the background is John Barron.* (Courtesy of the Antony Wallace Archive, BAPRAS)

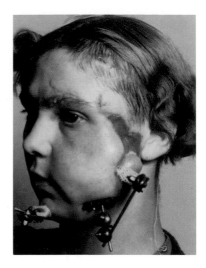
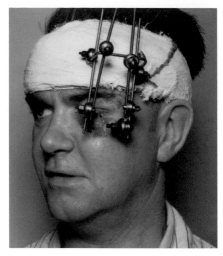

PLATE 26. LEFT: *Case treated by Major DO Brown (David Officer Brown) of the Australian Army Medical Corps and Mr FA Walker. Mandible fractured in three places following a bomb blast during the Blitz; three fragments were pinned (anterior displacement of the condyle was ignored) on 25 June 1941 within 24 hours of the injury. The patient was taking semi-solids within two days and the pins were removed after 4 weeks. Plastic surgery was then performed. Photograph taken 22 days after the operation on 18 July 1941 and used by Gillies to illustrate his 1941* British Dental Journal *article; it was later included in* The Principles and Art of Plastic Surgery.*
RIGHT: *Cranio-maxillary fixation designed to support a depressed fracture of the cheek. The photograph is not dated, but must have been early in the war as the method was later abandoned because of the thinness of the malar (cheek) bone. Both photographs were taken by Percy Hennell of the Metal Box Company.* (Courtesy of the Gillies Archives, Frognal Centre, Queen Mary's Hospital, Sidcup)

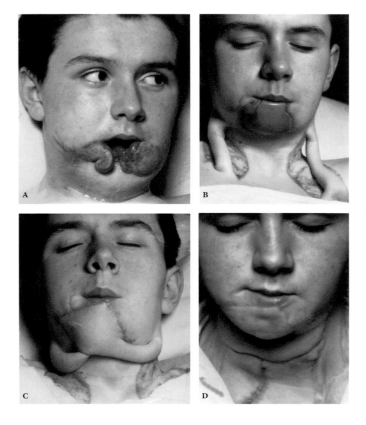

PLATE 27. (A) *Merchant seaman Campbell on admission.*
(B) *Vulcanite prosthesis to maintain and measure the defect and stop saliva dribbling out of his mouth, plus tubed pedicles raised from the neck.* (C) *Double pedicle, two-layered cross-over repair; one pedicle with the skin surface facing inwards to provide the new lip with an epithelial lining, and the other to restore the surface defect.*
(D) *Pedicles divided and returned to the neck. Photographs taken by Percy Hennell of the Metal Box Company.* (Courtesy of the Gillies Archives, Frognal Centre, Queen Mary's Hospital, Sidcup)

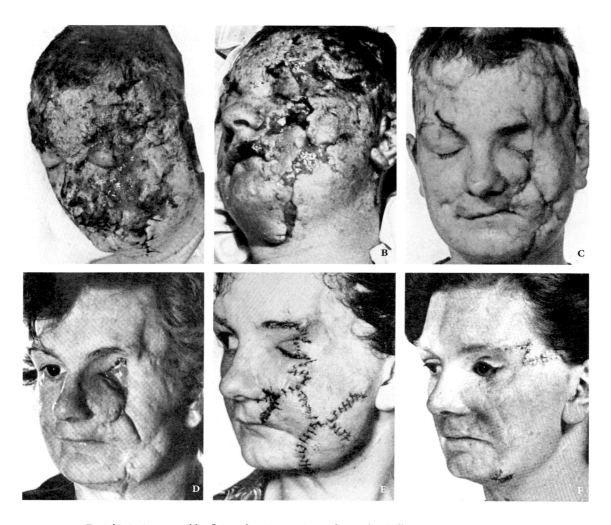

FIGURE 10.2. *Facial injuries caused by flying glass in a patient admitted to Hill End.* (A) *The major pieces of glass have been removed, but the face was a mass of minute fragments responsible for much tissue breakdown as she progressed through stages* B–D. (E) *Shows the early stages of secondary repair; because of the numerous fragments of glass, 11 surgical knives were required.*
(F) *Not the completed stage, but getting close. The series of operations performed by Mowlem in carrying out the secondary repair in this patient can be viewed in Part 1 of* Techniques in Plastic Surgery *on the DVD inside the back cover.* (Photographs from History of the Second World War: Surgery (1953), edited by Sir Zachary Cope)

This difference of opinion still had some mileage several years later. During the annual meeting of the British Dental Association at the University of Reading in August 1941, a number of papers were presented at a symposium entitled *Methods of Fixation* by representatives of the various EMS maxillofacial units in the southeast of England. The aim was to enable dental practitioners to learn at first hand about the work of the 'Jaw Centres' and the latest methods that had evolved from recent wartime experience for treating maxillofacial injuries.[6–10]

Alan McLeod and Rae Shepherd, two of the dental surgeons at East Grinstead, discussed the use of cap splints for fixing mandibular fractures in the tooth-bearing area.[7] However, cap splints cast in silver–copper alloy required skilled technical help and dental laboratory facilities, and could be rather bulky and unhygienic (Figure 10.3). (Anyone who has served time as a dental house surgeon will remember the joys of cementing cap splints to teeth with black copper cement, and the even more joyous task of cleaning up the mouth after their removal.) Wiring the jaws together for the immediate fixation of fractures of the mandible had the advantage of simplicity, but joints are designed to move, and any method which immobilised the jaws for periods of several weeks could lead to joint adhesions and reduced mobility.[8] Furthermore, both of these methods required the presence of sound teeth, and where the fracture involved the mandible behind the last molar tooth, neither method was able to prevent displacement of the posterior fragment by contraction of the powerful masseter and temporal muscles that closed the lower jaw.

To avoid this complication, Mowlem and his colleagues had adapted the technique of external pin fixation to immobilise jaw fractures. Pairs of crossed Kirschner pins – originally described by Roger Anderson to treat fractures of the radius and ulna[11] – were inserted into the mandible in the form of an X: their external ends were locked together using a variety of designs to keep the fragments in position.[9,12,13] This had the advantage of eliminating the need to fix the mandible to the maxilla, thereby allowing the temporomandibular

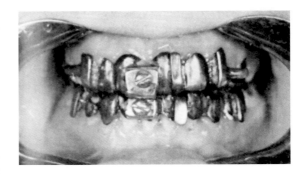

FIGURE 10.3. *Upper and lower cast cap splints cemented to the teeth to immobilise the jaws; the precision screw connecting bar provides for rigid fixation. Cast splints were made from silver–copper alloy containing a high proportion of silver.* (From History of the Second World War: Surgery (1953), edited by Sir Zachary Cope)

joints to function normally. Pin fixation could also be used to immobilise the recalcitrant posterior fragment (Figure 10.4), and the mandible in patients without teeth. By the end of 1941 the appliance had been used successfully in 14 patients at Hill End. Mowlem reported that residual facial scars were minimal, the mouth remained clean, and patients were able to eat relatively normal meals soon after reduction of the fracture. The technique was not without problems, however – the pins sometimes loosened, and skill was required in placing them in the correct position.

Gillies' contribution to the symposium was the last of the articles published in the *British Dental Journal*, and reading between the lines it is difficult to avoid the impression there may have been some disagreement as to which unit had first adapted the pin fixation method to the jaws. Gillies, no stranger to disputes over priority, firmly stakes a claim for two surgeons (Converse and Waknitz) in the American Hospital at Basingstoke as the first to adapt the method to stabilise mandibular fractures, adding that it was subsequently taken up by Mowlem and the other maxillofacial centres.[10] Pin fixation, in combination with various designs of headcap, was also used to immobilise fractures of the upper jaw, although these resulted in much more complicated arrangements (Figure 10.5).

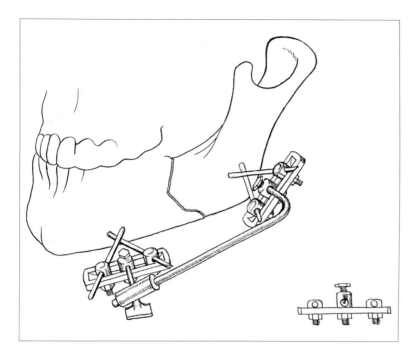

FIGURE 10.4. *Method of external pin fixation used at Hill End Hospital to immobilise fractures of the mandible. Each pair of pins was fixed to a single plate and joined by a sliding bar in a tube giving complete universality of movement. Pin fixation was ideally suited for immobilising the edentulous posterior fragment and at the same time allowing for jaw movement.* (Drawing by Diana Orpen, Antony Wallace Archive, BAPRAS)

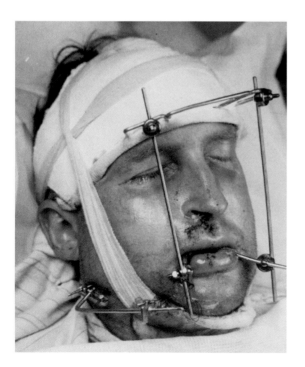

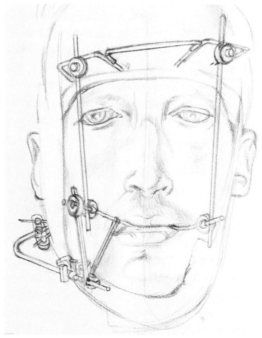

FIGURE 10.5. *Box-frame with two attachment bars fixed to a plaster head cap designed to provide support for the upper and lower jaws. In this example, the system of universal joints enables the frame to support the fractured mobile maxilla as well as the external pin fixation device inserted into the right side of the mandible.* (Photograph taken by Percy Hennell of the Metal Box Company; drawing by Diana Orpen, Antony Wallace Archive, Reference number BAPRAS/DSB 1/24)

It is also interesting to note that the arguments for and against the extraction of teeth in the fracture line or adjacent to it, debated at some length during the First World War by Valadier and Colyer (see Chapter 3), were still being waged fiercely. MacGregor, in a paper entitled 'Sepsis in relation to fractures of the mandible' – no doubt representing the view of Hill End – agreed with the general consensus that the extraction of a tooth in the fracture line was advisable, but pointed out among other things that it depended upon whether the tooth was loose or embedded firmly in the bone.[14] Furthermore, there had been a tendency in some units to remove two or three teeth on each side of the fracture line, in the belief this might be beneficial, but the movement involved in such a procedure may do more harm by pumping bacteria into the fracture area and collecting debris in the socket.

Fickling is likely to have been influential in Hill End adopting a more conservative approach – after all, he had recently completed a review with Warwick James of some of the cases treated at the 3rd London General Hospital, Wandsworth, during the previous war, which they had published in *Injuries of the Jaws and Face* (1940).[15] From their analysis of the surviving records, they had concluded that the extraction of teeth should be avoided as far as possible in the earlier stages of treatment. Warwick James and Fickling were also against extracting teeth on either side of a fracture: they were of the opinion that delayed union and non-union of a fracture were often associated with extractions, while numerous cases had demonstrated that union occurred in the presence of teeth and roots. More importantly, they had the radiographic and follow-up evidence to prove it.

Martin Rushton, who was clearly influenced by the dictum of Sir Frank Colyer regarding extractions, took a much more radical position. He pointed out that the policy at Rooksdown House was not only to extract any teeth in the line of fracture, but also, in severely infected cases, to open up the fracture site and explore it for separated pieces of bone and debris of all kinds. A drain was then passed down through the buccal sulcus and out through the skin, and this was left for a week. Rushton did add that such drastic methods were not used where there was little displacement and no comminution (fragmentation) of bone.

It would seem that Rushton and his colleagues at Rooksdown had either forgotten or chosen to ignore the advice of the Army Advisory Standing Committee's report on maxillofacial injuries.[5] The committee had expressed the view that, with jaw fractures, the dental officer should be most conservative in his outlook regarding extractions, bearing in mind the future treatment of the case and the importance of teeth in retaining dentures. On the controversial question of the extraction or retention of teeth on either side of the lines of fracture, the committee considered that, unless a tooth has actually been involved in the line of fracture, it should not usually be disturbed. The committee also added that given its recuperative powers, partly detached fragments of bone should, as a rule, be retained (p. 12). By the end of the war the availability of penicillin rendered much of this argument redundant, but the divergence of opinion expressed by the audience during the subsequent discussion was sufficient to convince one of the merits of evidence-based practice.

The grafting and regeneration of bone

Mowlem's most important contribution to reconstructive surgery was arguably in the field of bone grafting – work for which he was elected to a Hunterian Professorship by the Royal College of Surgeons of England in 1940: his Hunterian lecture on the use and behaviour of cartilage and bone transplants was published the following year in the *British Journal of Surgery*.[16] Bone has a unique capacity to renew itself – a property that allows it to be grafted with a high success rate, irrespective of whether the bone is autogenous or from another human donor. During the late nineteenth and early twentieth centuries one of the questions that exercised the minds of surgeons was whether the cells of transplanted bone survived and to what extent they contributed to new bone formation.

Sir William Macewen (1848–1924), Regius Professor of Surgery at the University of Glasgow, had conducted a series of experiments on dogs and concluded that small pieces of transplanted bone retained their vitality and that new bone originated from osteogenic cells contained within the grafted tissue.[17,18] Other investigators, however, suggested that most bone grafts were resorbed and gradually replaced by osteoblasts migrating from the surrounding bone – a process called creeping substitution. In other words, the graft functioned primarily as an osteoconductive substrate or scaffolding to support the ingrowth of osteogenic cells. This concept had become the established dogma.

Bone grafts of the jaws

Gunshot and shrapnel wounds of the face were often complicated by compound fractures of the jaws, involving the fragmentation and/or loss of bone. Nevertheless, the development of surgical techniques to replace lost bone, or to treat fractures of the mandible that had not united properly, was slow to evolve. At the beginning of the First World War, the success of a bone graft was regarded as being dependent on accurate carpentry and the precision techniques developed by Fred Albee[19] and EW Hey Groves,[20] and early operative technique largely followed their example. This was the procedure followed by Lindemann in the first large published series of mandibular bone grafts that appeared in 1916 (see Chapter 3). In all 97 cases the mandible was exposed via an external incision to minimise infection, and the defect was grafted with a piece of bone with periosteum attached, usually from the tibia.[21] No direct methods to secure exact reapposition of the graft to the bone ends were used – the ends of the graft were usually inserted or mortised into grooves cut in the bone ends, which was not only difficult, but also often unsuccessful.[22]

It was not until after the move to Sidcup that direct methods of fixation were used by British surgeons. This is surprising when one considers that the wiring and plating of fractures to secure the exact reapposition of the broken ends by osteosynthesis had been pioneered by none other than Sir William Arbuthnot Lane, who had even written a book on the subject: *The Operative*

Treatment of Fractures.[23–25] Eventually Lane was invited to give a demonstration of the use of wire fixation to secure bone grafts of the mandible, and the problem was solved.[22] The opposition to Lane's wiring and plating of fractures from some quarters was intense, however; the practice was widely condemned, with a president of the Royal College of Surgeons of England reputedly going so far as to say that any man who converted a simple fracture into a compound one was guilty of malpractice, and should be brought before the GMC.[26]

With improvements in understanding the biology of bone that had been published by Gallie and Robertson, showing that the more cancellous bone contained in a graft the more rapid the repair,[27] in 1918 Waldron and Risdon in the Canadian Section at Sidcup abandoned tibial bone grafts and began reconstructing osseous defects of the mandible with bone from the iliac crest.[28] Cortical or compact bone and cancellous bone behave differently when transplanted. Most of the cells in the dense outer cortical bone, particularly those osteoblastic cells enclosed in the bone matrix (osteocytes) will die – as will osteocytes in cancellous bone; however, surface osteoblasts lining the latticework of trabeculae in cancellous bone are capable of survival – a process aided by the associated bone marrow and rapid revascularisation of the graft from the adjacent tissues. In a paper delivered to the Surgery Section at the Royal Society of Medicine in January 1919, Waldron and Risdon reported on 10 cases they had treated successfully in this way. Autogenous bone from the hip of the patient was used in each case, and after trimming back the ends of the fragments by 1–1.5 cm until bleeding healthy bone was reached, the graft was then wired into place. At the same meeting, Gallie recommended splitting a graft into several portions so that a larger number of osteoblasts had a chance of survival.[29] However, the largest series of mandibular bone grafts involving patients at Sidcup was carried out by Gilbert Chubb, an ENT surgeon who joined the British Section at the end of 1918 and who continued to work with Gillies and Kilner for several years after the war. Following on from the work of Waldron and Risdon, all the grafts in

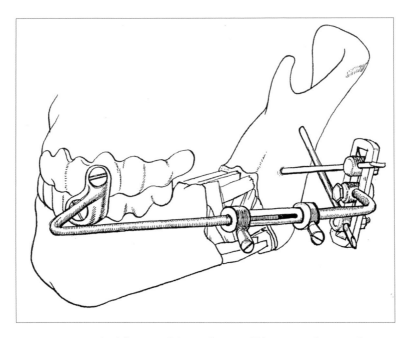

FIGURE 10.6. *Method for immobilising the mandible prior to bone grafting developed at Hill End Hospital using a combination of external pin fixation in the vertical ramus and cap splints cemented to the teeth. A rectangular-shaped supporting 'distance piece' of bone was inserted between the bone ends at the lower border of the mandible and cancellous bone chips layered on top. The connecting bar could also be used to distract the ends of the mandibular segments as and when necessary.* (Drawing by Diana Orpen, Antony Wallace Archive, BAPRAS)

Chubb's series were composed of autogenous bone taken from the iliac crest, and were wired into direct apposition with the jaw fragments: bony union was reported in 91 out of 100 patients.[30] It is not recorded in either of these series whether any deliberate fragmentation of the transplanted bone was carried out.

Although the principle of cancellous bone chip grafts had originally been used by Sir William Macewan in 1887, Mowlem reintroduced and developed the technique in 1940, filling bony defects with a cellular mass of bone chips from the iliac crest, which survived and produced the requisite amount of new bone within a matter of weeks.[31] As described in his 1963 Gillies Memorial Lecture, this was discovered inadvertently during the insertion of a mandibular bone graft when he was unfortunate enough to break it into three pieces.

With much reluctance these were tied together with catgut and inserted, and greatly to his surprise, the union was at least as rapid as it would have been had the graft been in one piece. This did not make sense if new bone had to invade the length of the graft from the cut mandibular ends and cross two fracture lines.[32] However, since fragmented bone grafts took no part in the provision of stability, it was necessary to devise alternative methods of fixation, and the technique of external pin fixation previously developed for fractures of the mandible was modified accordingly (Figure 10.6).

Bone from the iliac crest was deliberately fragmented to increase the exposed surface area, and in practice it was found that cancellous bone chips (1 x 0.5 x 0.2 cm) had two advantages over cortical bone grafts. First, small bone implants were rapidly vascularised which helped preserve the vitality of the tissues, and the greater the number of ossifying centres the more rapid the healing; second, they seemed to be more resistant to infection.[31] The bone marrow in cancellous bone is a rich source of osteoblast precursor cells, and an additional factor, not known until the 1960s, was that bone matrix contains bone morphogenetic proteins (BMPs) and other osteogenic growth factors.[33] These are released from the bone matrix by osteoclastic action and promote the proliferation and differentiation of mesenchymal stem cells into osteoblasts – a process referred to as osteoinduction. New bone from both these sources will be deposited on and eventually replace the old bone through the ongoing process of bone remodelling.

It is also clear from his Gillies Memorial Lecture that Mowlem understood the importance of exposing bone grafts to mechanical loading if their structural integrity was to be preserved – a bone deprived of mechanical stimuli slowly undergoes resorption and melts away. However, it would seem from his experience with bone onlays that he learned this lesson the hard way. It is worth noting that in 1919 Sir Arthur Keith had written in his celebrated historical critique of orthopaedic surgery, *Menders of the Maimed*, that a graft must be placed in contact with adjacent bony segments and should be exposed to mechanical stresses and strains if it was not to eventually disappear.[23] Perhaps Staige Davis was right when he claimed that surgeons did not know the literature (see Chapter 5).

Penicillin

At the end of the First World War, Alexander Fleming (1881–1955) returned to St Mary's Hospital and continued his work on the bacteriology of septic wounds begun at No 13 General Hospital in Boulogne (See Chapter 4). Having shown that antiseptics did more harm to the body's defences than they did to kill bacteria, he began searching for naturally occurring antibacterial agents. In 1921 he found the antibacterial enzyme lysozyme, first in his own nasal mucus and subsequently in tears. But his annus mirabilis was 1928, with his serendipitous discovery of the ability of the common mould

Penicillium notatum to inhibit bacterial growth in a Petri dish seeded with a culture of *Staphylococcus aureus*.[34] Fleming noted its therapeutic potential, but it was not until 1936, and the award of a grant of the princely sum of £250 from the American Rockefeller Foundation, that Howard Florey, Ernst Chain (a refugee from Hitler's Germany), Norman Heatley and their co-workers at the Dunn School of Pathology in Oxford began the research that eventually demonstrated the extraordinary power of penicillin to kill certain bacteria.[35,36]

Unable to interest the British pharmaceutical industry in penicillin production, and unable to produce sufficient quantities for clinical trials under wartime conditions with a minuscule budget and makeshift equipment (Heatley was growing penicillin in bedpans), in July 1941 Florey and Heatley travelled to the United States with a sample of *P. notatum* to try to persuade American drug companies to become involved. Eventually they were directed to the US Department of Agriculture's Northern Regional Research Laboratory (NRRL) in Peoria, Illinois, where Andrew Moyer, a government scientist, worked with Heatley to develop methods for mass production. Moyer's anti-British (isolationist) attitude, not unusual in the US at the time, plus his unwillingness to share details of his work, did not make for an easy collaboration. The secret eventually turned out to be corn steep liquor (a by-product of the starch industry) plus deep-vat fermentation, which led to a thirty-fold increase in penicillin production.[37] (The best source of *P. notatum* turned out to be a strain cultured from a mouldy cantaloupe picked up in a Peoria fruit market.) By 1942 penicillin was a hot topic. The large chemical corporations, Pfizer, Squibb and Merck, realised its financial potential, and for the last two years of the war commercial production of penicillin provided enough to save the Allied forces from sepsis and gangrene. During the First World War, wound infection claimed the lives of 15 percent of all injured soldiers; by the end of the Second World War this had fallen to less than 3 percent.

For their seminal discoveries, in 1945 Fleming, Florey and Chain shared the Nobel Prize for physiology or medicine. It is ironic, considering the role the Oxford team played in transforming an interesting laboratory observation into the first antibiotic (Fleming never extracted any penicillin or conducted clinical trials), that while Fleming became an international celebrity, Florey, Chain and Heatley remain virtually unknown outside the scientific community. To be fair, this was not due to self-publicity on the part of Fleming, who was modest about the part he had played in the story and gave full credit to the Oxford team.[38] Moreover, unusually for an Australian, Howard Florey happened to be a quiet man who hated publicity, avoided public attention and neglected to write his memoirs. When the benefits of penicillin came to the attention of the public, it has been suggested that Sir Almroth Wright and Lord Moran (former Dean of the Medical School and Churchill's personal physician) made sure it was Fleming and St Mary's that received the credit, not the Oxford team.[39] Whether this is true or not, Moran certainly understood the value of publicity for raising large financial donations and recruiting the most promising students to St Mary's, particularly from Wales for the hospital's rugby teams (as a student Moran had captained the St Mary's Hospital 1st XV and also played for Middlesex). By the 1920s and 1930s he had converted what had become a decrepit educational institution into one of the finest medical schools in the country, and he aimed to keep it that way.[40] In his personal memoir, Moran has left some interesting observations about Fleming's career and character (p. 489):

Alexander Fleming had lived in obscurity and some disfavour. His research into the acne bacillus and the Wassermann reaction had been generally discredited. He seemed to his profession to be disgruntled by criticism and by neglect; a sour, rather dour Scot. And then on the verge of old age, he discovered penicillin. He, too, had found a place in the sun, so that it was no longer necessary to stake a claim aggressively. For he knew now that his name had a place in history. Fleming seemed to spend the rest of his days travelling over the world, making modest little speeches implying that there had been a great element of luck in his discovery. Famous universities were proud to give him an honorary degree, and everywhere he went he won men's hearts by his happy simplicity.[2]

Another enduring myth of the penicillin story is that Moyer published a paper written jointly with Heatley under his name alone, regardless of a contract which stipulated that any publications should be jointly authored. Despite the claims of several historians, Norman Heatley (1911–2004), the last surviving member of the Oxford team, who was interviewed by Peter Neushul in September 1991, said he had never seen a published version of the paper he and Moyer had worked on. If Moyer did publish this paper it is not included in his CV, nor is it listed as a basis for any of his patent applications.[37] Moyer was in fact a reluctant author, although his name did appear on some of the papers that came out of the work at the NRRL.[41] What is certain, however, is that in 1948 Moyer took out British patents for the method of production (as a government employee he was barred from doing so in the US), which meant that royalties on penicillin manufactured in the United Kingdom had to be repatriated to the United States. While perfectly legal, this did not endear him to the British. It is unclear whether any royalties were ever paid.

Penicillin trials at Hill End

When sufficient but still limited quantities of penicillin became available, responsibility for its distribution in the United Kingdom devolved to the MRC and the Penicillin Clinical Trials Committee that had been established in 1943. The committee allocated supplies to four main centres, one of which was Hill End, where most of the work testing the clinical effectiveness of penicillin was carried out in the special orthopaedic, thoracic and maxillofacial units. The results were published in the *British Medical Journal* in April 1944. One hundred and ninety-eight patients had been treated by the local application of penicillin, and 18 by systemic administration. Most fell into the following groups: skin diseases (75 cases), wounds of the skin and soft tissues (70 cases), breast abscesses (15 cases),

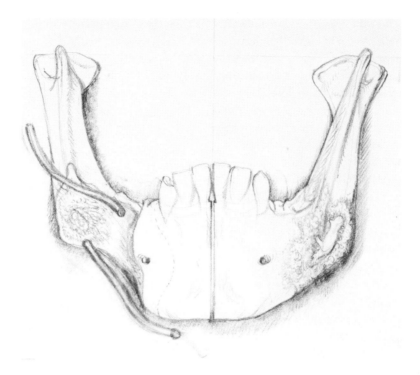

FIGURE 10.7. *Osteomyelitis of the mandible treated by radical surgery in combination with penicillin. The illustration shows the extent of the excision required to eliminate all infected bone with saucerisation of the edges and the position of the penicillin tubes – one running along the upper border of the residual bone and the other along the lower edge. Bacteriological swabs were taken during the operation for penicillin-sensitivity testing – within 18 hours a bacteriological report was available and penicillin administered, the usual dosage being 1000 units injected into each tube every 24 hours.* (The original drawing by Diana Orpen used to illustrate Mowlem's 1944 report in the British Medical Journal. *Reference number BAPRAS/DSB 20/45)*

infections of the mandible (20 cases), and other infections of bone (34 cases).[42]

In his report on the series of 20 cases of mandibular infection treated with a combination of surgery and penicillin, Mowlem divided the cases into two groups.[43] Group I consisted of four postoperative cases in which infection was either anticipated following surgery or had caused an early reaction; two were bone-graft cases and two involved resection of part of the body of the mandible, one being restored by a graft of bone chips. In each case a penicillin tube was inserted along the upper margin of the operative area. In all four cases, immediate bacteriological and clinical control was obtained by injections

of penicillin, followed by satisfactory healing. Group II comprised 16 cases of osteomyelitis of the mandible, a relatively rare condition usually resulting from the extraction of teeth or, in children, from blood-borne infection. In every case the infection had been gross and well established, and penicillin treatment was used in combination with radical surgery (Figure 10.7). The surgery consisted of subperiosteal excision of the lower border of the mandible together with the outer buccal plate of bone and the infected cancellous or spongy bone. This was followed by closure of the soft tissues, which Mowlem felt had three advantages: (1) the soft tissues could be closely approximated to the underlying bone and expected to contribute to vascular ingrowth; (2) the closed cavity not only excluded secondary infection but also retained the penicillin, permitting it to exercise a continuous action; and (3) primary instead of delayed healing was obtained. Bacteriological swabs were taken during the operation for culture and penicillin-sensitivity testing, and two small-bore tubes were inserted through two stab incisions made with a scalpel. Within 18 hours a bacteriological report was available and penicillin treatment was begun: the usual dosage was 1000 units injected into each tube every 24 hours. Immediately before each injection, the cavity was aspirated via the tubes and any fluid was sent for bacteriological investigation and penicillin-inhibition testing. Treatment was continued until the wound was healed – on average about 10 days.

The report by Barron and Mansfield dealt with the local application of penicillin in surgical cases involving the reconstruction of various types of tissue loss where control of infection had always been a problem.[44] Group A included seven cases of Thiersch graft donor sites infected with haemolytic streptococci, staphylococci or both, which were treated with a cream containing 400 units of penicillin in a base composed of equal parts of Lanette wax (sodium lauryl sulfate), paraffin and water. All except one cleared up in 10–14 days, but some relapsed (in closed lesions), and two patients had developed eczema. In Group B, penicillin solution in a concentration of 1000 units/ml was injected into five abscess cavities; two were successful, one was doubtful and two were failures. They concluded that early application was desirable and that penicillin in the presence of necrotic tissue did not have much effect. Group C comprised five patients with acute cellulitis under skin flaps treated by early penicillin solution, and in all cases the infection was halted. In a second series of eleven patients with infected tubed pedicle graft inserts, the results were mixed. Six of the inserts survived, but in five cases loss of tissue necessitated further surgery. Barron and Mansfield concluded that although the infection had been controlled, intravascular thrombosis continued with progressive tissue loss. In the final Group

D, 15 cases of superficial wounds with skin loss were treated with penicillin cream. They reported that while penicillin could sterilise a wound and prevent its reinfection with sensitive organisms, it may be invaded by penicillin-resistant organisms – an early sign, as it was to turn out, of things to come.

Art and surgery at Hill End Hospital

The wartime patient notes of the Plastic and Jaw Unit at Hill End (the name was changed from Maxillofacial Unit in 1943) have been destroyed. Fortunately, two unique records of the surgery performed at the hospital still exist. The first record comprises more than 2500 pencil and pen drawings

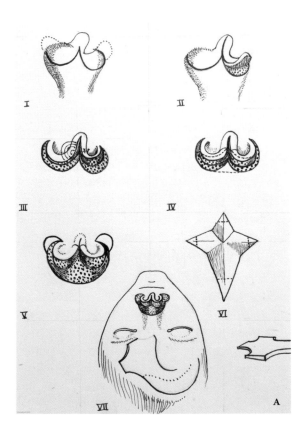

by Diana 'Dickie' Orpen[†], faithfully recording in great detail the surgery carried out by Mowlem and the other members of his surgical team (Figures 10.8–10). These are held in the Antony Wallace Archive of the British Association of Plastic, Reconstructive and Aesthetic Surgeons (BAPRAS) at the Royal College of Surgeons of England, and may be viewed online at www.bapras.org.uk.

Diana 'Dickie' Orpen was the youngest of three daughters of the Irish portrait painter Sir William Orpen (1878–1931), who had studied at the Slade School of Art under Henry Tonks. His view of art was as serious as Tonks' – he forbade his children to paint or draw – and Orpen grew up under the dictum 'one damn good painter in the family and

no bloody amateurs'. Quite by chance her father found some drawings she had brought back from boarding school and sent them around to Tonks, whose response was, 'Send her to the Slade on Monday.' She was 15 years old.[45] Knowing of Tonks' association with Aldershot and Sidcup in the previous war, in 1942 Orpen wrote to Gillies asking if she could assist in any way with her drawing. The letter was passed on to Mowlem, and from 1942 to 1945 she was the artist attached to the Plastic and Jaw Unit at Hill End. In addition to a large number of loose drawings, the Orpen collection comprises 36 Windsor and Newton sketchbooks of drawings made in the operating theatre, each with the name of the patient, the surgeon's initials and the date of

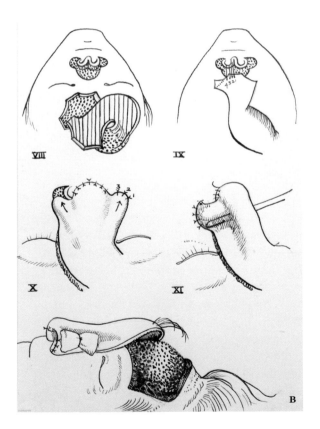

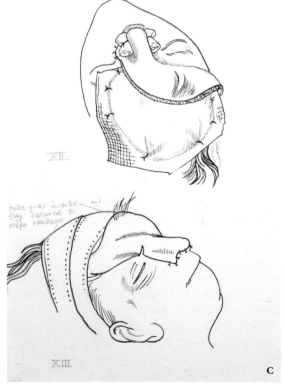

FIGURE 10.8. *Rhinoplasty: Sequence of events involved in reconstructing the tip of the nose with a rotational forehead flap. A similar operation being performed by Mowlem can be viewed in Part 3 of the instructional film* Techniques in Plastic Surgery, *on the DVD inside the back cover. (Drawings by Diana Orpen, Antony Wallace Archive, Reference number BAPRAS/D891–D893)*

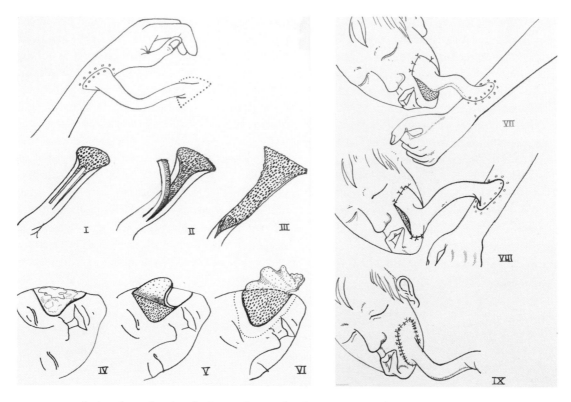

FIGURE 10.9. *Series of pen drawings by Diana Orpen, dated 15 June 1942, showing a full-thickness tubed pedicle graft previously raised from the skin of the left forearm, being transferred from the wrist to the left side of the face to reconstruct the soft tissues of the chin.* (Antony Wallace Archive, Reference number BAPRAS/D200; D201)

the operation, annotated with explanations of the procedures carried out.

The second record of the surgery at Hill End consists of a series of four 16-mm cinematographic instructional films, *Techniques in Plastic Surgery*, produced in 1945 by the J Arthur Rank Organisation Ltd for the British Council, showing Mowlem performing a variety of plastic operations. Originally made for trainee surgeons to show how various plastic operations are performed, the films are accompanied by a commentary describing in some detail the sequence of steps involved in each procedure – demonstrating the power of visual media as a form of instruction. When the Plastic Unit moved from Mount Vernon Hospital, they

were saved from the skip by Brian Morgan, and are reproduced courtesy of the Antony Wallace Archive on the DVD inside the back cover of this book. The films are entitled as follows: Part 1: 'Primary repair and secondary suture' – the latter illustrating the revision of scar tissue from a previous attempt at repair. Part 2: 'Full thickness grafts' includes examples of cosmetic grafting, grafting for function and a combination of both. Part 3: 'Local flaps' describes Z-plasty and a variety of rotational flaps including a reconstruction rhinoplasty by means of a forehead flap. Part 4: 'Direct flaps' – illustrates cross-leg and abdomen-to-arm flaps. However, be warned – they are not for the squeamish, or those disturbed by the sight of blood.

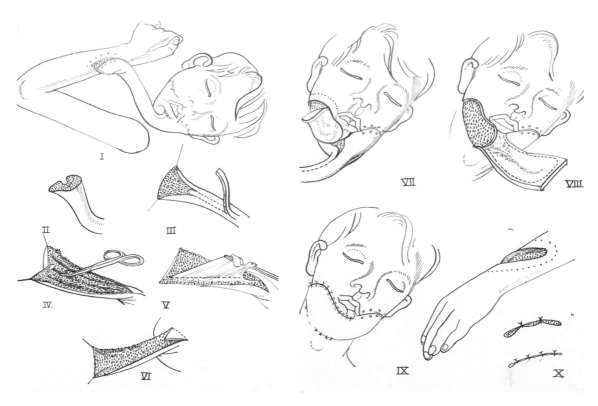

FIGURE 10.10. LEFT: *Pen drawing by Diana Orpen, dated 30 July 1942, six weeks later – the end of the pedicle sutured to the face has successfully taken.* RIGHT: *Drawings dated 8 October 1942. The pedicle is divided and used to reconstruct the chin. Any osseous defect in the mandible can now be made good with a bone graft.* (Antony Wallace Archive, Reference number BAPRAS/D202; D204)

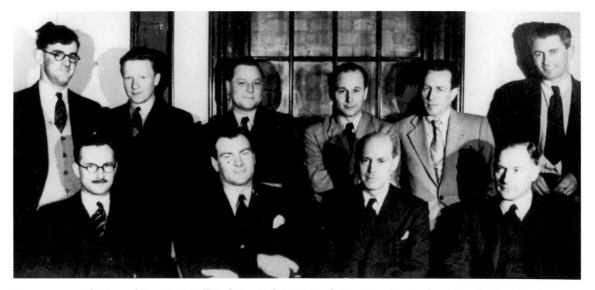

FIGURE 10.11. *Plastic and Jaw Unit, Hill End Hospital, 1951. Back Row: Gordon Fordyce, Charles Dundas, Louis Rouillard (South Africa), M Derganc, Klementek (both from Yugoslavia), RLG Dawson. Front Row: Stewart Harrison, Alex McGregor, Rainsford Mowlem, Benjamin Fickling.* (Courtesy of the Antony Wallace Archive, BAPRAS)

Chapter 11

Gillies chooses Rooksdown House

Written in collaboration with Andrew N Bamji

Rooksdown House was the last of the plastic and jaw units to be established in the southeast of England. One Sunday in September 1939, several days after war had been declared, Gillies and Kelsey Fry motored down from London to take a look at a mental institution near Basingstoke in Hampshire, the Park Prewett Hospital – so-called because it was situated on 300 acres that had originally formed part of the Park Prewett farm. Construction of Park Prewett had begun in 1912, but progress was slow and during the First World War it had been requisitioned for use as a military hospital, No 4 Canadian General. After the war it was converted back to its original purpose as a psychiatric hospital, and the first patients were admitted in 1921. A week before the outbreak of the Second World War, all but 80 of the patients had been evacuated and the hospital taken over by the EMS to provide 2000 beds for civilian and service casualties.

Looking around the grounds, Gillies noticed a building set off by itself. Rooksdown House had opened in 1930 as the private wing. Unlike the rest of the hospital it was comfortably furnished with reading rooms, private suites and a billiard room; at the time it was being used as temporary quarters for nurses from St Mary's and Westminster Hospitals who had been evacuated from London. Gillies

and Kelsey Fry went up to have a look and as they entered one of the rooms a young nurse looked up and was heard to sigh, 'Ye gods – a man at last!' Gillies, never one to be lost for words, turned to Kelsey Fry and remarked, 'Obviously this is the place for us.' They recommended that Rooksdown be taken over by the Ministry of Health as an EMS plastic and jaw unit.[1]

Rooksdown House was rapidly converted into a 200-bed maxillofacial unit, complete with open fireplaces and decorative mantelpieces in all the rooms. The largest was converted into the main operating theatre and the wings into wards. Scrubbing was carried out with all due care and attention, but the operating theatre had dust-laden cornices, the plaster ceiling of a prewar drawing room, and opened more or less directly onto a busy corridor. In spite of the lack of sterility, wound infection seemed to be no more of a problem at Rooksdown than anywhere else.[2] As Gillies was consultant–adviser to the Ministry of Health and was busy organising the new plastic units in Birmingham, Liverpool, Manchester and Leeds, in his absence the unit was opened by the orthopaedic surgeon James Cuthbert, with Martin Rushton[†] as dental surgeon and Patrick Shackleton as physician–anaesthetist.

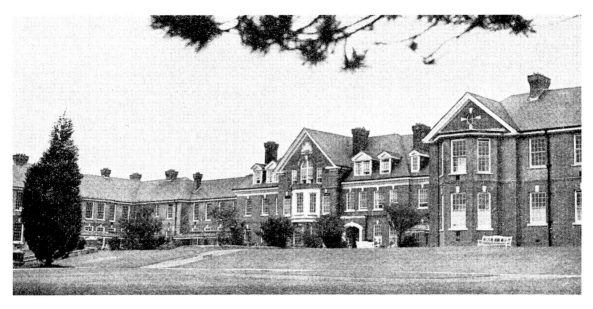

FIGURE 11.1. *Rooksdown House, the private wing of the Park Prewett Hospital, Basingstoke, Hampshire. The Plastic and Jaw Unit opened in February 1940 and remained in use until 1957 when it was moved to Queen Mary's Hospital, Roehampton. After the war the main hospital returned to its original purpose as a psychiatric hospital for the second time, but 'care in the community' rendered it obsolete and it was finally closed in 1997.* (Photograph courtesy of the Gillies Archives, Frognal Centre, Queen Mary's Hospital, Sidcup)

The evacuation of Dunkirk

At first there were few patients. By the end of the 'Phoney War' in April 1940 only 11 beds were occupied. The numbers increased, however, following the Battle of Dunkirk. In the nine days from 26 May 1940, under the code name Operation Dynamo, 338,226 men were evacuated from the beaches of Dunkirk (including 139,997 French, Polish, Belgian and Dutch troops) aboard an armada of more than 800 warships, merchantmen and small pleasure-boats, of which 243 were sunk.[3] This was followed two weeks later by Operation Aerial: between 15 and 25 June 1940 the Royal Navy evacuated the three remaining divisions of the BEF, plus Allied troops and civilians, from the northwestern ports of Le Havre, Cherbourg, St Malo, Brest, St Nazaire and La Pallice – a total of 191,870 fighting men (144,171 British, 18,246 French, 24,352 Polish, 4938 Czechs and 163 Belgians) were successfully rescued.[4] In the circumstances, it is therefore scarcely believable

that after the fall of France and the signing of an armistice on 22 June 1940 between Maréchal Pétain and Hitler in the Forest of Compiègne, of the more than 100,000 French troops evacuated from Dunkirk and other ports, fewer than 10,000 joined General de Gaulle's Free French Forces to continue the fight against the Germans – the rest elected to return home to France, and Britain ended up fighting Vichy French forces in North Africa, the Middle East and Madagascar.[5]

The largest loss of life during the entire evacuation operation occurred on 17 June with the sinking of the troopship RMS *Lancastria* off Saint-Nazaire by four Junkers Ju 88 bombers. Three direct hits – including one bomb which penetrated the funnel and exploded deep inside the hull – caused the ship to roll over, and it sank within 20 minutes. Over 1400 tons of fuel oil leaked into the sea, which was set partially ablaze, and many of the survivors who had leapt overboard were drowned or severely burned. The official death toll was 1738, but since

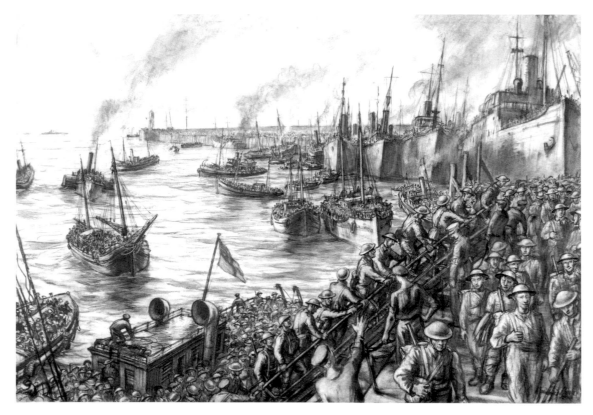

FIGURE 11.2. *The Return from Dunkirk: Arrival at Dover* by Sir Muirhead Bone, 1940. Charcoal, chalk wash on paper, showing the disembarkation of troops evacuated from Dunkirk by ships moored in Dover Harbour. Bone (1876–1953) was appointed Britain's first official war artist in May 1916 and arrived in France during the Battle of the Somme. (IWM ART LD 251. By kind permission of the Imperial War Museum)

no one knew how many people were on board, the number is thought to have been much higher. It was Britain's greatest maritime disaster; Churchill banned all news coverage of the catastrophe. In the aftermath of these demoralising events, the wards at Rooksdown soon filled with marine, navy and army casualties, plus the occasional airman who had parachuted into the Channel – aerial combat over the sea was particularly dangerous, because ditched air crew were unable to survive more than a few hours in the icy and treacherous waters of the Channel, and the RAF had yet to develop an efficient air–sea rescue service.

An additional worry for Gillies at the time was that his eldest son John, a fighter pilot with 92 Squadron, had been reported missing presumed dead. On the evening of 23 May 1940 the squadron

had set off from RAF Hornchurch on an evening patrol over Dunkirk when they encountered a formation of Heinkel He 111s, heavily protected by Messerschmitt Bf 109s and Bf 110 Zerstörers. Squadron Leader Roger Bushell, a South African-born barrister, ordered an attack and plunged into the bomber force with John Gillies and Paul Klipsch. All three were shot down – Klipsch was killed; Bushell and Gillies were captured. (It was three weeks before the Gillies family was notified he had survived and was a prisoner of the Germans.) Bushell was one of the masterminds behind the 'Great Escape' from Stalag Luft III on the night of 24–25 March 1944, and one of the 50 escapees summarily executed by the Gestapo on the orders of Hitler after being recaptured.[6] (The character named Roger Bartlett, played by Richard

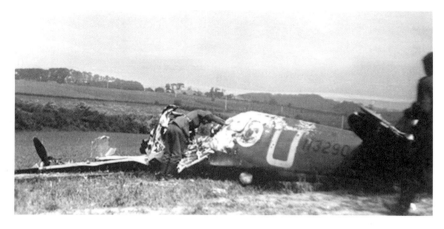

FIGURE 11.3. *The Supermarine Spitfire Mk I of 92 (East India) Squadron (GR-U, serial number N3290), piloted by Flying Officer John Gillies, lies burnt out in a French field after being shot down by a Messerschmitt Bf 110 in combat over Dunkirk on the evening of 23 May 1940. The identification code for 92 Squadron was changed from GR to QJ at the end of May 1940.* (Photograph kindly provided by Kelvin Youngs and Aircrew Remembered: www.aircrewremembered.com)

Attenborough in the film *The Great Escape*, was modelled on Bushell.) John Gillies remained a POW until the end of the war.[7]

The Battle of Britain

The scene was now set for the next big test. As Winston Churchill declared in a speech to the House of Commons on 18 June, shortly after taking over as Prime Minister: 'What General Weygand has called the Battle of France is over, I expect that the Battle of Britain is about to begin.'[8] The objective of Unternehmen Adler (Operation Eagle), the code name for the air campaign waged by Reichsmarschall Göring and the Luftwaffe during the summer and autumn of 1940, was to gain air superiority over the RAF and enable Hitler to launch an amphibious and airborne invasion of Britain.

The initial phase, known as the *Kanalkampf* (Channel battle), lasted from 10 July until early August. This involved running battles over the English Channel between the Hurricanes and Spitfires of RAF Fighter Command and the Luftwaffe, which was undertaking photo reconnaissance missions and the bombing of coastal shipping, radar stations and the Channel ports. On 16 July 1940, having grown impatient with Churchill's rejection of his peace overtures, Hitler issued Führer Directive 16, Unternehmen Seelöwe (Operation Sea Lion), setting in motion preparations for the invasion of England. This was followed on 1 August by Führer Directive 17, Unternehmen Adlerangriff (Operation Eagle Attack), for the all-out attack on Britain to destroy the RAF. However, the attack was delayed by bad weather and the first main battle phase was not officially launched until 13 August – Adlertag (Eagle Day) – when the Luftwaffe began a series of concentrated aerial attacks on RAF airfields and infrastructure, aircraft factories and industrial centres throughout the British Isles. Göring thought it would take four days to cripple the RAF.

On Saturday 7 September in the afternoon there was a change of tactics (code-named Unternehmen Loge, after the Norse God of Fire), when 364 bombers escorted by 515 fighters switched the attack to London in an attempt to demoralise the civilian population. The offensive developed into a terror bombing campaign, targeting London and other major cities across the country – the

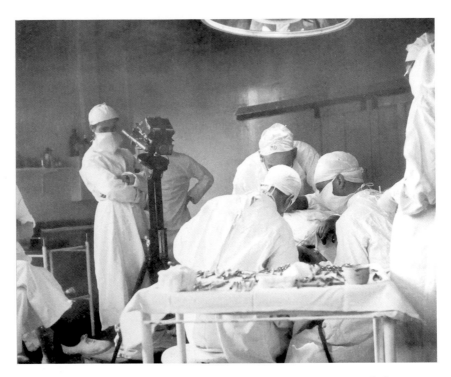

FIGURE 11.4. *Gillies (standing) with two other surgeons operating at Rooksdown House. To the left is Percy Hennell waiting to take photographs.* (Courtesy of the Gillies Archives, Frognal Centre, Queen Mary's Hospital, Sidcup)

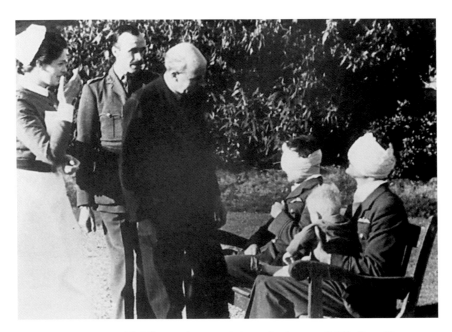

FIGURE 11.5. *Sir Harold Gillies on his rounds interviewing two RAF pilot officers with severe head wounds at Rooksdown House in 1941 – not all RAF casualties were treated at East Grinstead.* (Courtesy of the Gillies Archives, Frognal Centre, Queen Mary's Hospital, Sidcup)

'Blitzkrieg' had arrived, heralding the second main battle phase and 57 consecutive nights of bombing. The climax occurred on 15 September when the Luftwaffe made its largest daylight attack on London and was repulsed, suffering its greatest losses (56 aircraft lost, with 136 air crew killed or captured), although at the time the numbers were greatly exaggerated. The RAF lost 29 aircraft, with 12 pilots killed. By 17 September, realising the RAF could not be defeated, Hitler postponed Operation Seelöwe indefinitely and the imminent threat of an invasion was over. The Führer could now focus his attention on Eastern Europe: on 18 December he issued Führer Directive 21, Unternehmen Barbarossa, the invasion of the Soviet Union that began on 22 June 1941 – the largest military operation in human history. Although the Blitz continued until May 1941, when the Luftwaffe spearheaded the attack on Russia, the official British dates for the Battle of Britain are from 10 July to 31 October 1940, and the 15th of September is commemorated each year as Battle of Britain Day.[9]

The RAF had several specialist centres of its own for the treatment of maxillofacial injuries and burns (East Grinstead, Ely, Cosford, Halton and Wroughton) but no special centres were established by the army or navy – their casualties were treated at the regional EMS units. As a result, in addition to several airmen (not all were admitted to East Grinstead), the wards at Rooksdown were filled with marine, navy and army wounded from the campaign in France – and, following the Blitz, a growing number of civilians. Later, service casualties came from North Africa, the Middle East and Italy and, after the D-Day landings in 1944, from Europe via the army maxillofacial units discussed later in the chapter. As Gillies observed, 'On the front lawns could be found burned pilots and soldiers, cleft lip and palate babies, bombed housewives, half a dozen Army gunshot wounds to the face, and several German prisoners of war.'[1] Throughout the war he continued to train surgeons from all over the world, and frequently the only Englishman present in the doctors' mess was Martin Rushton, chief dental surgeon; 34 nationalities had served on the medical staff by 1944.

During the period 1939–46, 4665 patients were admitted and 10,128 operations performed at Rooksdown.[2] Regrettably, the records of many of the patients treated by the unit (and transferred to the Gillies Archive from Queen Mary's Hospital, Roehampton, in 2001), particularly from the wartime years, have either gone astray or been cannibalised, and few have complete case notes – most of the records are in fact postwar. Fortunately, there are some colour photographs taken by Percy Hennell[†] during his visits to Rooksdown in the archives, but many of the photographs and the case notes of patients used to illustrate Gillies' *Principles and Art of Plastic Surgery* have not survived.

The American Hospital in Britain

With Britain involved in another European war, Dr Philip D Wilson, Surgeon-in-Chief at the oldest orthopaedic hospital in the United States, the Hospital for Special Surgery in New York City, felt there was a need for the Americans to support the British with medical personnel, as they had done in the First World War. To achieve this he personally organised the American Hospital in Britain, a privately funded voluntary unit to help care for the wounded. The objectives of creating the American Hospital were: (1) to give surgical assistance to the British; (2) to provide moral support in time of need; and (3) to gain experience in the treatment of war injuries. On 20 May 1940 Wilson telegraphed (Sir) Harry Platt (1886–1986), Professor of Orthopaedic Surgery at Manchester Royal Infirmary, offering to set up an orthopaedic hospital in England – a generous offer which was accepted by Platt on behalf of a grateful British government. On 22 August 1940 a small advance group of seven doctors and five nursing staff sailed from Brooklyn on the steamship *Western Prince* through the submarine-infested waters of the North Atlantic, arriving safely in Liverpool on 1 September.[10]

The American Hospital in Britain was assigned a block of six wards with 300 beds and a separate operating theatre at the Park Prewett Hospital. By the end of the year the unit had performed 254 operations, mainly on soldiers, sailors and airmen,

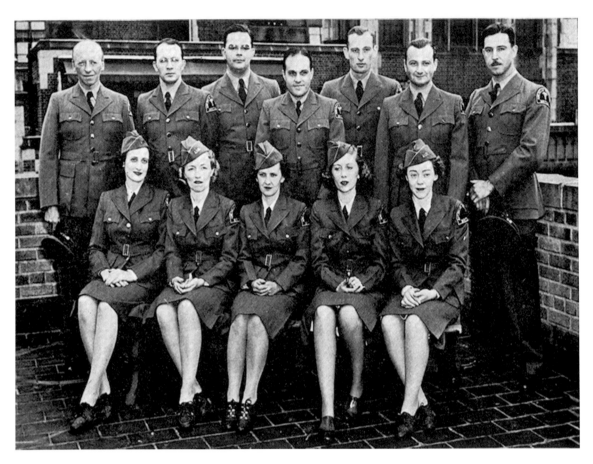

FIGURE 11.6. *The first unit of the American Hospital in Britain sailed on 22 August 1940 for Liverpool. Standing: Dr Philip D Wilson, Dr Donald E Dial, Dr Charles H Bradford, Dr W Richard Ferguson, Dr Frederick W Waknitz, Dr John M Converse, Dr Norman Egel. Seated: Miss Miriam L Knight, Miss Adelbert E Overman, Miss Mildred L Lewis, Mrs Sheila M Converse, Mrs Helen D Dial.* (Published with the kind permission of the Hospital for Special Surgery, New York, and SpringerLink)

but also on an increasing number of civilians after the Luftwaffe bombing campaign of the docks and shipping at Southampton and Portsmouth. The American Hospital remained at Basingstoke until January 1942, when its staff, now grown to 12 doctors and 140 personnel, was moved to the Churchill Hospital in Oxford.

Fractures of the facial skeleton
The significance of the American Hospital Unit at Park Prewett is that Gillies, writing in the *British Dental Journal*, claims that two of its surgeons, John Converse[†] and Frederick Waknitz, were the

first to adapt the Roger Anderson pin fixation method to stabilise mandibular fractures; he goes on to say that the method was subsequently taken up by Mowlem and other maxillofacial centres (see Chapter 10).[11] At the time of Gillies' article, 10 patients had been treated by this method at Rooksdown (Colour plate 26). To set the record straight, Converse and Waknitz subsequently reported the management of the first patient in the January 1942 issue of *The Journal of Bone and Joint Surgery* – a soldier aged 21, who had been admitted to the maxillofacial unit at Rooksdown for the treatment of a non-united fracture through the left angle of the mandible. The posterior fragment was displaced laterally, upwards and forwards, and a third molar had been left in the fracture line. On 8 January 1941, two weeks after extraction of the third molar, the fracture site was exposed via a small incision below the angle of the mandible, the fibrous tissue between the ends of the bones resected, and fixation obtained by the two-pin method. The pins were removed after five weeks with a good anatomical and functional result.[12]

The second case treated at Rooksdown by Gillies and Rushton, was a bilateral fracture of an edentulous jaw that had been previously treated by circumferential wiring. Healing was satisfactory on the left side, but non-union resulted on the right side because the Gunning splint was unable to control the short posterior ramal fragment. The problem was solved with a bone graft and stabilisation of the posterior fragment by pin fixation. In May 1942 Rushton and FA Walker reported on a series of 21 cases that had been treated at Rooksdown by pin fixation over the previous year, and described in detail three cases using the Clouston–Walker appliance,[13] an improved form of fixation developed in conjunction with Clouston, an engineer.

Burns at Rooksdown

It is clear from the cases used to illustrate *The Principles and Art of Plastic Surgery* that many of the burns patients treated by Gillies and his team at Rooksdown were particularly severe – in many cases a good deal more severe than the airmen being treated by McIndoe and his colleagues at East Grinstead and other RAF units. Gillies had a long history of treating naval and civilian burns, dating back to Able-Seaman Vicarage in 1917 (discussed in Chapter 5), and the explosion of a phosphorus bomb on the Danish cruiser *Gejser* in 1923, in which 17 naval officers and men had been badly burned (for his services in treating the Danes, many of whom required long-term management, Gillies was awarded the Order of Dannebrog by a grateful King Christian X).

In the early days of the Second World War, burns patients were mainly servicemen who had been evacuated from the ill-fated campaigns in Norway and France, or rescued from the burning sea after the sinking of the *Lancastria*. During the Battle of Britain and the Blitz the patients were mainly RAF and civilian casualties, and since this was the heyday of tannic acid therapy (the malign consequences of which have already been discussed in Chapter 8), burnt faces, bodies and hands were liberally coated with the stuff. Eventually the maxillofacial units became flooded with burns victims.[1]

It has been alleged that Gillies and McIndoe had different approaches to the resurfacing of skin defects: whereas Gillies favoured full-thickness flaps, McIndoe was a leading advocate of free skin grafts. John Mustardé, who spent some of his training with Gillies, has left an interesting account of joint meetings between the Rooksdown and East Grinstead trainees shortly after the war: 'The respective entourages of the two Masters followed their leader with a blind acceptance to the exclusion of all others that was almost religious in its bigotry.' The meetings usually ended up in a state of war between the two groups.[2] Whether the views of Gillies and McIndoe were as polarised as their disciples' seems doubtful; differences in technique were likely to have been tailored to the individual needs of the patients admitted to their respective units. Since McIndoe was consultant plastic surgeon to the RAF, many of the air crews with burns, particularly in the early years of the war, came under his care, and commonly required free skin grafts to resurface second- or third-degree burns of the face and hands. The priority was the preservation of sight and maintenance of function, but the area affected was localised and relatively small. In other words, while the *mortality* in this type of burn was small, the *morbidity* was great.[14] In contrast, naval personnel, with their open uniforms, received burns of the entire face including the ears and neck, and any of the occupants of a tank who survived a direct hit from a 75-mm armour-piercing shell fired from a Wehrmacht Panzer were likely to have had more than their hands and eyelids singed.

Gunshot wounds to the face

Campbell was a merchant seaman whose ship had been bombed (Colour plate 27). His primary treatment, which Gillies noted was right up to hospital standards, had been carried out on board – the skin was sewn to mucous membrane and the bony parts were retained in their normal position. When he arrived at Rooksdown, the gap in the chin including the bone was obvious, so to maintain and measure the defect and stop saliva dribbling out of his mouth, the first procedure undertaken was the construction of a vulcanite prosthesis. After careful planning by Gillies with a number of colleagues, the repair was carried out by James Cuthbert and David O Brown.

The solution was a double-pedicle, two-layered cross-over repair; one pedicle with the skin surface facing inwards to provide an epithelial lining, and the other to restore the surface defect. However, as Gillies explains in *The Principles and Art of Plastic Surgery* (pp. 503–04), the method always results in a temporary fistula as only three edges of the lining flap can be joined until its pedicle can be divided, and although the method has the advantage of two independent lifelines, it does use an extravagant amount of skin. One solution was to make the end of a single pedicle large enough to be folded back on itself – there is less donor scarring and the buccal fistula stage is avoided.[1] Unfortunately the photographs in colour plate 27 are not dated.

One soldier with a deep penetrating wound of the neck and lower jaw for which there is a complete history is shown in Figure 11.7. The case was fortuitously included in *Fractures of the Facial Skeleton* (1955) by Rowe and Killey (pp. 570–03),[15] and there is also an abbreviated version in *Principles and Art of Plastic Surgery* (p. 524). The patient had suffered a shell wound in France on 8 October 1944, aged 34. A stitch had been inserted at a regimental aid post to stabilise the tongue, and he was then admitted to No 10 CCS. The wound beneath the mandible appeared to have penetrated the trachea and breathing was difficult; there was also a large transverse wound of the upper neck, severing the tip of the epiglottis and exposing the larynx; and the mandible had a compound comminuted fracture of the right angle.

Operation 8.10.1944: *Pharynx repaired and wound closed in layers with drainage. Tracheotomy and gastrostomy (surgical opening into the stomach) performed; 100,000 units of penicillin given. 9.10.1944: Interdental wiring applied to support the jaw. 11.10.1944: Evacuated to 79th British General Hospital in Normandy and transferred later the same day to Maxillofacial Unit No 5 (see below), attached to No 8 British General Hospital.*

Second operation 12.10.1944: *Upper Gunning-type splint (the patient had no upper teeth) secured to the alveolus with peralveolar wires. Cast metal cap splints cemented onto the anterior teeth of the lower jaw and loose fragments of bone removed. Exploration of a foul sloughing cavity extending forwards to a septic opening into pharynx at the base of the epiglottis. Rubber drain inserted into the lingual aspect of the symphyseal region and cavity left open to drain. Fixation of jaws applied.*

Third operation 13.10.1944: *Reinsertion of gastrostomy tube which had been removed by the patient during sleep.*

Fourth operation 19.10.1944: *Gastrostomy not functioning properly. Tube reinserted and passed as far as the duodenum. Lower splints localised and two pints of blood were transfused.*

Fifth operation 25.10.1944: *Gastrostomy closed and jejunostomy performed; one pint of blood transfused. 31.10.1944: Evacuated to the UK.*

1.11.1944: *Admitted to Rooksdown House where he was encouraged to sit up and sip liquids. 10.11.1944: Consultation with Brigadier Miles Formby who advised conservative rehabilitation prior to further surgery.*

Sixth operation 15.12.1944: *(Sir Harold Gillies and FA Walker). Exposure of the fracture site by an external approach and necrotic fragments of bone removed.*

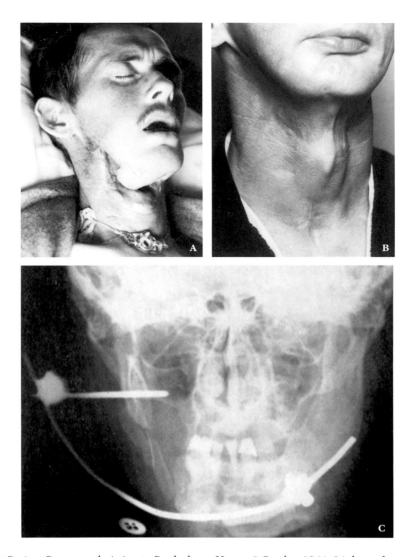

FIGURE 11.7. (A) *Patient Bone on admission to Rooksdown House, 8 October 1944, 24 days after receiving a shell wound, showing exposure of the larynx and tracheotomy tube still in position;* (B) *Final appearance 24 March 1950 after nine operations and several other procedures, the last of which was carried out in April 1945.* (*Photographs taken by Percy Hennell. Courtesy of the Gillies Archives, Frognal Centre, Queen Mary's Hospital, Sidcup*); (C) *Pin fixation of the mandibular fragments after insertion of a bone graft. No limitation was placed on the movement of the mandible.* (*From NL Rowe & HC Killey (1955), Fractures of the Facial Skeleton*)

Seventh operation 10.1.1945: (*Commander Matthew Banks*). *This involved the exploration of a sinus leading down to the posterior fragment of the mandible with a probe, followed by exposure and removal of loose pieces of bone. Bone ends were trimmed with rongeurs; soft tissues sutured into place with drainage.*

Eighth operation 31.1.1945: (*Sir Harold Gillies and Brigadier Formby*). *A pharyngeal fistula was closured by a flap from neck.*

Ninth operation 12.4.1945: (*Commander Banks and FA Walker*). *Bone graft to the mandibular defect at the right angle of 2½ inches utilising bone from the iliac crest. Medullary chips packed into the defect and fragments immobilised by external pin fixation (c). 4.6.1945: Pins removed: anterior pin was loose, but the posterior firm; good clinical union. Full upper and lower dentures subsequently constructed with satisfactory result. No difficulty in swallowing or speaking. The anaesthetics at Rooksdown were given by Dr Patrick Shackelton.*

The Rooksdown Club

Unlike McIndoe, who encouraged press visits to East Grinstead arranged by the Ministry of Information and the Air Ministry, Gillies was less cooperative with the press and studiously avoided publicity – he often disappeared when he saw them on the horizon. He was by now in his late fifties and had already established his reputation as the doyen of modern plastic surgery – not to mention keeping the specialty alive in Britain between the wars – and he did not see the need to interrupt his work at the hospital to accommodate the interference of tiresome journalists.

As a result, very little is known about the role of Rooksdown House and the Rooksdown Club in rehabilitating injured servicemen and civilians during the war years. An additional reason for this is that the Rooksdown Club – the equivalent of the Guinea Pig Club – was not formed under the War Charities Act (1940) until May 1945, and did not achieve charitable status until July 1947. Its aims were similar to those of the Guinea Pig Club: to enable former patients to keep in touch with each other, to establish a support network to help ease them back into society, and to educate the public into accepting the injured and mutilated without comment or prejudice. Anyone who had an association with Rooksdown House either as a patient or staff was eligible for membership. Gillies was president, and a committee was made up of former patients. In 1958 the club had an active membership of over 800, and it continued to function after the unit was transferred to Roehampton. The club had its own magazine, and two principal gatherings were held each year – a garden party in June at Rooksdown and a dinner in December, first held in 1950. Over the years the

membership inevitably declined and the last issue of the Rooksdown Club magazine was published in February 2005, the sixtieth anniversary of the club's foundation.

The main difference between the two clubs was that the Rooksdown had a much more diverse membership. The only thing the army, navy, air force and civilian patients at Rooksdown had in common was their injuries. This meant they were not as likely to have the close personal relationships or that special bond that defined the Guinea Pig Club, best described by Brian Kingcome, the Spitfire pilot who was a patient of Gillies and McIndoe in the 1930s (see Chapter 7). McIndoe made Kingcome an Honorary Guinea Pig and after the war invited him as his guest to one of their annual dinners. Kingcome, who had never been an patient of Ward III at East Grinstead, felt like an interloper and never went again. As he observed in his autobiography (p. 31):

Whenever those who have had a shared common horrendous experience gather together, they have a special bond, an intimacy, an invisible but almost intangible barrier that outsiders can never penetrate, however warmly they may be welcomed.[16]

The British Army had recognised this more than 300 years earlier with the introduction of the regimental system – regimental loyalties were essential to the development of corporate identity, esprit de corps and an efficient fighting unit: anyone who has ever played team sports or is old enough to have done national service will understand what Kingcome meant. The Rooksdown patients had acquired their scars in a tank, a merchant marine tanker, a warship, naval aircraft, or an air raid – almost anywhere except in an RAF aircraft. What they found most irritating after the war, according to James 'Rusty' Russell in the Rooksdown Club magazine of February 2005, was being greeted by prewar friends with, 'You must be one of those Guinea Pig chaps from East Grinstead.'

Another important difference between the two groups is that very little has been written about Rooksdown House and its patients – with

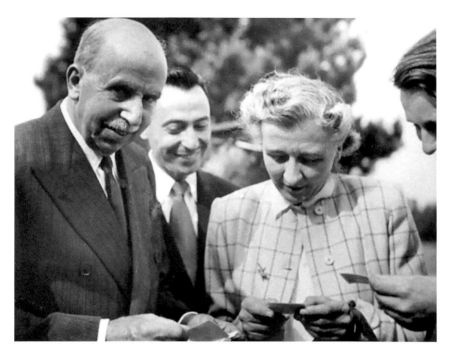

FIGURE 11.8. *Sir Harold and Lady Gillies at a garden party at Rooksdown House in 1956 or 1957; between them is Dr JP Szlazak from Canada. (Courtesy of the Gillies Archives, Frognal Centre, Queen Mary's Hospital, Sidcup)*

the exception of Gillies' *Principles and Practice of Plastic Surgery*, which was hardly suited to public consumption – whereas there have been numerous books and newspaper articles published about East Grinstead and McIndoe's work. Perhaps airmen had more interesting wartime stories to write about and these generated plenty of public interest and publicity. Just one former patient at Rooksdown felt motivated enough to write a book, and he left it until he was in his late sixties.[17] Ironically, he happened to be a fighter pilot, Wing Commander RFT Doe DSO, DFC and Bar. And to add insult to injury, his obituaries in both the *Daily Telegraph* (22 February 2010) and *The Times* (3 March 2010) reported that Doe had been a patient of McIndoe's at East Grinstead, although he later became a post-war member of the Guinea Pig Club.[18]

Wing Commander Bob Doe

Pilot Officer Bob Doe[†] was the antithesis of the popular image of the public school-educated Battle of Britain hero – a modest, unassuming man who had left school at 14 to work in an office. He joined the RAF Volunteer Reserve and after being accepted for flying training became the fifth-highest-scoring RAF Ace in the Battle of Britain, with 15 enemy aircraft destroyed (the top four were Josef Frantisek (Czech; 17), Eric Lock (UK; 16.5), Brian Carbury (NZ; 15.5) and James 'Ginger' Lacey (UK; 15.5)).[19] His first successes came on 15 August 1940 when Doe, flying Spitfires with 234 Squadron from RAF Middle Wallop in Hampshire in his first engagement with the Luftwaffe, shot down and destroyed two Messerschmitt Bf 110s; the next day he destroyed a Bf 109 and a Dornier Do 18 flying boat, and two days later destroyed a Bf 109 and damaged another before running out of ammunition – not a bad start for someone who, by his own admission, lacked confidence, disliked flying upside down and was no good at aerobatics.

In January 1941, having been transferred to 238 Squadron, Doe was flying a night sortie when the

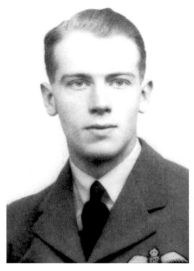 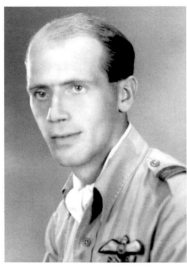 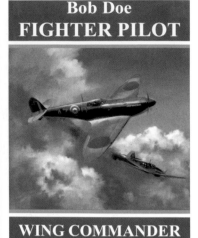

FIGURE 11.9. LEFT: *Pilot Officer RFT Doe, November 1939.* MIDDLE: *Squadron Leader Doe DFC and Bar in 1943 after 22 operations at Rooksdown House. The right eye is still visibly lower than the left. (Photographs from Bob Doe (1999),* Fighter Pilot: The story of one of the few) RIGHT: *The cover of the only book written by a patient at Rooksdown House. It is from an original painting by Frank Wootton showing a Messerschmitt Bf 109 in flames after being attacked by Bob Doe in Spitfire AZ-D, August 1940. During the Battle of Britain 234 Squadron was stationed at RAF Middle Wallop in Hampshire.*

oil in the cooler of his Hurricane (V6758) froze and, after losing height, the engine stopped completely at 5000 feet. He attempted to land on the snow-covered airfield at RAF Warmwell in West Dorset, but the aircraft crashed into a heap of oil drums. The Sutton harness snapped and Doe smashed his face against the reflector gunsight. He was taken to the local cottage hospital, where an army surgeon put his right eye back in the socket and sutured his nose into the correct position. After a couple of weeks he was transferred to Rooksdown House and into the care of Gillies, where he endured another 22 operations.

In the words of Thomas Hardy, 'More life may trickle out of a man through thought than through a gaping wound,'[20] and Gillies had a long history of dealing with the psychological effects of facial mutilation, both on his patients and in the wider community. In much the same way as at East Grinstead, the good folk of Basingstoke took a while to adjust to the new inhabitants of the nearby mental asylum, and some longer than others. Doe

describes in *Fighter Pilot: The story of one of the few*[17] how, after being at Rooksdown for a few weeks and undergoing a number of operations that enabled him to eat and speak normally, it became clear the patients were encouraged to go into Basingstoke to shop, socialise and go to the pubs (p. 53):

> *A favourite haunt was the Red Lion where the attraction was a big, busty, blonde barmaid, who everyone swore was paid by Gillies … Can you imagine five or six chaps, some of whom were in a ghastly state with severe burns … walking into a large comfortable bar full of people (who tended to edge away from this frightful sight) and being greeted by – 'My darling – how lovely to see you!' and being given a big kiss. She deserved a medal if anyone did.*

Eventually, after some 20 operations, Gillies called on Doe one evening with a book of noses and a bottle of scotch, to talk about reconstructing his nose. The plan involved taking a bone graft from the hip, dovetailing it into his forehead and stitching

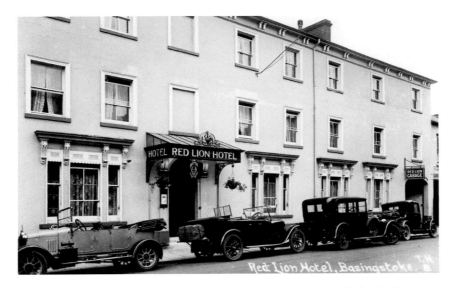

FIGURE 11.10. *The Red Lion Hotel, Basingstoke, favourite watering-hole of Bob Doe and the patients of Rooksdown House, taken around the late 1920s by local photographer Terry Hunt. The licensees during the war were William and Kathleen Sweetman.* (Photograph kindly provided by their granddaughter, Deborah Reavell, whose mother remembers Sir Harold and the Rooksdown patients at the hotel.)

the skin over it. The outcome was successful, but unfortunately, two days later he walked into a door and this dislodged the bone. Nevertheless, judging by the photograph of Doe taken in 1943 (Figure 11.9) the result wasn't too bad, although his right eye is lower than the left – this resulted in double vision (diplopia) if he looked up. However, because all vision tests were conducted at eye level, Doe was still able to pass his flying medical – no doubt with the collusion of the examining MO – and he returned to active duty until the end of the war.

Army maxillofacial units

The first plastic surgeon to serve abroad in the British Army during World War II was Captain RJV Battle RAMC[†], who arrived in Dieppe in December 1939. Although there was no established maxillofacial unit at the time, patients with face and jaw injuries were being sent to No 1 General Hospital at Dieppe where the Senior Dental Officer, Major J Wren, was an Army Dental Corps specialist. Arrangements had been made for those

with maxillofacial injuries to receive preliminary treatment before their evacuation to England, and Battle was posted to No 1 General as the surgeon. However, with the fall of France they were all back in England by the end of May.[21]

With the opening up of military campaigns in North Africa in the summer of 1940, followed by those in Italy, India and Burma, delays in the repatriation of patients to England for specialist care were inevitable. The obvious solution was to train teams that could operate closer to the fighting. Since the army still had no plastic surgeons other than its civilian consultants, Gillies together with Colonel John M Weddell (1884–1966), consulting surgeon to the British North African Force, made plans to train a number of maxillofacial teams for service abroad. Each team consisted of plastic and dental surgeons, anaesthetists, nurses and orderlies.[1] Gillies and the Army Dental Corps selected all the surgeons and dental consultants. Eventually six British maxillofacial units and two Indian units staffed by British officers were formed and trained

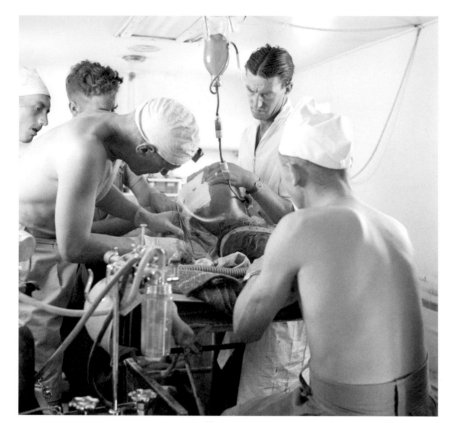

FIGURE 11.11. TOP:
Emergency operation being carried out in a mobile operating theatre, North Africa, 28 July 1942. (Photographer: Lt Mayne; No 1 Army Film & Photographic Unit, IWM: E 14996. Published with the kind permission of the Imperial War Museum, London.)

BOTTOM: *Emergency operation being performed at an advanced dressing station, North Africa, 5 November 1942.*
(Photographer: Sgt Mapham; No 1 Army Film & Photographic Unit, IWM: E 18997. Published with the kind permission of the Imperial War Museum, London.

In the Second World War the medical chain of evacuation was little changed from the First. Casualties went from regimental aid posts or advanced dressing stations where emergency treatment was carried out, then to CCSs and general hospitals in the various theatres of operation for major surgery.

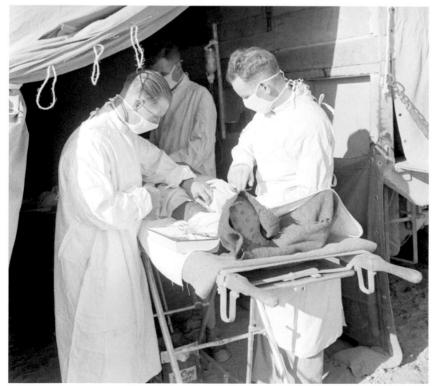

at Rooksdown House, with the exception of No 6, which trained at Hill End Hospital with Rainsford Mowlem.[21] Few of the trainee surgeons had any previous experience of plastic operations; the names of the plastic surgeons and dental surgeons attached to each of the overseas maxillofacial units are listed in Appendix IV.

Maxillofacial Unit (MFU) No 1, under the command of Major Randall Campion, was formed in Alexandria in the early part of 1941. It treated casualties from the North African desert, Sudan, Eritrea, Greece and Crete. It moved via Tripoli to Sicily, where Richard Battle took command. By 1943 it had split into advanced and rear sections, which operated in Sicily and on the Italian mainland. (Among the unit's surgical staff was (Sir) Reginald Sydney Murley 1916–1997), who returned to general surgery after the war and became president of the Royal College of Surgeons of England (1977–80).)

MFU No 2, under Michael Oldfield, was mobilised late in 1940 and posted to Jerusalem in August 1941. After treating casualties from the Syrian campaign, the unit was transferred to Heliopolis, a Cairo suburb, where it was attached to No 9 General Hospital. Both units received patients from the desert fighting, and sent patients they could not return to active service back to Rooksdown.

MFU No 3 was mobilised at Aldershot in March 1942, under the command of Charles Heanley and with John Hovell as the dental consultant (he later established a reputation in both orthodontics and maxillofacial surgery). The unit was sent to Ranikhet, United Provinces, India – a Himalayan military hill station situated at an altitude of 6000 feet, which provided an ideal climate for plastic surgery. Here the unit treated casualties from the whole of India, the Burma campaign and the Middle East.

MFU No 4 was formed at Rooksdown in August 1942. Three months later, under Patrick Clarkson[†] and with Rex Lawrie as a surgical trainee, the unit was posted to Algiers to function as the specialist unit for the First Army in North Africa, treating casualties from the Tunisian and Italian campaigns.

At the beginning of 1944 an advanced section, led by Rex Lawrie, proceeded to Naples in preparation for the Battle of Monte Cassino – two plastic surgeons, two general duty medical officers and two specialist dental surgeons treated 221 maxillofacial injuries, performing 200 operations in 12 days. The unit split again into two sections: one advanced on Rome, while the other remained in Naples, treating casualties from the Mediterranean coast of Italy, until it was transferred to the British Liberation Army in June 1945.[21,22]

Both MFU No 5 (with Geoffrey Fitzgibbon and Tom Gibson, formed early in 1944 from a team working at Rooksdown) and MFU No 6 (attached to Hill End Hospital, led by William Hynes) served in France, Belgium and Holland and were sending back casualties to Rooksdown from Normandy 12 hours after the D-Day landings. The earliest maxillofacial casualties were sent back to Portsmouth in the returning tank-landing ships (LSTs) to the Royal Naval Hospital at Haslar, and then on to Rooksdown House or other centres.

The Ad Hoc Unit was a small unit that worked in close liaison with MFU No 1. It was located at Andria, near Bari, and was created to deal with casualties from Yugoslavia and Albania. After the war, two civilian teams were sent from Rooksdown House and Hill End Hospital – at the instigation of Gillies – to Belgrade, where there were a considerable number of maxillofacial injuries requiring long-term reconstructive surgery.

In addition to the six British units, two Indian units were formed. Indian MFU No 1 was formed in Calcutta in 1943 under the command of FW Pickard. It moved the following year to Barrackpore in Bengal, where it worked in conjunction with No 3 British MFU. Indian MFU No 2, led by Eric Peet, was raised in Poona in 1943 and in December 1944 moved to Secunderabad. Both the Indian units dealt with large numbers of casualties from the South East Asia Command under particularly trying conditions – an adverse climate, long lines of communication and the poor physical health of the wounded, who had received little if any initial treatment.

Maxillofacial Unit No 4

Although nominally maxillofacial units, in reality their case mix in the field was much broader, and most of the patients with burns came into their care. MFU No 4, for example, during its two-and-a-half-year period in Algiers and Italy, treated nearly 5000 patients: 3000 cases were maxillofacial, 1000 were burns, and the remainder large chronic wounds and hand injuries. They managed nearly 200 acute burns from naval catastrophes in the Mediterranean, and also a number of acute maxillofacial injuries from terrorist-style antipersonnel devices in Algiers. In 1943 Howard Florey visited the unit and produced a box of small vials of brown powder, which turned out to be early samples of penicillin, and the treatment of maxillofacial injuries was transformed. Penicillin proved to be particularly effective in increasing the rate of skin-graft healing,[22] and experience gained in resurfacing serious burn injuries with split- and full-thickness grafts was later reported by Clarkson and Lawrie in the *British Journal of Surgery*.[23]

Clarkson *et al* also published an account of the treatment of 1000 jaw fractures at MFU No 4.[24] Seven hundred of the cases were open-missile wounds, usually involving comminution of the jaws with scattering of bone and tooth fragments into the surrounding soft tissues. The remaining 300 were closed injuries – a third of which were due to brawls! Their priority was primary closure of face wounds, which not only shortened healing times – to the relief of the patients – but also diminished the incidence of bone infection. The jaw was fixed at the same operation, if possible, or within two days of the injury – except when there was an associated wound of the tongue and pharynx, with danger of suffocation. Intermaxillary fixation (wire was preferred to elastics) was delayed in these cases for about a week, and then done preferably without an anaesthetic. Their preferred method of fixation was sectional cap splints fitting closely around the gum margin (over 800 were fitted). Pin fixation was used in only 15 cases, when it was required to control edentulous posterior fragments or compound fractures opening into the mouth. The

unit followed a conservative policy regarding tooth extraction. Thirty-three patients in the series died – 14 from an associated injury of the brain or spinal cord, and 15 from the maxillofacial injury. The chief causes of early death (within the first week) with maxillofacial casualties were the same as they had been in the First World War – haemorrhage and suffocation; as in the First World War, later death was most commonly caused by pulmonary complications.

The army MFUs played a vital role in saving the lives of injured soldiers by early intervention. They also left an invaluable postwar legacy of a group of well-trained and experienced plastic and maxillofacial surgeons, who were available to transfer their clinical skills to civilian practice in the newly established National Health Service. This meant that, together with those trained at the various RAF maxillofacial units, instead of just four specialists at the outset of the war – Gillies, Kilner, McIndoe and Mowlem – the first meeting of the British Association of Plastic Surgeons in 1947 was attended by 36. Plastic surgery was now on the threshold of becoming accessible to all.

Rooksdown and the advancement of maxillofacial surgery

Gillies and the Rooksdown unit played an important role in the advancement of postwar maxillofacial surgery in two ways: first, by applying principles gained from the treatment of wartime facial injuries to the treatment of civilian patients; and second, by helping train the next generation of maxillofacial surgeons. Of these, two stand out: Paul Tessier (1917–2008) and Hugo Obwegeser (1920–), both of whom were to revolutionise the treatment of congenital facial deformity.

In 1942 a 14-year-old girl was referred to Gillies from the Isle of Wight.[25] She was not a casualty of the war but was suffering from what Gillies referred to as oxycephaly, an inherited abnormality resulting from craniosynostosis (premature closure of the joints between the bones of the cranial vault, thereby distorting the shape of the skull). She also had associated abnormalities of the eyes and upper jaw. (Today she would be classified as having Crouzon syndrome: genetic analyses have shown that despite their characteristic facial appearance or phenotypes, the eponymous syndromes of Crouzon, Apert, Pfeiffer and Jackson-Weiss are all due to gain-of-function mutations in the same gene – the fibroblast growth factor receptor-2 (FGFR2) gene on chromosome 10.)[26] To improve her appearance, Gillies carried out the first recorded Le Fort III osteotomy,[27] which enabled the bones of the middle third of her face to be surgically repositioned forwards in one piece (Figure 11.12). After three and a half years some relapse in the advancement had taken place, but as Gillies later reported, 'In the light of subsequent experience,

even this small loss could have been avoided by packing chip grafts into the strategic osteotomy chinks.'[1]

The significance of the operation – although Gilllies never repeated it – was to anticipate the revolutionary methods developed years later by the French surgeon Paul Tessier to treat similar cases of severe facial deformity. After the war Tessier spent time with Gillies at Rooksdown for periods of up to two months, twice a year from 1946 to 1949, gaining experience in soft and hard tissue reconstruction. He was familiar with Gillies' Le Fort III osteotomy patient, but it was not until 1958 and a particularly severe case of Crouzon syndrome that Tessier abandoned the standard procedures for treating

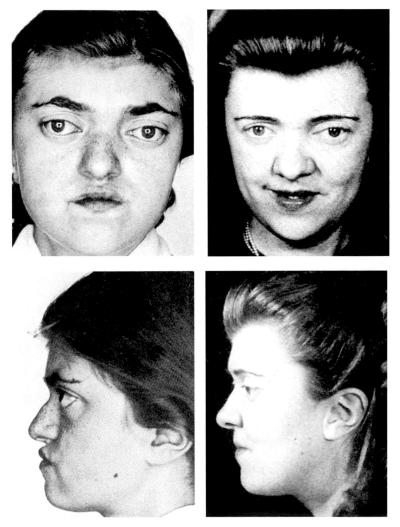

FIGURE 11.12. *Pre- and post-operative photographs of the Crouzon syndrome (oxycephaly) patient on whom Gillies performed the first Le Fort III osteotomy to advance the bones of the middle third of the face. Although a relatively mild case, she shows the characteristic facial features of the syndrome: increased distance between the eyes (hypertelorism); midface (maxillary) hypoplasia; prominence of the eyes (proptosis); relative mandibular prognathism.*

(From Gillies HD & Millard DR (1957), The Principles and Art of Plastic Surgery, vol 2, pp. 551–53, published with permission of Lippincott Williams & Wilkins)

craniofacial anomalies – only bone grafting and other camouflage operations – and adopted a much more radical approach. In close cooperation with Gérard Guiot, a neurosurgeon, Tessier combined a Le Fort III osteotomy with an operation inside the skull to separate the orbits from the cranial base, which enabled the eyes and forehead also to be repositioned, stabilising the advancement with bone grafts, and in doing so created a new sub-specialty – craniofacial surgery.[28]

When Hugo Obwegeser started his training in maxillofacial surgery at the University of Graz Dental School in 1947, orthognathic surgery to reposition the jaws was virtually nonexistent, consisting of a series of largely unsatisfactory operations to correct prominence of the lower jaw. A Le Fort I (Guerin-type) operation had been used at Rooksdown since 1941 to mobilise and reduce traumatic impactions of the bones of the middle third of the face, and subsequently adapted for use in patients with cleft lip and palate and other craniofacial anomalies.[29,30] According to Obwegeser, who spent a year with Gillies courtesy of the British Council in 1951–52:

> He used horizontal vestibular incisions to approach the maxilla, despite the palatal surgery and concern for blood supply. But he only rotated the collapsed cleft segments with a green-stick fracture at the pterygoid-maxillary junction, as did Schmid to correct the cross-bite, and I had never seen him advance the maxilla. He fixed them in the new position using cast cap splints fixed to a vertical bar to a head cap. He then placed cancellous bone grafts on the steps of the canine fossa open to the maxillary sinus. The grafts were covered on the vestibular side only. The sagittal discrepancy he corrected by setting the mandible back. The patients retained their dish face or at best a flat appearance.[31]

Several examples of cleft lip and palate surgery included in *Principles and Art of Plastic Surgery* support this, although at least one case suggests the maxilla might have been advanced.[1] However, without accurate cephalometric radiographs – a technique not widely available at the time – it is impossible to tell, and the records have not survived.

Operations to mobilise the maxilla had been around since the time of von Langenbeck (1810–1887) but at the time a reliable procedure for advancing the maxilla did not exist; it was not until 1964 when Obwegeser introduced what became the standard Le Fort I osteotomy that the problem was solved. Obwegeser had earlier revolutionised mandibular surgery with the invention of the bilateral sagittal split osteotomy in the late 1950s, an operation performed inside the mouth designed to produce a broad contact between the two bone surfaces of the split vertical ramus. This innovation meant it could be used to reposition the tooth-bearing body of the mandible forwards or backwards.[31,32] With these two operations, the fertile and energetic mind of Obwegeser enabled orthognathic surgery to evolve into the reliable double-jaw procedure it has become today. In later years both Tessier and Obwegeser were to acknowledge their debt to Gillies, as Obwegeser recalled:[31]

> I was equally fortunate to have had Sir Harold Gillies and Eduard Schmid as my teachers. Each taught me that it was not so much knowledge of what came before, but the imagination of solving problems as the patients presented themselves. In the middle of difficulty lies opportunity. The surgeon today can disassemble each of the elements of the craniofacial skeleton and then reassemble it. He only is limited by his imagination to seek the solution.

CHAPTER **12**

Epilogue

Pickerill

In 1927 Pickerill resigned as Dean of the Dental School and moved to Sydney with the intention of specialising in plastic surgery, leaving his wife and four children behind in Dunedin. The attempt by a 47-year-old Englishman to gain acceptance in Macquarie Street and break into the Sydney surgical scene was bound to be something of a gamble, and so it proved: he wrote to the University of Otago asking if he could have his old job back and his request was declined.[1] The usual reason given for Pickerill's resignation is his disagreement with his wartime colleagues Hunter and Rishworth over proposals to meet the national shortage of dentists by introducing a School Dental Service. The scheme, which was Hunter's brainchild, was designed to provide free dental care for children in clinics attached to primary schools. The service was to be staffed not by university-trained dentists, but by young women (dental nurses) who had been through a limited training programme of just two years, and this no doubt played a part. But having participated in the vast surgical enterprise that had spawned the new specialty of plastic surgery, the petty jealousies of academic and professional life in a provincial university must have made his return to civilian status seem something of an anticlimax. This was further compounded by his failure to understand the importance of making friends on

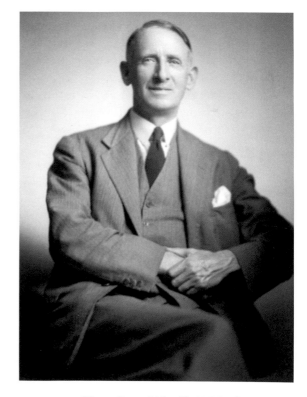

FIGURE 12.1. *Henry Percy Pickerill, 23 March 1935. The photograph was taken by Stanley Polkinghorne Andrew after Pickerill returned from Sydney. (By kind permission of the Alexander Turnbull Library, Wellington, SP Andrew Collection, Reference number F-018390-1/1)*

the way up who might be helpful on the way down.

However, there was an additional and rather more compelling reason for his resignation. Dr Cicely Clarkson, who had worked as a house surgeon with Pickerill at Dunedin Hospital in 1926, later joined him in Sydney as his pupil and associate; in 1934, after Pickerill had divorced his wife, they were married – the age difference was 24 years. One doesn't need exceptional insight to work out what had transpired, and the eyebrows their relationship must have raised in a small community with its roots in the Free Church of Scotland.

In 1930 Pickerill was elected a Fellow of the recently established (1927) Royal Australasian College of Surgeons, and in 1933 was appointed plastic surgeon to the Royal North Shore Hospital in Sydney. Nevertheless, he must have felt the Sydney surgical scene was uncongenial and returned to New Zealand the following year to set up practice in Wellington. The Pickerills continued to be close surgical associates for the rest of their working lives – at Lewisham Hospital in Wellington and later as visiting plastic surgeons to Middlemore Hospital in Auckland. In 1939 they established Bassam Hospital in Lower Hutt, where they specialised in the treatment of children with cleft lip and palate and other congenital defects.[1] Pickerill was appointed CBE in 1923 for his wartime service but never knighted, although Cecily Pickerill was made a Dame of the British Empire in 1977, the first female doctor in New Zealand to be so honoured. He died in Upper Hutt on 10 August 1956, aged 77.

Whatever one might think about Pickerill's character – and he clearly was a difficult man – he had been responsible for establishing dentistry as a university discipline in New Zealand, and played a leading role in the renaissance of plastic and maxillofacial surgery at Sidcup during the First World War. He was also the first surgeon in Australia and New Zealand to limit his practice to plastic surgery. Nevertheless, his contributions appear to have been largely forgotten by the present generation of plastic surgeons in Australasia – and for understandable reasons. Unlike Gillies and

McIndoe, he did not train a cohort of admiring disciples to carry on his name – apart from his wife, and her career was ultimately disadvantaged by the narrowness of her clinical training and the lack of a surgical fellowship. Without wishing to detract from the achievements of the next generation, it must be pointed out that plastic surgery in New Zealand did not begin after the Second World War with Jack Manchester and Frank Hutter as popularly believed. It is perhaps sad to note that after almost 50 years of living in the Antipodes, Pickerill still felt like an exile. After his death, Cecily and their daughter Margaret carried his ashes back to England and scattered them from a bridge at Holme Lacy into the River Wye near Hereford where he was born.[1]

McIndoe

After the war the famous partnership of Gillies, McIndoe and Mowlem was wound up. The junior partners were no longer prepared to do most of the work without a corresponding share of the profits, and McIndoe, like most of his contemporaries, had finished the war in a relatively poor financial position. With the election of a Labour government in 1945 that was committed to the introduction of a national health service, he concentrated on building up his civilian practice (his specialty was the 'McIndoe nose') and became increasingly involved in medical politics. He was elected to the council of the Royal College of Surgeons of England in 1948 (as chairman of the finance committee he was reputed to have raised over £2.5 million for the college), was made vice-president in 1957, and had designs on the presidency, due to become vacant in 1960. As Lord Porritt wrote, 'By a strange twist of fate the two most favoured candidates were two New Zealanders, Archie and I. I had told him that if it came to a choice, I would prefer to step down.'[2] In the event, Porritt was not required to test his resolve – McIndoe died three months before the election and Porritt was chosen as president by the College Council. Arthur Porritt, in addition to being a distinguished surgeon, was the 100-metres bronze medallist at the 1924 Olympic Games in Paris behind Harold Abrahams (GB) and Jackson

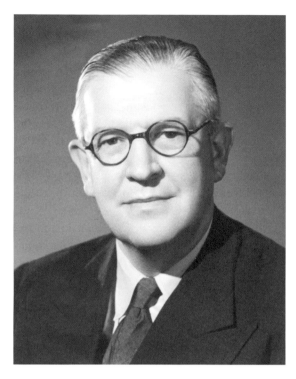

FIGURE 12.2. *Sir Archibald Hector McIndoe with trademark horn-rimmed spectacles. (Courtesy of the Antony Wallace Collection, BAPRAS)*

Scholtz (US), in a race immortalised in the film *Chariots of Fire*. (Many who were familiar with the story were puzzled to find that, unlike Abrahams and Scholtz, Porritt was portrayed by a fictional character by the name of 'Tom Watson'. Apparently this was due to that most elusive of traits in a surgeon – a sense of modesty.)

McIndoe was appointed CBE in 1944, knighted in 1947 and received numerous foreign decorations. He was a founder member of the British Association of Plastic Surgeons, and the association's third president in 1949. Unfortunately, the years of unrelenting work had taken their toll: on 11 April 1960 he died of a heart attack in his sleep at his home, 84 Albion Gate, London, aged just 59. His ashes were buried at the RAF church of St Clement Danes in the Strand – a unique honour for a civilian. An indication of how successful his private practice had been is that on his death his estate was worth £142,901 – a prodigious sum

of money for the time, given the punitive rates of personal taxation introduced by the postwar Labour government.

McIndoe's extraordinary career was attributable to a combination of factors. He was clearly ambitious, determined to get what he wanted even if it meant treading on other people's toes, and had an infinite capacity for hard work. More importantly, he was a first-class surgeon, an outstanding administrator and a powerful personality – so powerful that, as Richard Battle has pointed out, there was no share of the limelight even for his immediate colleagues.[3] While this is unlikely to have been intentional, one hopes the present narrative has shed some light on their contributions to the wartime success story of East Grinstead. McIndoe's enduring legacy is the Blond McIndoe Research Foundation at the Queen Victoria Hospital, East Grinstead, and indeed the continued survival of the hospital itself.

Gillies

As the war came to a close, Gillies' colleagues were surprised to find he could not afford to retire. During the war his private practice had all but vanished, and with no partners willing to work for him while he went fishing or played golf, he was left with little choice. He was not a saver and had made no plans for his eventual retirement, so he was obliged to continue working until shortly before his death. In 1947, at the age of 65, he was made Emeritus Consultant to the South-West Metropolitan Regional Hospital Board and allowed to continue his clinical commitment to the Plastic and Jaw Unit at Rooksdown House – but on a non-salaried basis – and on attaining the age of 70 he was informed that his appointment was to be terminated on 17 June 1952.

The formation of a British Association of Plastic Surgeons – an idea that Gillies had proposed at a meeting at Hill End Hospital in 1944 – came to fruition in 1946. Thirty-six surgeons attended the first meeting and elected Gillies president, crowning his pioneering work of thirty years. There was further recognition from the Royal College of Surgeons of England in its president Sir Alfred Webb-Johnson's foreword to the first issue of the

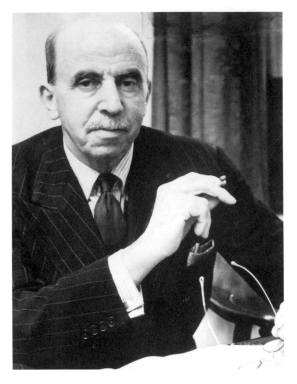

FIGURE 12.3. *Sir Harold Delf Gillies at his Harley Street consulting rooms in 1946 with ubiquitous cigarette.*

(Courtesy of the Antony Wallace Collection, BAPRAS)

British Journal of Plastic Surgery. Plastic surgery had proved its worth and could no longer be regarded as a Cinderella specialty.

During these postwar years, in addition to continuing to train surgeons from around the globe at Rooksdown, Gillies also fulfilled the role of roving ambassador and distinguished elder statesman of plastic surgery, touring the world giving lectures and consultations and performing operations. Always the innovator, in 1946 he found an unexpected use for the tubed pedicle when he performed the first ever female-to-male sex reassignment surgery on Laura/Michael Dillon, a Dublin medical student; and in 1951 he carried out the first male-to-female transgender surgery in the United Kingdom on Robert/Roberta Cowell, a former Spitfire pilot and racing-car driver.

Gillies' second mammoth autobiographical work, *The Principles and Art of Plastic Surgery*,

written in association with the American surgeon Ralph Millard, was published in 1957. It was peppered with amusing asides, anecdotes, advice and cartoons from a man who never let the serious subject of plastic surgery interfere with his sense of humour or the absurd. He enjoyed being the centre of attention and at times could be an exasperating friend and colleague, with a fondness for schoolboy practical jokes. These included turning up to functions in disguise, or disappearing under the table at formal dinners where he was the principal guest, just as the chairman was about to propose his health. He also had no concept of punctuality and was famous for being late, particularly for afternoon operating sessions after a long lunch; on one memorable occasion he turned up exactly one day late for his operating list at Saint Andrew's Hospital, Dollis Hill, and was furious to find no one still waiting for him.[4] Despite being loved and admired by his colleagues, it seems likely his unpredictable behaviour at occasions that demanded strictly correct behaviour was the reason his ambition to be elected to the council of the Royal College of Surgeons of England remained unfulfilled.[5]

On 3 August 1960, after undertaking a major operation on a girl of 18 whose right leg had been shattered in an accident, Gillies suffered a slight cerebral thrombosis and was advised not to operate again. Predictably he turned out to be a difficult patient. He died at the London Clinic, 20 Devonshire Place, Marylebone, on the evening of 10 September 1960, aged 78. His estate was assessed by probate at just £21,161[6] – and this was a man who between the wars had been earning an estimated £30,000 per annum.

Of the New Zealand-born trio of Gillies, McIndoe and Mowlem, Gillies was the only one to revisit his homeland – he returned for the first time in 51 years in 1956, at the age of 73. One reason was to present three papers at the annual congress of the Royal Australasian College of Surgeons in Christchurch. Another was 'to smell the New Zealand bush on a wet day … I want to hear the tui, catch a brown trout, do a little painting, and perhaps play three or four holes of golf. And I want to see the pohutukawas in full bloom.'[7]

Mowlem

After the war, Mowlem became an NHS consultant and returned to private practice at the London Clinic, as well as serving as adviser in plastic surgery to the Ministry of Health. When the Hill End unit moved to Mount Vernon Hospital in 1953 Mowlem transferred his appointment while retaining his post at the Middlesex Hospital, where he had been consulting plastic surgeon since 1936.[8] In 1950 he became the fourth president of the British Association of Plastic Surgeons, after Gillies, Kilner and McIndoe, and in 1959 he was elected president of the association for a second term in order to preside over the International Congress in Plastic Surgery in London. In addition to his Hunterian Professorship from the Royal College of Surgeons of England, his contributions to the specialty were recognised internationally by the award of an honorary Doctorate of Science by Trinity College in Hartford, Connecticut, and an honorary fellowship of the American Society of Plastic and Reconstructive Surgeons.

Mowlem was regarded as an artist and craftsman in handling live tissues. He had a deep concern for patients, particularly those with serious diseases as a result of malignancy and its treatment, and he had to be convinced there were valid reasons for undertaking 'cosmetic' surgery.[9] At the outbreak of war (Sir) James Paterson Ross (1895–1980), Professor of Surgery at St Bartholomew's Hospital, moved with his unit to Hill End, and in 1948 paid tribute to the stimulus and inspiration provided by Mowlem and the EMS plastic surgery unit to him and his general surgical colleagues.[10] Mowlem was described by RLG Dawson as being exacting, a superb surgeon and not one to suffer fools gladly – also not above telling his colleagues to take a patient back to the operating theatre if he was not satisfied with the result:[11]

> *Rainsford always knew exactly where he was going. He drove his Bentley and Aston Martin rapidly, but in a controlled way. He operated rapidly, but with absolute control of all his incisions and manipulations. He made his plans and kept to them. He was the fastest surgeon that I have*

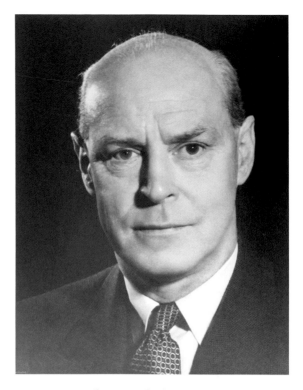

FIGURE 12.4. *Arthur Rainsford Mowlem. (Courtesy of the Antony Wallace Collection, BAPRAS)*

> *known, and like many good and fast surgeons, his infection rate was very low.*[12]

In 1963 Mowlem took early retirement, sold his house at Great Missenden, Buckinghamshire, and moved to Spain, where he bought La Morena, a villa in Mijas, Andalusia. He and his wife Margaret lived quietly there with five servants, including two to look after the garden.

It has often been asked why Mowlem retired at the age of 60. He was a strong individualist and did not take kindly to the bureaucracy, red tape and conditions surrounding the NHS. When the opportunity arose he chose early and complete retirement; the loss of two of his former partners in the space of six months in 1960 probably helped make up his mind, and it seems unlikely he needed the money. He had also been involved in an unfortunate sequence of events related to a case brought before the GMC by a malcontent in an allied branch of the profession, naming the leaders of the British Association of Plastic Surgery at the time. The case was dismissed with a reprimand to the defendants, but he was upset by the whole business.[13]

Mowlem was a quiet, thoughtful man who did not have the extrovert personality of Gillies or McIndoe, and, like Pickerill, did not appear to have been blessed with that most priceless of gifts – a sense of humour. He died on 5 February 1986 at home in Andalusia at the age of 83. In 1990 the residue of the Mowlem estate, dating back to Durand de Moulham and William the Conqueror, was gifted to the town of Swanage.[14]

Postscript

What can one learn from this tale? First, the enormous energy, ambition and spirit shown by the early Scottish settlers of Dunedin, who carved a city out of the wilderness and within 21 years had founded the first university in New Zealand with a medical and a dental school.

Second, the impact that war has had on the development of surgery. War provides the catalyst for change in many fields, and the treatment of battlefield casualties has always provided an important impetus for the advancement of medical knowledge dating back to Hippocrates of Kos (ca 460–370 BC) ('War is the only proper school for a surgeon'), Ambroise Paré (1510–1590) and John Hunter (1728–1793). War enables a lifetime's surgical experience to be telescoped into a few months, and information gained during the First World War, particularly in neurosurgery, orthopaedics and maxillofacial surgery, had an enormous impact on later civilian practice. Indeed, war could be seen as the catalyst for the greatest advance of them all, when Fleming returned to St Mary's Hospital from No 13 General in Boulogne, continued his work on the bacteriology of wound infection and in his search for natural anti-bacterial agents discovered penicillin.

And third, the role that luck plays in all our lives and the development of most professional careers. It helps to be in the right place at the right time. As Sister Catherine Black observed[15] (pp. 84–85):

The Cambridge Hospital at Aldershot, like most military hospitals in those early days of the War, was in a state of confusion … The surgeons had for the most part been drafted to casualty clearing stations, and their places taken by elderly general practitioners unfit for active service, and young men who had only recently qualified, fresh from walking the hospitals. In every hospital in the country was the same rather motley crowd, yet out of it emerged some of the foremost doctors and surgeons of our time and some of the greatest medical discoveries, for the Great War in which millions of lives were sacrificed was indirectly responsible for saving millions of others. It revolutionized both medicine and surgery. In its desperate emergencies experiments which would never even have appeared possible in time of peace were tried out … and tried out successfully … and the young and unknown men who would ordinarily have been buried in small general practices were given their opportunity.

One of them was Harold Gillies, the man who put plastic surgery on the map and made life worth living again for thousands of despairing war-disfigured men. Now he has one of the most fashionable practices in Europe, for the knowledge gained in repairing the frightful ravages of war has raised the plastic surgeon's work to a new level, and made it as important in its own way as any other branch of surgery.

A good deal has been written about the dominant position occupied by surgeons from the dominions and particularly New Zealand in the establishment of plastic surgery, with much emphasis being placed on the colonial temperament and willingness to experiment. I think the reason is altogether rather more prosaic. The key figure in the story is unquestionably Gillies, one of the beneficiaries of the wartime assignment of ENT surgeons to treat gunshot wounds of the face that so captured his imagination. Had fate not intervened in the guise of a sick Welsh surgical registrar, Mowlem would not have been asked to look after Gillies' patients at the Hammersmith Hospital and returned to Auckland and general surgical practice as he had originally planned. And had McIndoe not decided to resign his position at the Mayo Clinic and take his chances on a surgical career in London on the strength of a conversation with Lord Moynihan, he would in all likelihood have remained an abdominal surgeon, albeit a very distinguished one. Luckily for McIndoe and the RAF, he happened to be Gillies' cousin, and Gillies persuaded him otherwise. The irony, of course, is that with the wartime publicity surrounding East Grinstead and the Guinea Pig Club, a steady stream of books and, more recently, a series of television documentaries (including the 1991 six-part TV mini-series *A Perfect Hero* based on the story of Hillary),[16] it is the name of McIndoe, not Gillies, that is synonymous with plastic surgery in the mind of the public both in the United Kingdom and in New Zealand.

APPENDIX I

Dramatis personae

(Marked in text with a †)

Albee, Fred Houdlette (1876–1945) MD, FACS was born in Alna, Maine, on 13 April 1876 and educated at Bowdoin College and Harvard Medical School. After internship at Massachusetts General Hospital he specialised in orthopaedic surgery. Albee pioneered the routine use of bone-grafting (applying the principles learned from Grandfather Houdlette while helping him to graft fruit trees), particularly the use of autogenous bone from the tibia for spinal fusion and reconstructing fractured limbs. Inventor of the 'Albee Bone Mill', a power-driven saw which greatly reduced operating time. During the summer of 1916 he operated at the military hospital at Ris-Orangis and other centres in France, returning to the US to open US Hospital Number 3 at Colonia, New Jersey, for rehabilitating the wounded. He died on 15 February 1945. (With acknowledgements to: FH Albee (1943), *A Surgeon's Fight to Rebuild Men: An Autobiography*, EP Dutton and Co, New York)

Allaway, Joseph John (1922–2009) was born in Worcester on 15 August 1922. He joined the RAF in January 1941 and trained as a wireless operator/gunner. He flew on 27 operational flights with No 521 Squadron from RAF Docking, Norfolk until 10 October 1943, when the Hampden in which he was a crew member was shot down by a Junkers Ju 88 intruder as it was about to land and crashed in flames. Allaway and his skipper, Flight Lieutenant Jack Maxwell RCAF, were the only survivors. He was taken to RAF Ely where he spent six months before

being transferred to East Grinstead; after a long series of operations to reconstruct his face and hands he was discharged in August 1947. On his return to civilian life he took over the Faraday Avenue Stores and Post Office in Birmingham, before moving into the hotel business, and following the death of Edward Blacksell served as welfare officer of the Guinea Pig Club. He died on 12 September 2009. (With thanks to Bob Marchant and the Queen Victoria Hospital, East Grinstead)

Barron, John Netterville (1911–1992) MB ChB, MS (S'hampton), FRCS (Edin & Eng) was born on 23 December 1911 in Napier. He was educated at Wanganui Collegiate School and the University of Otago Medical School, graduating MB ChB (NZ) in 1936. He arrived in England in 1938, and during the Second World War joined Mowlem at Hill End and then Gillies at Rooksdown House. In 1949 he founded the Wessex Regional Plastic and Maxillofacial Surgery Centre, Odstock Hospital, Salisbury. He received professional honours including presidency of the BAPS and the Yugoslav Flag with Golden Wreath, Yugoslavia's highest honour. In 1981 Barron edited the two-volume *Operative Plastic and Reconstructive Surgery* with MN Saad. He died on 7 July 1991. (With acknowledgements to the 1992 obituary by Magdy N Saad in the *British Journal of Plastic Surgery*)

Battle, Richard John Vulliamy (1907–1982) MBE, MA, MChir (Cantab), FRCS (Eng) was born on 21

January 1907. He was educated at Gresham's School, Norfolk, Trinity College, Cambridge (BA 1928; MChir 1935) and St Thomas' Hospital (MRCS, LRCP 1931). A member of the Territorial Army before the war, he served with the RAMC in France (1939–40) and Italy (1943–46), retiring with the rank of lieutenant-colonel. Postwar he was consultant plastic surgeon to St Thomas' and several other hospitals in London, and to the British Army (1955–71), and was twice elected president of the BAPS (1952 and 1967). In 1964 he published *Plastic Surgery* and in 1970 was recipient of the Gillies' Gold Medal. He died on 26 May 1982. (With acknowledgements to the obituary in the *British Medical Journal*)

Blacksell, James Edward (1912–1987) MBE was born in Sheffield, Yorkshire. He was educated at Torquay Grammar School and the University of Reading where he read geography, becoming an assistant schoolmaster. In 1939, after being turned down on medical grounds by the Royal Navy, he was accepted by the RAF as a physical training instructor. Posted to QVH, where he was quickly dubbed 'Blackie', he became welfare officer to the Guinea Pigs, a role he fulfilled in one way or another for the rest of his life. After the war he became headmaster of Barnstable Boys' Secondary Modern School and devoted much of his time to the arts, including the theatre, and was a founder and director of the English Stage Company. He died on 16 October 1987 aged 75. (With acknowledgements to the obituary by Tom Gleave entitled 'Tribute to Blackie' that appeared in the July 1988 *Guinea Pig* magazine)

Blair, Vilray Papin (1871–1955) AM, MD, FACS was born in St Louis, Missouri on 15 June 1871, a descendant of some of the original French founders of St Louis. He was educated at Christian Brothers College (AB, 1890; AM, 1894) and Washington University School of Medicine (MD, 1893) and became Professor of Oral Surgery in the School of Dentistry and Associate in Surgery in the School of Medicine, Washington University. In 1912 he published *Surgery and Diseases of the Mouth and Jaws*, and from February 1918 to June 1919 served as chief consultant in maxillofacial surgery to the AEF in France. On his return to St Louis, Blair founded one of the foremost training programmes for plastic and reconstructive surgery in the US, and was the

driving force behind the formation of the American Board of Plastic Surgery. He died on 24 November 1955. (With acknowledgements to JP Webster (1956), 'In memoriam: Vilray Papin Blair 1871–1955', *Plastic and Reconstructive Surgery* 40, pp. 1144–47)

Buxton, John Leycester Dudley (1893–1980) LDS, LMSSA, FDSRCS (Eng) was born on 20 January 1893 in Hertfordshire, England. He was educated at University College Hospital and the Royal Dental Hospital, London, and obtained the LDSRCS (Eng) in 1915 and the LMSSA in 1917. He was the author of *Handbook of Mechanical Dentistry* (1921) and two volumes in the *Outline of Dental Surgery* series published in 1927: *Dental Pathology* (vol VII) and *Dental Surgery* (vol IX). He practised dentistry at 38 Harley Street and was honorary dental surgeon at the Royal Dental Hospital and UCH. In 1939, together with Rainsford Mowlem, Buxton established the EMS Maxillofacial Unit at Hill End. In retirement he toured the world as a ship's surgeon. (With acknowledgements to Glyn Wreakes and James Moss in response to a letter in the *British Dental Journal*)

Capka, Josef (1916–1973) DFM, Croix de Guerre, Czech War Cross was born in Olomouc, near Brno in 1916. After leaving school at 15 he became an electrical apprentice and was accepted for training as a pilot in the Czech Air Force. Following the German occupation of Czechoslovakia he fled to Poland and after their surrender joined the French Foreign Legion. In 1940 he reached England and was posted to the RAF's all-Czech 311 Squadron, flying 56 bombing missions in Wellingtons. In 1941 he was awarded the DFM and Czech War Cross and commissioned as a pilot officer. In 1944 during a suspected 'friendly-fire' incident he was blinded in his left eye and sent to East Grinstead, where his left orbit was reconstructed. After the war Capka returned to Czechoslovakia, but following the communist coup in 1948 was charged with high treason and sentenced to 10 years in prison. He was released in May 1957, and rejoined his wife in the UK. His inhumane treatment in prison, however, had undermined his health and he died in 1973 at the age of 57. (With acknowledgements to Vítek Formánek (1998), *The Stories of Brave Guinea Pigs*, J&HK Publishing, Hailsham, East Sussex)

Clarkson, Patrick Wensley (1911–1969) MBE, MB (Lond), FRCS (Eng) was born in New Zealand. He was educated at Christ's College in Christchurch, the University of Edinburgh Medical School and Guy's Hospital, where he was awarded the Gold Medal in both medicine and surgery. As a student he was also the United Hospitals heavyweight boxing champion. He joined the RAMC in 1940, and after training with Sir Harold Gillies was appointed surgical specialist and officer commanding MFU No 4 in Algiers and Italy; for his wartime service he was awarded the MBE. After the war he returned to Guy's in charge of the accident services. He died on 28 December 1969 at the age of 58. (With acknowledgements to the obituary in *The Lancet*)

Cleminson, Frederick John (1878–1943) MA, MChir, FRCS (Eng) was born in Hull. He was educated at Kingswood School in Bath, and Gonville and Caius College, Cambridge (BA, 1901). After clinical training at University College Hospital he took the MB, BChir (Cantab) in 1909 and MChir in 1913 and after several clinical posts at UCH was a clinical assistant in ENT at the Hospital for Sick Children, Great Ormond Street. During the First World War he served in Salonika and in France with Valadier's unit at No 83 General Hospital, Wimereux, and later specialised in otolaryngology at the Middlesex Hospital. He died of pneumonia on 21 August 1943. (With acknowledgements to the obituary in the *British Medical Journal*, 4 September 1943, p. 315)

Cole, Herbert Robert (1890–1962) was born on the Isle of Wight, England, 22 September 1890. In 1906 the Coles immigrated to New Zealand and settled in Dunedin where his father Reuben established an art studio at Clarence House, 2 Scotland Street. Herbert later joined his father as a teacher of drawing and painting. In 1916 he left for Europe as a sub-lieutenant with the Motor Boat Patrol Service, but, following illness and convalescence at No 1 NZ General Hospital in Hampshire, was transferred to the NZ Section at Sidcup as staff artist with the rank of sergeant. He returned with the unit to Dunedin and in the 1930s moved to Auckland, where he painted under the improbable alias of *Rix Carlton*, and was best known as a marine artist working mainly in watercolours and as a muralist. He died in Auckland on 29 July 1962. (With acknowledgements to

Donald Gordon, Ross Grimmett, Ralph Body, Lyndal Kilgour and Hugh Tohill)

Converse, John Marquis (1909–1981) AB, MD was born in San Francisco on 29 September 1909 and educated at the Lycée Janson de Sailly (AB, 1928) and the University of Paris (MD, 1935). He trained in maxillofacial surgery with Kazanjian at Massachusetts General and during the Second World War with Gillies at Park Prewitt, later treating French troops in North Africa and after the liberation in Paris. After the war he returned to New York and established a plastic surgery unit at Bellevue Hospital, and in 1963 the Institute of Reconstructive Plastic Surgery at New York University, where many well-known plastic and craniofacial residents were trained. In 1949 he co-authored *The Surgical Treatment of Facial Injuries* with Kazanjian. He died in Southampton, New York, on 31 January 1981. (With acknowledgements to 'John Marquis Converse 1909–1981', *Annals of Plastic Surgery* 8, pp. 342–58)

Davies, Russell Maddox (1914–1991) MRCS, LRCP, FFARCS (Eng), DA was born at Ponthir, Monmouthshire, in Wales on 6 June 1914. He was educated at Newport High School, King's College London and the Westminster Hospital. He joined QVH in 1940 as assistant anaesthetist to John Hunter, and when the Guinea Pig Club was founded in 1941 served on the founding committee. After the war he declined a partnership in private practice with McIndoe, being committed to the NHS, and remained at East Grinstead until his retirement in 1974. He died in 1991 aged 77, the last surviving member of the Guinea Pig Club medical and welfare committee of McIndoe, Blacksell and Davies. (With acknowledgements to Bob Marchant and the *Guinea Pig* magazine)

Davis, John Staige (1872–1946) MD, FACS was born in Norfolk, Virginia, on 15 January 1872. He was educated at Yale University (AB, 1895) and Johns Hopkins University (MD, 1899). Early in his career he limited his practice to plastic surgery, publishing a total of 78 papers; his first in 1907 concerned scar contracture following a burn, and its treatment by a full-thickness skin graft. In 1919 he published the first modern textbook on plastic surgery entitled *Plastic Surgery: Its principles and practice*. Staige

Davis was the first chairman of the American Board of Plastic Surgery (1938) and president of the American Association of Plastic Surgeons (1946). He died in Baltimore, Maryland, on 23 December 1946. (With acknowledgements to: WB Davis (1978), 'The Life of John Staige Davis, MD', *Plastic and Reconstructive Surgery* 62, pp. 368–78.)

Doe, Robert Francis Thomas (1920–2010) DSO, DFC & Bar was born in Reigate, Surrey, on 10 March 1920. Educated at Leatherhead School, he left at 14 and became an office boy at the *News of the World*. In 1937 he joined the RAF Volunteer Reserve and was accepted for pilot training, going solo after 9¾ hours. In March 1939 he passed the entrance exams for a short service commission and was sent to the Flying Training School at Redhill. In November 1939 he was posted to 234 Squadron flying Spitfires, and became one of the most successful RAF fighter pilots in the Battle of Britain, with 14 kills and two shared. On 22 October 1940 he was awarded the DFC and a month later a Bar. In January 1941, during an attempt to land at RAF Warmwell, he crashed, smashing his face, and was taken to Rooksdown House where he had 22 operations under Sir Harold Gillies. In 1945 he was awarded the Indian DSO following service in Burma with the Indian Air Force, one of only two men to be so honoured. He died on 21 February 2010 aged 89. (With acknowledgements to: Bob Doe (1999), *Fighter Pilot: The story of one of the few*, CCB Associates, Selsdon, Surrey)

Fickling, Benjamin William (1909–2007) CBE, FDSRCS, FRCS (Eng) was educated at Framlingham College, Suffolk, the Royal Dental Hospital (LDSRCS, 1932) and St George's Hospital Medical School (MRCS, LRCP, 1934). At the outbreak of the Second World War he was drafted into the EMS at St George's Hospital during the Blitz and at Hill End Hospital. After the war he played an important role in the development of oral and maxillofacial surgery in the UK as an independent specialty. Awarded the FDS by the newly established Faculty of Dental Surgery of the RCSEng in 1947, he was elected to the Board of Faculty in 1957, serving as dean from 1968 to 1971, and in 1973 was honoured with the CBE for services to dental surgery. He died on 27 January 2007. (With acknowledgements to the *British Dental Journal*)

Gleave, Thomas Percy (1908–1993) CBE, US Legion of Merit, was born in Liverpool on 6 September 1909 and educated at Westminster High School and Liverpool Collegiate School. He learned to fly in 1929, joined the RAF in 1930 and when war was declared was Fighter Command's Bomber Liaison Officer. Appointed supernumerary commanding officer of 253 Squadron in June 1940, on 31 August 1940 during an attack on a formation of Junkers Ju 88 bombers, he heard a 'click' and the plane blew up. Badly burned, he became one of the first pilots to receive treatment at QVH. With skin grafts to his face and legs, and a new nose, he returned to operations within a year as commanding officer of RAF Manston in Kent, and ended the war as Chief of Air Plans at SHAEF (Supreme Headquarters Allied Expeditionary Force). He died in hospital at Ascot near his home in Bray, Berkshire, on 12 June 1993. Tom Gleave was the first and only Chief Guinea Pig. (Information kindly provided by Angela Lodge, Tom Gleave's daughter, and his obituary in *The Times*)

Harding, John Robert (1919–2002) DFC was born in London, Ontario. He served as a navigator with RAF Bomber Command from the end of 1942 to mid-1944, rising from the rank of sergeant to flight lieutenant. He completed two tours of operations on Lancasters with 103 (Elsham Wolds) and 550 (North Killingholme) Squadrons and was awarded the DFC. In January 1945 he was a member of the crew of a DC-3 (Dakota) of 168 Squadron RCAF which crashed on take-off at Biggin Hill in Kent. Badly burned, he was treated first at Orpington and then moved to the Canadian wing at East Grinstead. In 1946 Harding joined Air Canada, serving for 30 years as a navigator on trans-Atlantic and Caribbean routes. He died on 15 May 2002. (With acknowledgements to: John Harding (1988), *The Dancin' Navigator*, Asterisk Communications, Guelph, Ontario, and the *Guinea Pig* magazine)

Hett, Geoffrey Seccombe (1878–1949) MB, FRCS (Eng) was born on 14 August 1878 in Bayswater, London. He was educated at St Paul's School, University College London and University College Hospital. He qualified MRCS, LRCP in 1903, MB BS (Lond) the following year and in 1908 FRCS. He undertook postgraduate study at several European centres and in 1912 was appointed assistant surgeon in the ENT department at UCH. During the First World War he served in the British and French Red Cross and later with the RAMC. He was the officer-in-charge of the Middleton Park Red Cross Hospital for head injuries and joined Gillies and the British Section at Sidcup in 1917. After the war he returned to UCH and private practice and died in London on 3 May 1949. (With acknowledgements to: *Plarr's Lives of the Fellows*, Royal College of Surgeons of England)

Hillary, Richard Hope (1919–1943) was born in Sydney on 20 April 1919 and arrived in England aged three when his father, an Australian government official, was posted to London. He was educated at Shrewsbury School and Trinity College, Oxford, where he read PPE (philosophy, politics and economics) before changing to modern history, stroked the Trinity VIII to Head of the River (1938–39) and joined the University Air Squadron. During the Battle of Britain Hillary was credited with five enemy aircraft until being shot down on 3 September 1940. After being rescued from the Channel, he spent three months at the Royal Masonic Hospital in London before being transferred to East Grinstead. In 1941 he went to the USA on a speaking tour and while there wrote *The Last Enemy*. He returned to operational flying against the wishes of McIndoe, and on 8 January 1943, while on a night flying exercise, crashed his Bristol Blenheim, killing himself and his radio operator, Cambridge-educated Wilfred Fison. (With acknowledgements to: Richard Hillary (1942), *The Last Enemy*, Macmillan & Co Ltd, London; Lovat Dickson (1950), *Richard Hillary*, Macmillan & Co Ltd, London)

Hodgkinson, Colin Gerald Shaw (1920–1996) was born at Wells, Somerset, on 11 February 1920. He was educated at Pangbourne Nautical College, Berkshire, and in 1938 was accepted for pilot training as a midshipman in the Fleet Air Arm. After training on the aircraft carrier *Courageous*, while practising blind flying he collided with another aircraft and crashed, killing his instructor and sustaining injuries that resulted in both legs being amputated. In 1940 McIndoe had Hodgkinson transferred to QVH and used him to successfully challenge the 90-day rule. By 1942, equipped with 'tin legs', he was flying Spitfires on bomber escorts as a PO with the RAF and in 1943 joined 611 Squadron at RAF Coltishall, Norfolk. However, while he was on high-altitude

weather reconnaissance his oxygen failed and he crashed in France, becoming a POW. After 10 months Hodgkinson was repatriated, and following further surgery ended the war flying with a ferry unit at Bristol. (With acknowledgements to the *Daily Telegraph*)

Hunter, John Truscott (1898–1953) MRCS, LRCP, FFARCS (Eng), DA was born on 4 September 1898. He was educated at St Bartholomew's Hospital (MRCS, LRCP, 1925) and after some years in general practice, specialised in anaesthesia. As an anaesthetist he was remarkably successful, above all at QVH where he was appointed consultant anaesthetist in 1939 and together with Jill Mullins formed part of McIndoe's surgical team. He obtained the Diploma of Anaesthetics in 1944 and was elected a Fellow of the newly formed Faculty of Anaesthetists of the RCSEng in 1948. Hunter was a large, jovial man whose geniality and generosity were legendary; he enjoyed the good life but his health was undermined by diabetes and he died on 9 August 1953 at the age of 54. (With acknowledgements to *The Lancet*; the *Guinea Pig* magazine)

Hunter, Sir Thomas Anderson (1863–1958) KBE was born in Dunedin on 10 February 1863 and educated at Otago Boys' High School. He trained as a pupil-dentist with Alfred Boot in Dunedin and became registered in 1881. Politically astute, Hunter was influential in the formation of (1) the NZDA in 1905 (he was its second president), (2) the Dental School in 1907, (3) the NZDC (Director 1916–30), and (4) the School Dental Service in 1920. He was knighted in 1946 for services to dentistry. A keen sportsman, he played rugby for the Union Club in Dunedin and captained the Otago provincial side of 1887. He died at Heretaunga near Wellington on 29 December 1958. (With acknowledgements to: TV Anson (1966), 'Hunter, Sir Thomas Anderson (1863–1958), Dentist, public health administrator', in *An Encyclopaedia of New Zealand*, vol 1, ed. AH McLintock. RE Owen, Government Printer, Wellington)

Ivy, Robert Henry (1881–1974) DDS, MD, ScD, FACS was an influential figure in the development of plastic surgery in the US. He was born in Southport, Lancashire, on 21 May 1881 and educated at Emanuel School on Wandsworth Common and the University of Pennsylvania (DDS, 1902;

MD, 1907). In 1917 he was appointed assistant to Vilray Blair in the Office of the Surgeon-General and in 1918 posted to Base Hospital No 115 at Vichy in France. On his return to Philadelphia, Ivy established a plastic surgery training programme at the University of Pennsylvania, which trained over 35 residents. He died at Skytop, Pennsylvania, on 21 June 1974. Contrary to widespread belief, there is no record of Ivy ever having been stationed at the Queen's Hospital, Sidcup. (With acknowledgements to: RH Ivy (1962), *A Link with the Past*, Williams & Wilkins Co, Baltimore)

Kazanjian, Varaztad Hovannes (1879–1974) CMG, DMD, MD was born in the city of Erzincan in Turkish Armenia on 18 March 1879. At the age of 16 he was smuggled out of the country to escape the Armenian genocide by the Ottoman Turks and settled in Worcester, Massachusetts, where he worked for several years in a wire mill. He took evening classes and at 22 passed the entrance exam to Harvard Dental School, and after graduating DMD in 1905 went into practice. He served with the Harvard Surgical Unit at Dannes-Camier 1915–19 and was awarded the CMG. After graduating MD from Harvard in 1921, he became Head of Plastic Surgery at the Massachusetts Eye and Ear Infirmary, Massachusetts General Hospital, Professor of Clinical Oral Surgery, and in 1941 Harvard's first Professor of Plastic Surgery. In 1949 he published *The Surgical Treatment of Facial Injurie*s with JM Converse. Kazanjian's life was an extraordinary immigrant success story, a personification of the American dream. (With acknowledgements to: H Martin Deranian (2007), *Miracle Man of the Western Front*, Chandler House Press, Worcester, Massachusetts)

Kelsey Fry, Sir William (1889–1963) CBE, MC, MDS, DSc, FRCS, FDSRCS was born on 18 March 1889 and educated at Hurstpierpoint College in West Sussex and Guy's Hospital, London, qualifying MRCS, LRCP (1912) and LDSRCS (1913). In 1914 he joined the RAMC, serving as RMO to the 1st Battalion, Royal Welch Fusiliers, and was invalided home in 1916 having been awarded the MC at the Battle of Festubert. Subsequently he was appointed to the Cambridge Hospital, Aldershot, and then to the Queen's Hospital, Sidcup. During the Second World War Kelsey Fry was consultant dental surgeon

to the RAF at QVH, East Grinstead. After the war he was closely involved in establishing the Faculty of Dental Surgery of the RCSEng and elected its second dean (1950–53). Appointed CBE (1946) and KBE (1951), Kelsey Fry had a life-long passion for growing carnations for which he enjoyed a national reputation. (With acknowledgements to: MA Rushton (1963), 'Obituary: Sir William Kelsey Fry', *British Dental Journal* 115, pp. 422–23; FC Wilkinson (1963), 'In Memoriam: Sir William Kelsey Fry', *Annals of the Royal College of Surgeons of England* 33, pp. 390–92)

Kilner, Thomas Pomfret (1890–1964) was born in Manchester on 17 September 1890 and educated at Queen Elizabeth Grammar School, Blackburn, and the University of Manchester (MB ChB, 1912). During the First World War he served with the RAMC, first at a CCS in France and later at base hospitals, and in 1919 joined Gillies at Sidcup. At the outbreak of the Second World War Kilner was appointed first to Queen Mary's Hospital, Roehampton, and later to Stoke Mandeville Hospital, Buckinghamshire. In 1944 he was appointed Nuffield Professor of Plastic Surgery at the University of Oxford, an appointment he held until his retirement in 1956. His chief clinical interest was the treatment of cleft lip and palate and other congenital deformities. He died on 2 July 1964. (With acknowledgements to: RJV Battle (1964), 'Thomas Pomfret Kilner, CBE, DM, FRCS', *British Journal of Plastic Surgery* 17, pp. 330–34)

Kingcome, Charles Brian Fabris (1917–1994) DSO, DFC & Bar was born in Calcutta on 31 May 1917. He was educated at Bedford School and in 1936 won a place as an officer cadet at the RAF College at Cranwell. Soon after beginning pilot training, however, he received serious facial injuries when he crashed his car. Gillies and McIndoe straightened his nose, but more importantly corrected his diplopia and he was able to complete his training. He served with 92 Squadron during the Battle of Britain and later in Malta, North Africa and Italy with the Desert Air Force. By the end of the war his personal tally was eight enemy aircraft destroyed, three shared, five probable and 13 damaged, a number always thought by his fellow airmen to be an underestimate. He died on 14 February 1994. (With acknowledgements to: Brian Kingcome (1999), *A Willingness to Die*. Tempus Publishing Ltd, Stroud, Gloucestershire)

Lane, Sir William Arbuthnot (1856–1943) Bart, CB, Légion d'honneur, MB, MS (Lond), FRCS (Eng) was born at Fort George, near Inverness, on 4 July 1856, the son of an army doctor. After a somewhat peripatetic education he entered Guy's Hospital aged 16 in 1872 as a medical student; he was appointed full surgeon at Guy's in 1903 and was also a consultant surgeon at Great Ormond Street Hospital for Sick Children (1883–1916). At his peak he was regarded as one of the leading surgeons in England, and one whose operations a patient could be expected to survive. During the First World War he continued at Guy's as well as being consulting surgeon to the Aldershot Command, and helped organise the Queen's Hospital, Sidcup. After the war he retired from medicine to pursue other interests and died in London on 16 January 1943, aged 86. (With acknowledgements to: TB Layton (1956)*, Sir William Arbuthnot Lane*, E&S Livingstone Ltd, Edinburgh; AAG Morrice (2004), 'Lane, Sir William Arbuthnot, first Baronet (1856–1943), surgeon and health campaigner', in *DNB*, Oxford University Press)

Lindemann, August (1880–1970) MD was a surgeon who worked for Professor Dr Christian Bruhn (1868–1942), a dentist by training, who decided to open a clinic for the treatment of war injuries, Die Düsseldorfer Lazarette für Kieferveletzte (The Dusseldorf hospital for the facially injured), at his own expense. During the First World War the hospital had over 600 beds and Lindemann, who had experience of treating the facial injuries of miners in Essen, was encouraged by Bruhn to join him. In 1917 the clinic became the Westdeutsche Kieferklinik, part of the Medical Academy where dentistry and maxillofacial surgery were taught. In 1926 Lindemann was made Dozent (Reader) for 'Surgery of the Jaws and Face', the first person to receive such a title in Germany. He was later promoted to professor and was head of the Westdeutsche Kieferklinik 1935–50. (With acknowledgements to Dr Dirk Bister)

Lindsay, Sir Daryl (1889–1976) was born on 31 December 1889 into a distinguished family of artists and writers at Creswick, Victoria, and educated at Creswick Grammar School. He joined the Ballarat branch of the English, Scottish and Australian Bank, but left to become a jackeroo (farmhand). During the First World War he served in France as a driver

before his talent for drawing was noticed and he was posted as artist to the Australian Section at Sidcup, where he was befriended by Henry Tonks. Lindsay became keeper of prints (1939) and then director of the National Gallery of Victoria (1941–56). On retirement he was knighted for services to Australian art, and he died on 25 December 1976. (With acknowledgements to: B Smith (1986), 'Lindsay, Sir Ernest Daryl (1889–1976)', *Australian Dictionary of Biography*, vol 10, Melbourne University Press, pp. 106–15)

MacGregor, Alexander Brittan (1909–1965) MA, MD, BChir, FDSRCS (Eng) was born on 25 January 1909. He was educated at Marlborough College, Trinity Hall, Cambridge, and St Mary's Hospital, London (MB, BChir, (Cantab), MRCS, LRCP). He then studied dentistry part time at the Royal Dental Hospital while undertaking dental research for the MRC, qualified in 1936 and joined consulting dental staff at St Bartholomew's Hospital. Throughout the Second World War he served in the plastic and jaw unit at Hill End and on demobilisation continued at Bart's, Hill End and Royal Dental Hospitals. In 1953 he was invited to become Director of Dental Studies at the University of Birmingham, an appointment he held until his death. MacGregor was a member of the Board of the Faculty of Dental Surgery, RCSEng, and elected dean in 1962. He died suddenly at home on 12 January 1965 aged 55. (With acknowledgements to *The Times*)

Marshall, Angus McPhee (1892–1927) was born in Dunedin on 11 November 1892. He was educated at Waitaki Boys' High School, Oamaru (1905–10; *Dux,* 1909) and the University of Otago, graduating MB ChB in 1915. During the First World War he was a captain in the NZMC serving in Egypt and CCSs on the Western Front, before being appointed specialist anaesthetist to the NZ Section Sidcup (1918–19). From 1921 he was senior anaesthetist at Dunedin Hospital and lecturer at the Medical School. Marshall died on 31 July 1927 by his own hand from an overdose of hyoscine: a brilliant scholar, his premature death was a tragic loss to the medical profession and the development of anaesthesia in New Zealand. (Information kindly provided by Dr Basil Hutchinson of Auckland, Waitaki Boys' High School, and the NZ Defence Force Archives)

Morestin, Hippolyte (1869–1919) was born on 1 September 1869 at La Basse-Point, Martinique, in the Antilles. He studied medicine in Paris and submitted his doctoral thesis to the Faculté de Médicine in 1889. In 1914 he became chief of surgery at the Hôpital Saint-Louis, Paris, and during the First World War at the Hôpital Val-de-Grâce and Hôpital Rothschild, where he concentrated on treating the facially mutilated. Although world famous during his lifetime, he has largely been forgotten. Morestin wrote an astonishing 634 medical articles, but since they were published in French the English-speaking world did not read them, and he trained no disciples. Morestin, a Creole, was a controversial character with a difficult and fiery temperament. He died from pneumonia during the influenza epidemic of 1919. (With acknowledgements to: JP Lalardrie (1972), 'Hippolyte Morestin 1869–1919', *British Journal of Plastic Surgery* 25, pp. 39–41; BO Rogers (1982), 'Hippolyte Morestin (1869–1919), Part I: A brief biography', *Aesthetic Plastic Surgery* 6, pp. 141–47)

Newland, Sir Henry Simpson (1873–1969) Kt, CBE, DSO, MB, MS, FRCS (Eng), FRACS was born in Adelaide on 24 November 1873. He was educated at St Peter's College and the University of Adelaide, graduating MB ChB in 1896. After further study in London and passing the FRCS (Eng) in 1899, he returned to Adelaide. During the First World War he served with the AAMC at Gallipoli, Ypres and Passchendaele and in 1917 was awarded the DSO and appointed head of the Australian Section at Sidcup (CBE, 1919). After the war he returned to Adelaide and practice as a general surgeon. Knighted in 1928, Newland was an energetic medical politician active in the BMA and the foundation of the Royal Australasian College of Surgeons in 1927, serving as its second president 1929–34. He died on 13 November 1969. (With acknowledgements to: N Hicks, E Leopold (1988), 'Newland, Sir Henry Simpson (1873–1969)', *Australian Dictionary of Biography*, vol 11, Melbourne University Press, pp. 8–9)

Orpen, Diana 'Dickie' (1914–2008) was a daughter of the Irish portrait painter Sir William Orpen (1878–1931). At the age of 15 she began studying at the Slade School of Art under the direction of Henry Tonks as well as attending the Byam Shaw School of Art, now part of Central Saint Martin's College of Art and Design. From 1942 to 1945 she was the artist to the Plastic and Jaw Unit at Hill End, producing pencil and pen drawings showing in great detail the surgery being performed by Rainsford Mowlem and his surgical team. After the war she lived in Nyasaland (now Malawi) where her husband was the provincial commissioner. In the 1960s she taught painting and drawing at Silverwood, a centre for people with poliomyelitis in Surrey, and was involved in illustrating *Operative Plastic and Reconstructive Surgery* (1981) edited by JN Barron and MN Saad. (With acknowledgements to Brian Morgan)

Page, Alan Geoffrey (1920–2000) DSO, OBE, DFC & Bar was born at Boxmoor, Hertfordshire on 16 May 1920. He was educated at Dean Close School, Cheltenham, and Imperial College London, where he studied engineering, and joined the University of London Air Squadron at RAF Northholt. An uncle was the aircraft manufacturer Sir Frederick Handley Page. In 1939 he was posted to 56 Squadron flying Hurricanes at RAF North Weald, Essex. On 12 August 1940 Page was shot down, badly burning his hands and face; picked up from the Channel he was transferred to the Royal Masonic Hospital, Hammersmith, followed by RAF Halton and eventually QVH. In 1943 he returned to flying, earning a Bar to his DFC on his tenth kill, and in September 1944 after a crash arrived back at East Grinstead with a fractured cheek bone. By that time Page had achieved 17 kills and been decorated with the DSO. He died on 3 August 2000. (With acknowledgements to the *Daily Telegraph*)

Pape, Richard Bernard (1916–1995) MM, Polish Air Force Eagle, was born in Yorkshire and worked as a journalist on the *Yorkshire Post*. He trained as a navigator in the RAFVR and posted to 15 Squadron at RAF Wyton, Cambridgeshire. While returning from a night raid on Berlin on 7 September 1941 in a Short Stirling bomber he was shot down. The aircraft crashed near the Dutch border and Pape became a POW in Stalag VIIIB. He escaped twice but was recaptured and moved to Stalag Luft VI. Eventually he was repatriated to Britain on health grounds and returned to flying duties, but was again involved in a crash, spending two years at QVH. Awarded the MM in 1947, Pape wrote several books including the best-seller *Boldness Be My Friend* (1953), which eventually sold 160,000 copies. He died in Australia on 19 June 1995. (For a no-holds barred and amusing account of Richard Pape's character, see the obituary by Anthony Blond in *The Independent* of 12 July 1995)

Philippi, George (1890–1962) MC, First Royal Dragoons and the RFC served in both the First and Second World Wars. Educated privately and at Exeter College, Oxford, Second Lieutenant Philippi, a member of 60 Squadron, was awarded the MC for conspicuous gallantry in November 1916, the citation reading: 'He dived at a hostile balloon under heavy fire, and brought it down in flames. Though wounded in the head, he brought his machine back at a low altitude, and landed safely in his aerodrome.' He was a flying instructor at Gosport with Smith-Barry, and helped train the Escadrille Lafayette in Virginia. In 1918 Philippi was Assistant Private Secretary to the Secretary of State for the RAF, and during the Second World War provided the link between the Air Ministry, QVH and industry. An excellent shot, for a time he was shooting correspondent for *The Times* and a successful polo player (handicap 6).

Rhind, Sydney Devenish (1894–1956) MC, MB BS (Lond), MRCS, LRCP, FRCS (Eng), FRACS was born in Christchurch on 18 July 1894. He was educated in New Zealand and Belgium prior to being awarded a scholarship by Berkhamsted School, Middlesex. He studied medicine at UCH, London, graduating in 1916. From June 1916 he served with the NZMC as an RMO with the Canterbury Regiment and in October 1917 was awarded the MC. In August 1918 he was posted to Sidcup as assistant surgeon to Pickerill from No 1 NZ General Hospital, Brockenhurst, Hampshire, where he had been a patient after being gassed for the second time. On his return to New Zealand in 1919 he was transferred to Hanmer Military Hospital, first as a patient and then as a member of staff for two years. Rhind then returned to England for postgraduate training at St George's Hospital, London (FRCS, 1923) followed by appointments at Wellington and Hutt Hospitals (1924–53). He died in Wellington on 1 September 1956 in his 61st year. (Information kindly provided by Gillian Martin, SD Rhind's daughter, the *NZ Medical Journal* (1956) 55, p. 411, and the NZ Defence Force Archives)

Risdon, E Fulton (1880–1968) DDS, MB, FRCS (C) was born in St Thomas, Ontario, on 21 March 1880 and educated at the University of Toronto, where he studied dentistry (DDS, 1907) and then medicine (MB, 1914). In 1915 he was commissioned in the CAMC and in 1917 joined Carl Waldron in the Canadian Section at Sidcup. After the war Risdon became a staff member at the Toronto Western Hospital, Professor of Oral Surgery at the University of Toronto, and the first surgeon in Canada to limit his practice to plastic surgery. A founder member of the American Association of Oral and Plastic Surgeons (predecessor of the American Association of Plastic Surgeons), he died in Toronto on 16 November 1968. (With acknowledgements to: RH Ivy (1969), 'E Fulton Risdon', *Plastic and Reconstructive Surgery* 44, pp. 214–16)

Rishworth, John Norman (1876–1946) MBE was born in Blenheim on 13 December 1876. He was educated at Nelson College and trained as a pupil-dentist with Tatton, Son and Black in Nelson, passing the qualifying examination in 1897. At the time he was in practice in Gore in Southland, moving to Onehunga (1900) and Auckland (1902). He was president of the NZDA in 1912 and deputy director of the NZDC, NZEF (1917–19), including four months with the NZ Section at Sidcup. On returning to Auckland he confined his practice to oral surgery and from 1930 to 1934 was director of the NZDC. He died in Auckland in February 1946. (Information kindly provided by the NZDA, Nelson College and the NZ Defence Force Archives)

Rushton, Martin Amsler (1903–1970) CBE, MD, LLD, DSc, OdontD, FDSRCS, FRCS (Eng) was educated at Gresham's School, Holt, Norfolk, Gonville and Caius College, Cambridge, and Guy's Hospital. After obtaining medical and dental qualifications he combined dental practice with part-time teaching at Guy's. At the outbreak of the Second World War he became chief dental surgeon at Rooksdown House. After the war he returned to Guy's as Professor of Oral Medicine, where he took an active role in promoting dental research and was the first person outside of North America to be elected president of the International Association of Dental Research. Rushton received many honorary degrees and awards including the CBE in 1960. A founder member of the Faculty of Dental Surgery of the RCSEng, he was elected Dean for 1961–64. He died in London on 16 November 1970. (With acknowledgements to: NM Naylor (1971), 'Martin Amsler Rushton 1903–1970', *Journal of Dental Research* 50, p. 327)

Seed, William Stanley (1887–1954) BDS, DDS was born in Christchurch on 17 April 1887. He was educated at Christchurch Boys' High School (1901–04), the University of Otago Dental School (BDS (NZ), 1911) and the Chicago College of Dental Surgery (DDS, 1913). During the First World War he served with the NZDC and was a member of the NZ Section at Sidcup, accompanying the unit when it was transferred to Dunedin. In 1920 he returned to Christchurch where he practised dentistry until his retirement in 1952. An excellent all-round sportsman, he played rugby for Otago University, NZ Universities, and in 1913 for Canterbury following his return from Chicago. He was president of the Canterbury Rugby Union in 1935 and in 1937 vice-president of the NZ Rugby Union. He died in Christchurch on 18 February 1954. (With acknowledgements to Dr Brian Adams of Christchurch, and the NZ Defence Force Archives)

Simpson, William (1914–2005) OBE, DFC was born in Glasgow on 9 October 1914. He was educated at King's School, Canterbury, and in 1931 joined an advertising agency in London. Disenchanted with life in an office, in 1935 he applied for a short-service commission in the RAF and was posted to 12 Squadron in Aden. The squadron returned home in 1936 and in 1939, equipped with the Fairey Battle, flew to France. On 10 May 1940 the Germans invaded the Low Countries and Simpson's task was to bomb a motorised column. Hopelessly slow, his aircraft was hit by ground fire and crashed; Simpson was enveloped in flames and badly burnt, but his crew pulled him clear. After treatment in French hospitals, in October 1941 he was repatriated to QVH to begin his long recovery with McIndoe. He returned to RAF service with the Air Ministry and as a war correspondent for the *Sunday Express*. Simpson was awarded the DFC and Croix de Guerre for his war service in 1940 and an OBE for his life-long service to the disabled. He died on 15 November 2005 aged 91. (With acknowledgements to *The Times*)

Siska, Alois (1914–2003) was born at Lutopency, Moravia, on 15 May 1914. After training as a commercial pilot he did his national service with the Czech Air Force. Following the German occupation he fled to Hungary where he was imprisoned, but escaped and joined the French Foreign Legion. When they realised he was a pilot, he was sent to a Czech unit in France. After the French capitulated he escaped to England and joined the RAF's all-Czech 311 Squadron flying Wellingtons. In December 1943 he was shot down and ditched in the North Sea and was washed up on the Dutch coast; his legs had been severely frostbitten. After being moved to Germany and several POW camps he eventually ended up in Colditz Castle. After two years at QVH Siska returned to Czechoslovakia, but when the communists came to power in 1948 was dismissed from the Czech Air Force, exiled from Prague and forced to do menial jobs. His rank was restored in 1991 on the collapse of the communist regime. He died on 9 September 2003 and was posthumously awarded the country's highest military decoration: the Order of the White Lion. (With acknowledgements to the *Daily Telegraph*)

Tilley, Albert Ross (1904–1988) OBE, CM, MD, FRCS(C), FACS was born in Bowmanville, Ontario, Canada. He studied medicine at the University of Toronto (MD, 1929) and was one of the first doctors in Canada to train in plastic surgery. At the beginning of the Second World War he was transferred from the CAMC to the RCAF Medical Branch and in 1942 was posted to QVH. Such was the number of Canadians requiring treatment that the Canadian government was persuaded to build a 49-bed Canadian wing at the hospital staffed by Canadians. In 1944 he was awarded the OBE, and in 1945 returned to practice in Toronto and Kingston, Ontario, where he taught plastic surgery at Queen's University. He was made a member of the Order of Canada (CM) in 1981 and died in Toronto on 19 April 1988. In 2006 he was posthumously inducted into Canada's Aviation Hall of Fame. (With acknowledgements to QVH Archives, East Grinstead)

Tonks, Henry (1862–1937) FRCS was born in Solihull, Warwickshire, on 9 April 1862. He was of Dutch descent on his father's side, the name being a corruption of Toncques. He was educated at Clifton

College, Bristol, and in 1880 became an in-pupil at the Royal Sussex County Hospital, Brighton. After 18 months he transferred to the London Hospital, Whitechapel, qualifying MRCS in 1886. Appointed house surgeon to Sir Frederick Treves (of Elephant Man fame), he passed the FRCS (1888) and was appointed SMO at the Royal Free Hospital. In his spare time Tonks studied with Frederick Brown at the Westminster School of Art. When Brown was appointed Slade Professor of Fine Art at University College London, he appointed Tonks Professor of Drawing. Tonks gave up practising medicine and in 1916 after meeting Gillies at Aldershot, he began recording the facial wounds of Gillies' patients both there and later at Sidcup. Tonks was appointed Slade Professor of Fine Art in 1918 and on his retirement in 1930 was offered a knighthood, which he declined. He died at his home in Chelsea on 8 January 1937. (With acknowledgements to: Joseph Hone (1939), *The Life of Henry Tonks*, William Heinemann Ltd, London; L Morris (2004), 'Tonks, Henry (1862–1937)', *Oxford Dictionary of National Biography*, Oxford University Press, Oxford)

Turner, James MacDougall (1890–1975) BDS, DDS was born in Oamaru on 5 April 1890. He was educated at Otago Boys' High School (1903–06) and the University of Otago Dental School, where he graduated BDS (NZ) in 1912, and went into practice in Invercargill. During the First World War he joined the NZDC, serving with the NZ Field Ambulance in Rouen, and as a member of the NZ Section at Sidcup. After the war he enrolled at the University of Pennsylvania (DDS, 1920), the same year a letter was received by the NZDA informing them he intended to remain in England. From 1920 until his retirement in 1965 he practised dentistry in Torquay, Devon, where he died in May 1975. (Information kindly provided by the University of Otago Alumni Office, University of Pennsylvania, and the NZ Defence Force Archives)

Valadier, Sir Auguste Charles (1873–1931) KBE, CMG was born on 26 November 1873 in Paris. He trained as a dentist at Philadelphia Dental College (DDS 1901) and established a dental practice in New York City. In 1910 he returned to France and studied part time at the École Odontotechnique in Paris, which enabled him to practise in France. In October 1914 Valadier was attached to the RAMC and assigned to No 13 General Hospital in Boulogne. Early in 1915 he organised a 50-bed unit for facial injuries at No 13 Stationary Hospital on the Gare Maritime. In September 1915, No 13 Stationary became a hutted hospital on the road to Wimereux and in May 1917 was renamed the 83rd (Dublin) General Hospital. Appointed CMG in 1916, he was knighted in 1921 for his wartime service after obtaining British citizenship. Postwar, Valadier ran a successful and fashionable practice in Paris, but lived extravagantly; he died on 31 August 1931, leaving his wife and family in straitened financial circumstances. (With acknowledgements to the Army Medical Services Museum Aldershot, and Sue Light)

Waldron, Carl William (1887–1977) MB, DDS, FACS was born on 24 September 1887 in Waubaushene, Ontario. He was educated at the University of Toronto (MB, 1911; DDS, 1913) followed by a residency in otolaryngology and maxillofacial pathology at Johns Hopkins. He enlisted in the CAMC, organising a facial injuries service at Westcliffe Canadian Eye and Ear Hospital, Folkstone, the Ontario Military Hospital, Orpington, and in 1917 was head of the Canadian Section at Sidcup. After the war Waldron returned to Canada where, together with Fulton Risdon, he continued the late care of war casualties. In 1920 he moved to Minneapolis and in 1926 became a naturalised US citizen. He was a founder member of both the American Association of Oral Surgeons (1921) and the American Board of Plastic Surgery (1937), Clinical Professor of Oral Surgery in the Dental School and Clinical Professor of Surgery (plastic and maxillofacial) at the University of Minnesota Hospitals. Waldron died in Scottsdale, Arizona, on 3 January 1977. (With acknowledgements to: Conrad I Karleen (1977), 'Obituary, Carl William Waldron MD, DDS 1887–1977', *Plastic and Reconstructive Surgery* 60, pp. 317–19)

Warwick James, William (1874–1965) OBE, FRCS, MCh, FDSRCS, FLS was born on 20 September 1874 at Wellingborough, Northamptonshire. He was educated at Wellingborough School and apprenticed to a dental practitioner in his home town. He then studied at the Royal Dental Hospital and Middlesex Hospital Medical School, qualifying LDSRCS (Eng) and MRCS (Eng), LRCP (Lond) in 1902, and in 1905 FRCS (Eng). Warwick James was elected to the honorary staff of the Royal Dental and Middlesex Hospitals, appointed dental surgeon to the Hospital for Sick Children, Great Ormond Street, and acquired a large private practice. During and after the First World War he treated facial injuries at the 3rd London General Hospital, Wandsworth, for which he was awarded the OBE. In 1940 with BW Fickling he wrote *Injuries of the Jaws and Face*. He died on 14 September 1965. (With acknowledgements to the obituary by ZC (Sir Zachary Cope) in the *Annals of the Royal College of Surgeons of England* (1965) 37, pp. 318–19)

Whale, George Harold Lawson (1876–1943) MD (Cantab), FRCS (Eng) was born at Woolwich on 23 August 1876. He was educated at Bradfield College, Berkshire, and Jesus College, Cambridge (BA, 1898), followed by clinical training at St Bartholomew's Hospital (MB, BChir (Cantab), 1902; MRCS, LRCP, 1902). He joined the Indian Medical Service (IMS) in 1902, but in 1906 was invalided home with coeliac disease (sprue), the subject of his 1907 Cambridge MD thesis. He then specialised in ENT surgery (FRCS, 1912). During the First World War he was a captain in the RAMC serving at the Val de Grâce French Army Hospital; as a surgeon-specialist at the 53rd General Hospital; at the Face and Jaw unit headed by Valadier at No 13 Stationary/No 83 General Hospital; and finally at Sidcup. Lawson Whale was a prolific author and wrote several books, his name gradually metamorphosing from GHL Whale at Cambridge to GH Lawson Whale on a *Lancet* paper in 1915, and finally, as author of *Injuries to the Head and Neck* (1919), to H Lawson Whale. He died at St John's Wood, London, on 17 June 1943. (With acknowledgements to *Plarr's Lives of the Fellows*, Royal College of Surgeons of England)

APPENDIX II

Officers holding appointments at the Queen's Hospital, Sidcup

THE FOLLOWING OFFICERS held appointments at the hospital during various periods until its closure in 1929. The list is an updated version of the names and post-nomial letters in the Appendix to *The Queen's Hospital Sidcup*, a small brochure tracing the origins and history of the hospital.

Captain HC Apperly LDS, MRCS, LRCP
Captain P Ashworth ADC
Captain JL Aymard MRCS, LRCP
Captain GE Beaumont DM, FRCP
Dr E Bellingham Smith MD, FRCP
Captain ACB Biggs MC, FRCS
Captain GC Birt LDS, MRCS, LRCP
Captain TW Bleakley CAMC
Dr WE Bond MRCS, LRCP
Captain NHM Burke MRCS, LRCP, DMRE
Captain AHL Campbell CADC
Dr I Campbell MRCS, LRCP
Captain WF Christie (Registrar)
Captain GC Chubb FRCS
Captain JC Clayton MRCS, LRCP
Captain FJ Cleminson MCh, FRCS
Dr FH Cleveland MRCS, LRCP
Mr L Colledge MB, FRCS
Lieutenant Colonel JR Colvin (Commandant)
Dr Corbett RAMC
Dr SD Craig MB, ChB
Dr GA Crowe LMSSA
Captain GL Cutts LDS, MRCS, LRCP
Major R Davies-Colley CMG, MCh, FRCS

Dr GW Davis MD
Major JC Duff (Quartermaster)
Captain JPS Dunn MB, ChB
Captain RS Dunning
Dr TH Edey MRCS, LRCP
Lieutenant JW Edwards (Sculptor)
Dr ECT Emerson MD
Major GL Findlay MB (Medical Superintendent)
Captain FG Flanders
Captain AL Fraser LDS, MRCS, LRCP
Dr M Freeborough MB, DMRE
Dr RA Fuller MC, MRCS, LRCP
Dr W Garton MRCS, LRCP, DMRE
Major HD Gillies CBE, FRCS
Dr T Grainger Stewart MD, FRCP
Captain EA Hardy LDS, MRCS, LRCP
Captain LA Harwood LDS, MRCS, LRCP
Captain BJ Hawke
Captain EP Hawkshaw CADC
Lieutenant WJ Heathfield (Education officer)
Captain WI Henderson CAMC
Captain G Seccombe Hett MB, BS, FRCS
Captain GM Hicks
Lieutenant JH Hindle
Dr C Hodgson MRCS, LRCP
Dr HK Graham Hodgson, CVO, MB, DMRE
Dr DH Hubbs MRCS, LRCP
Dr E Hudson MRCS, LRCP
Captain C Hurford (Workshops Officer)
Captain AEW Idris MRCS, LRCP
Dr JG Ingouvill MRCS, LRCP

Dr GM Jackson MB BS
Captain T Jackson LDS, MRCS, LRCP
Dr HH Jenkins MRCS, LRCP
Captain FE Johnson
Captain FH Johnson
Captain Gordon Johnson
Lieutenant HM Johnson FRCS
Dr JT Johnson
Captain DJ Jones
Dr HB Jones MRCS, LRCP
Captain A Jupp LDSRCS
Captain W Kelsey Fry MC, LDS, MRCS, LRCP
Captain TP Kilner MB, ChB, FRCS
Captain FD La Touche AAMC
Captain H Lawson Whale MD, FRCS
Captain EW Lowe LDSRCS
Sub-Lieutenant WJ Lyttle MB, ChB, BAO, FRCS
Colonel F Maclure AAMC
Captain IW Magill MB, BCh BAO.
Captain HC Malleson LDS, MRCS, LRCP
Captain A McP Marshall MB, ChB, NZMC
Captain A Matthews
Dr AS McDonald MB
Dr MA McDonald MC, MB
Captain V McDonald
Mr G McNeill FRCS
Captain B Mendelson LDSRCS
Dr AJ Middleton
Dr L Middleton (Acting Medical Superintendent)
Dr E Miller MRCS, LRCP
Captain RM Montgomery MD
Dr CW Morris OBE, MRCS, LRCP
Major GT Mullally MC, MS, FRCS
Lieutenant SF Mullard
Dr LAC Murphy
Captain DA Murray CAMC
Lieutenant Colonel HS Newland OBE, MB, FRCS
Major MWB Oliver OBE, MB, BCh, FRCS
Dr GH Oriel MD
Dr JI Palmer OBE, MRCS, LRCP
Major KS Parker AAMC
Dr GL Parsons MRCS, LRCP
Major HP Pickerill LDS, MB, ChB, NZMC
Captain WL Post CAMC
Captain SD Rhind MC, MRCS, LRCP, NZMC
Captain WKA Richards MC, MB
Dr RAC Rigby MRCS, LRCP
Captain EF Risdon DDS, MB, CAMC
Major JR Rishworth NZDC

Captain EG Robertson
Captain ES Rowbotham MRCS, LRCP
Captain CF Rumsey LDS, MRCS, LRCP
Mr HG Bedford Russell MCh, FRCS
Major K Russell AAMC
Captain WS Seed BDS, DDS, NZDC
Mr JMcI Shaw MC, FRCS
Major AV Sinclair
Major Stapleton (Education Officer)
Lieutenant LA Swash (Workshops Officer)
Captain Ferris N Smith MD, RAMC
Captain JW Smith AAMC
Captain P Smuts
Lieutenant Spence (Education Officer)
Captain DH Tasker RN
Captain HCD Taunton RAMC
Lieutenant AC Thompson
Dr CJ Thompson MRCS, LRCP
Captain MG Thomson CAMC
Captain RWL Todd MB, ChB
Captain J M Turner BDS, NZDC
Dr WJ Vance MRCS, LRCP
Dr S Vatcher MB, MRCS, LRCP
Captain R Wade MRCS, LRCP
Major CW Waldron MB, DDS, CAMC
Major FW Watkyn-Thomas FRCS
Captain EO Watson
Dr H Wetherbee MRCS, LRCP
Major A Wheeler
Dr E White MB
Dr AS Woodwarke CMG, CBE, MD, FRCP
Dr HJ Wright MD

United States medical and dental officers attached for the postgraduate course
Captain MF Arbuckle
Captain HW Brent
Major VP Blair
Major GM Dorrance
Lieutenant JE Herlihy
Lieutenant-Commander LW Johnston
Lieutenant EJ Kelly
Captain EF Lafitte
Major Read P McGee
Lieutenant JJ Ogden
Lieutenant Schildwachter
Major WJ Scruton
Captain Eastman Sheehan
Captain TR Stellwagen

Captain HR Stone
Captain TM Terry
Captain JM Waugh
Lieutenant Colonel JD Whitham
Lieutenant RP Wildes

Honorary consultants
Sir James Frank Colyer KBE, LDS, FRCS
Sir Francis Farmer KBE, LDS, FRCS
Sir William Arbuthnot Lane CB, MS, FRCS

Members of the Guinea Pig Club

NAMES OF THE 642 members of the Guinea Pig Club listed on the honours board in the Canadian Wing at Queen Victoria Hospital, East Grinstead. Those with an asterisk (36 in total) were Hurricane and Spitfire pilots who fought in the Battle of Britain (10 July–31 October 1940).
† indicates the addition of a Bar to the decoration.

Adamczyk J, Poland
Adams James G, Canada
Adams Robert Roy, 'Chiefy', 106 Sqn
Adcock R, in Aust, 1948
Aldridge Herbert, Canada, 464 Sqn
Allard JA
Allaway Joseph John, 'Jack', 521 Sqn
Allen George Willoughby, Canada, 422 Sqn
Allen T, in Aust 1948
Allison Kenneth, Canada
Anderson Harry D, Canada, 427 Sqn
Anderson Ian G, 156 Sqn
Anderson J Cyril, Canada
Anderson John A, UK*, 253 Sqn
Anderson L
Andrew JR
Anglin William G, Canada, 168 Sqn
Angold JP
Armstrong Rodney I, in NZ 1948
Ashton JD
Aslin DJ, UK*, 257 & 32 Sqns
Atcherley Richard LR, Air Vice-Marshall, KBE, CB, CBE, OBE, AFC†

Atherton MR
Atkinson John C
Bacon Douglas R, Canada, 149 Sqn
Bagard R, in France 1948
Bain JH, Canada, 168 Sqn
Ball Alan R
Ball RJ
Ballentyne FA, 901 Sqn
Banham A John, UK*, 264 & 229 Squadrons
Banks V, Canada, 428 Sqn
Barber William D, Canada
Barker John S, 109 Sqn
Barrow AA
Barry Patrick 'Paddy', 467 Sqn
Base Keith M, 'Bottomly'
Beauchamp George E, Canada, 420 Sqn
Begbie W, 76 Sqn
Benbow James, 97 Sqn
Bennett GC
Bennions George H, UK*, 41 Sqn, DFC
Bernier Gerry H, Canada, 260 Sqn
Berrington-Picket NE, South Africa
Berryman LE, Canada, 412 Sqn
Biddle Gordon A, Canada
Biel Joseph, Poland
Bielawski F, Poland
Bird-Wilson Harold AC, UK*, 17 Sqn, Air Vice-Marshall, 'Birdy' DSO, DFC† AFC
Birks J Brian W, DFC
Bobitko M, Poland
Boissonas C, Free French Air Force

Bond David EB
Bonney H van D
Bourne William John, 454 Sqn, in SA 1948
Bowes Alan C, Canada
Bowyer Ward M, in US 1947
Boyd CIL
Bradley GP
Branch Paul Fisher, Canada, 614 Sqn
Brandon Thomas W, 192 Sqn
Branston Kenneth, Canada, 419 Sqn
Briggs C
Bristow Eric, Canada, 419 Sqn
Broadbent R, 61 Sqn
Bronski E, USA, 322 Sqn
Brooke Peter WS
Brooke RH
Brooks N, 450 Sqn
Broughton John
Brown T, 180 Sqn
Browne Andre HR, Belgium
Browne Kenneth
Browne T, in NZ 1948
Brunskill Eric
Bubb John Durham, 99 Sqn
Buckee JW
Buckle JW
Buckman Harold W, Australia
Bull VG
Buller Edward G, 86 Sqn
Bullock Frederick T
Burrell Graham
Burton WR, Canada
Butcher G
Butler John C, Canada
Butler Maurice W
Caddell Les Arthur, Canada
Cadman BS, 96 Sqn
Cain EA, Canada
Cameron Lorne M, Canada, 401 Sqn, DFC
Campbell B, Canada
Campbell C, in Aust 1948
Cap K
Capka Joseph, Czechoslovakia, 68 Sqn, DFM, Croix
    de Guerre, Czech War Cross
Carlier J, Belgium, 350 Sqn
Carlson Edward L, Canada
Carnall R, UK*, 111 Sqn
Cartwright Edward M
Catellier Louis-Philippe, Canada

Cecile Edgar G, Canada
Chapman E
Charbonneau Maurice JDR, Canada
Charles RWH
Chater C, in Canada 1948
Chiswell Lawrence
Chitham RG
Clarke George B
Clarke John R, in USA 1948
Clarkson R, in Aust 1948
Cleland R, Canada
Clifford John, in Aust 1948, 50 Sqn
Colbert J
Cole Adrian Trevor 'King', Air Vice-Marshall, CBE,
    DSO, MC, DFC, Australia
Cole John, Australia, 617 Sqn
Cole Leslie PH
Collier G
Collin Roy, 139 Sqn
Colver R, Canada
Condon James, 578 Sqn
Cooke Arthur G, Canada
Cooper Cecil, Canada
Cooper Kenneth G
Cooper W, Australia, 127 Sqn
Coote LEM, UK*, 600 Sqn, (killed 10 Oct 1943)
Coppock Frank, Canada, 613 Sqn
Corpe Alfred, 158 Sqn
Corrigan LR, Australia
Cowham W, 57 Sqn
Craig Ian W 'Jock, 103 Sqn
Crampton Stanley
Crane Derek
Crawford Derek, in Aust 1950
Crombie Harry R, 139 Sqn
Cruikshank William GJ, 612 Sqn
Cummins John Sydney, Canada, 404 Sqn
Cunningham Walter, 'Jock'
Curwain HNH, Canada
Dakin G, Canada, 245 Sqn
Dalkin RW, Australia
Dash ED
Davidson Charles Edward, DFC
Davidson Kenneth, Canada
Davies FS
Davies Kenneth J, Canada
David J
Davoud Paul Yettvart, b USA, Canada, 409 Sqn, OBE,
    DSO, DFC

Davy EJ

Davy FG

Day RLF, UK*, 141 Squadron, (killed 18 June 1944)

De Bruhn G, South Africa

De Lyon EJ, Netherlands

Dean Francis J 'Dixie'

Dean John L

Debenham KB, UK*, 151 Squadron, (killed 16 Dec 1943)

Dee Harold John

Deniall A

De Renzy David, New Zealand

Dermerdash Mohamed, Egypt

Devers F, 328 Sqn

Dewar William, Canada, 402 Sqn

Douglas WA

Dove George, 101 Sqn, DFM, CGM

Dove Orvel, Canada, 256 Sqn

Doyle E Arthur, 'Art', Canada

Doyle William A, 132 Sqn, in Canada 1948

Dredge Alan Sydney, UK*, 253 Squadron, (killed 18 May 1945)

Dufort Gerald, Canada, 78 Sqn

Duncan G aka 'Jock', in SA 1950

Duncan John Stuart, Canada

Dunscombe RD, UK*, 213 & 312 Squads, (missing 31 May 1941)

Edmond P

Edmonds Godfrey, South Africa

Edmonston W, 35 Sqn

Edwards GD

Edwards H

Elkes A

Ellis Peter R

Erakdogan Nedim, Turkey

Ernst Henry 'Hank', Canada, 420 Sqn

Evans John, Australia, 466 Sqn

Everett John, Canada

Fairclough H

Falkiner Fraser, Australia

Fawcett George R, Canada, 410 Sqn

Ferguson Everett, Canada

Ferguson James, Canada

Figuiere Gilbert, in France 1949

Finnemore SG

Fisher Kenneth R, Canada

Fitzgerald PH

Fleming John, NZ*, 605 Sqn, MBE

Forbes G, Canada, 168 Sqn

Forster Michael E

Fowler Gilbert Lewis, 'Gus'

Fowler Ray P

Foxley William J

Fraser Robert A, Canada

Fraser Robert, 'Bob', Canada

Fredericks Gordon, Canada, 405 Sqn

Freeborn Donald B, Canada, 153Sqn, DFC[†]

Friend H Marshall, 255 Sqn

Gallop Samuel R, OBE, CBE

Gambier-Parry R, 29 Sqn

Gambling AH, 217 Sqn

Garne TA

Garvin Robert, Canada, 427 Sqn

Gauvin R, in Australia 1949

Gerald VP, Canada, 427 Sqn

Gibbs FG

Gilkes Kenneth, Australia

Gillies John, 'Jack'

Gingles John, 'Paddy', 432 Sqn, DFC, DFM

Giradet GB, 144 Sqn

Given Stanley, Canada, 432 Sqn

Gleave Thomas Percy, UK*, 253 Sqn, CBE, Vice-President GP Club 1941–93

Glebocki Jerzy, 'George', Poland, 304 Sqn

Glossop Douglas R

Glover Neville W

Golding William H, Canada, 57 Sqn

Goodman CE, 296 Sqn

Goodson Les A, Canada, in NI 1951

Gourlay J Frank, 252 Sqn

Graham Robert

Graveley A

Green Henry T

Grill J, Canada

Grudzien Joseph Michael, Canada

Gunnis J Neville, Canada, Australia 1949

Gwardiak E, Poland

Haddock J, 68 Sqn

Haines L, Australia

Hall Dennis

Hall Kim

Halifax ND

Hanton Frank E, Canada, 400 Sqn, DFC[†]

Harding John Robert, Canada, 168 Sqn, DFC

Harper Cyril

Harrington J, Living in USA 1949

Harris Walter W, 'Wally', Australia

Harrison Reginald, Canada, 431 Sqn

Harrop K
Hart Paul R
Harvey D, in Australia 1950
Haslam FR
Hastings Lionel E, Canada, 98 Sqn
Hawksworth A John
Heine W, Poland, 300 Sqn
Helsby DA
Henderson Arthur James, Canada
Henry AC
Heslop John
Hewison George
Hewitt R John, in Trinidad 1950
Hibbert WR, 168 Sqn, in Canada 1950
Hicks Cyril F, Canada
Hicks Douglas J, Canada, 550 Sqn
Hicks James L, Canada
Higgins William J, Canada
Hiley Frederick S, Canada, 420 Sqn, DFM
Hill John P, in Australia 1950
Hill N
Hill W
Hillary Richard Hope, UK* 603 Sqn, (killed 18 Jan
    1943)
Hills A John
Hindley George J, 'Little'
Hitchcock C, in NZ 1950
Hobbs Victor R, 35 Sqn
Hocken WW, Canada
Hodgkinson Colin, 'Hoppy', Fleet Air Arm
Holdsworth R, in Australia 1950
Holland Robert Hugh, UK*, 92 Sqn
Holmes N, 65 Sqn
Holmes NPC
Holmes William, 149 Sqn
Hood J, in USA 1950
Hooper J
Houston R, Canada, 214 Sqn
Hubbard Frank, Canada, 401 Sqn
Hughes J, in USA 1950
Hughes JDE, South Africa, 204 Sqn
Humphreys Ronald, 504 Sqn
Hunt DW, UK*, 257 Sqn
Hunter CO, in Australia 1950
Hurry CA 'Lyall', UK*, 43 & 46 Squads: AFC
Hutchinson GW, 432 Sqn
Hutchinson W John
Hyde Reginald HJ
Intepe Kemal, Turkey

Ireland NL
Jackson Gordon E, 42 Sqn
Jacob JWF, 88 Sqn
Jarman GT
Jarman J, New Zealand
Jenkins C Richmond
Johnston G Robin, South Africa
Jones B, in USA 1950
Jones IM
Jones I Wynne
Jones Jonah Stewart
Jones Owen J, Canada, 50 Sqn
Keene F
Keep J, 181 Sqn
Kemp John HF
Kerr John J, Canada, 427 Sqn
King FP
Kingcome C Brian F , UK*, 92 Sqn, DSO, DFC†
    (Hon GP)
Kirby John
Knott JJ
Knowles William Douglas
Korwell WP, Poland, 308 Sqn
Koukall Josef, Czechoslovakia* 310 Sqn
Krasnodebski E 'Kras', Poland*, 303 Sqn, in South
    Africa 1950
Kyd Peter S
Lacasse EM 'Bud', Canada, 30 Sqn
Lambell Neil, Australia
Lancaster E George, in Singapore 1950
Lanctot D, Canada, 419 Sqn
Lander A, Canada, in NZ 1950
Lane Roy 'Lulu', UK*, 43 Sqn (killed by Japanese 20
    June 1944)
Lane William, 103 Sqn
Langham-Hobart Neville C, UK*, 73 Sqn
Langlands Charles, 158 Sqn
Langley Stan
Lawson G, South Africa
Lea George T, 99 Sqn
Lee RGF
Lee SM, 147 Sqn
Lee Thomas M
Leitch Arthur K, Canada
Lestanges J, France
Leupp Ray Edward, USA, joined RCAF
Lever EJ, South Africa, 249 Sqn
Levi John E, Canada
Levin Bernard 'Barney', South Africa, 22 Sqn

Liddiard WH
Lightley Eric S, 158 Sqn
Lipsett C Maxwell, 'Maxie', Canada
Lloyd Robert T, Canada
Lock Eric Stanley, UK*, 41 Sqn, DSO, DFC† (MIA, 3 Aug 1941)
Loneon B, South Africa
Loosley S
Lord AJ, Canada
Lord Reginald C, 75 Sqn
Love James, Canada
Lowe Joseph, UK* 236 Sqn
Lugg S
Lunney David M, Canada, 405 Sqn
Lymburner Laurence 'Larry', Canada
McBride J
McCabe Owen James, Australia
McCallum Robert C
McConnell Allan 'Flash'
MacCormac Sidney
McCully G, Canada, 411 Sqn
McGovan T
McGowan Roy A, UK*, 46 Sqn, emigrated to NZ
McHolm Norman A, Canada
McIvor Ian CS
McKeown TD, Canada
McLaughlin John W, UK*, 238 Sqn
MacLean ACH
McLean Charles, 'Chuck', Canada
McLeod CA, Canada, 432 Sqn
McNally D, Australia, 127 Sqn
McNeill DC, Canada, 432 Sqn
MacPhail FJ, UK*, 603 Sqn
MacPherson WJ
McQuillan Sidney
McTavish Duncan, Canada
Major Robert
Mann John, 'Jackie', UK*, 64 & 92 Sqn, CBE, Hostage Beirut 1989–91
Marceau JA Henri Bernard, Canada, 434 Sqn
Marcotte Henri JA, 'Hank', Canada, 168 Sqn, DFC
Marjoram C
Marshall J
Martin Derek D, 210 Sqn, OBE
Martin James, Canada, 428 Sqn
Martin Stuart W
Martin William E, 'Bill', Canada
Martin W
Marygold D Cyril

Mathieson RM
Mattis J
Maxwell John Woer, Canada
May J
Melling L
Melvill JC, 264 Sqn
Methven W Reginald
Miles J
Miles NE
Mills WH, Australia
Mirchell Bruce S, Canada, 407 Sqn
Molivados Steven R, Greece, DFC
Monk EGS
Montgomery JF, 149 Sqn
Montpetit Marc, Canada
Moore Garnett, 'Tar', Canada
Moores FS, 'Dinty', DFC
Mordue J
Morgan Alan, 49 Sqn
Morris Ian CA, 'Jock'
Morson Harry J
Mounsden Maurice H, UK*, 56 Sqn
Mufford J Delmar, Canada, 432 Sqn
Munt JGE
Neale GD
Nelson Roy G
Nesbitt Alexander, 'Paddy'
Nettleton Basil P
Newman Noel 'Doc'
Newson William, Canada, 405 Sqn, DSO, DFC, CD
Nichols T, Canada, 199 Sqn
Nisbet N, South Africa
Nivison John, South Africa
Noble BR, UK*, 79 Sqn
Noble George Alistair, Canada
Noble WL
Noon-Ward Ronald Gordon, Canada, 199 Sqn
Norman CT, 57 Sqn
Noyes Sydney A, Canada
O'Brien J Bernard, New Zealand
O'Connell Desmond, 'Paddy', 502 Sqn
O'Connor Karl E, Canada
Ogden Harold, 'Hoagy', Canada
O'Halloran Terence, Australia
Orchel E, Poland
Orman Gilbert Henry
O'Sullivan D
Overeijnder Fritz, Netherlands
Owen E, Australia, 406 Sqn

Page Alan Geoffrey, UK*, 56 Sqn, DSO, OBE, DFC†
Pape Richard Bernard 'Ginger', 15 Sqn, MM,
    Polish AF Eagle
Parratt Hugh E, 'Pip', DFM
Paszkowski A, Poland
Payne Robert H
Peach TJ, Australia
Pearce Eric G, 26 Sqn
Pearce GH
Pearce Richard E
Pearson A, 207 Sqn
Peel H, 407 Sqn
Pelly John A, 816 Sqn
Penman F, New Zealand
Pereuse P
Perry EJ
Petit Donald, in NZ 1950
Phillips Howard L, USA, joined RCAF, 112 Sqn
Phillips L, Canada, 199 Sqn
Piercy Stewart A, 15 Sqn, in Canada 1951
Pike D
Pitts J
Platsko MA, 'Al', Canada, 422 Sqn
Podbereski Tadeusz A, 'Teddy', Poland, emig to
    Canada 1950
Poole E
Poole Malcolm J
Porter Kenneth L, Canada, 180 Sqn
Pretty Ronald
Price D
Propas B, Canada, 439 Sqn
Proudlove A, Canada, 408 Sqn
Pryor DM, South Africa
Quigley Frank J
Quilter Ian MacP, 811 Sqn, emig to NZ
Raby George H
Ralston Robert, 619 Sqn
Randall HJ, 408 Sqn
Raphael RFG
Rasumov Vladimir, 'Raz', USSR
Redekopp Jacob, Canada, 50 Sqn
Reece J, in Australia 1951
Reynolds CG, 101 Sqn
Reynolds George
Reynolds John A, Canada
Reynolds Stanley G, Canada, 410 Sqn, CM
Rhodes C, Australia
Richardson Desmond Brian
Richardson Walter

Rickard J, Canada, 224 Sqn
Ridding Bernard, Canada, 406 Sqn
Rix Frederick T, 625 Sqn
Robbins James E, 40 Sqn
Roberson John L, Australia
Roberts Edward D
Roberts R
Roberts T John, Canada
Robertson Alexander B
Rogers JH
Round S, Canada
Rowley A, 147 Sqn
Royds A, Australia
Russell James H
Russell K, 214 Sqn
St John JI, Canada, 411 Sqn
Sampson JFM, USA
Sandeman-Allen James A, DFM, MBE
Saunders Arthur C
Saunders RT
Schloesing Jacques Henri, France, GC
Scoffield Thomas J
Scott Edward E, 614 Sqn
Scott JE
Scott-Farnie GR
Scrivens DR
Shallis R
Shankland A
Shankland W
Simms W
Simpson Donald W, Canada
Simpson John Henry, 'Taffy'
Simpson William, 'Bill', 12 Sqn, OBE, DFC
Sims JA
Siska Alois, Czechoslovakia, 311 Sqn, Order of the
    White Lion
Skoczylas L, Poland
Smith BO (Bertram Owen Smith), 78 Sqn
Smith Edward W, 'Smithy', Canada, 102 Sqn,
    DSO, CD
Smith Dennis B
Smith John
Smith John Campbell, 'Jack', Canada, 36 Sqn
Smith PC
Smith PSS
Smith RJ
Smith TA
Smith Thomas CF
Smith TG, in NZ 1947

Smith-Barry Robert Raymond, AFC
Smyth Kenneth C, Canada
Snelling Alexander Benjamin
Snyder Karol
Somers Lawrence J, Canada
Southwell John, Canada, 426 Sqn
Spackman GL, Canada
Speedie WR
Spooner B, 268 Sqn
Spooner WHC
Squire JWC, UK*, 64 Squadron
Stafford John
Standen Henry H, 83 Sqn, MBE
Stangryciuk E (Black E), Poland
Stanley William M, Australia
Stannus Harold, Australia, 149 Sqn
Stansberg A
Stephen Douglas McCallum, Canada, 550 Sqn
Stewart DW Ross
Stickings HJ, 12 Sqn
Stoker P, USA, 328 Sqn
Stone Clifford, 'Rocky', Honorary GP
Strickland Freeman, Australia
Stroud George A, 249 Sqn
Struthers G, New Zealand, 180 Sqn
Stults D, Canada, 440 Sqn
Sullivan JB, Canada, 427 Sqn
Summerson AK
Sutton Percy W
Swain Frank G
Syrett Les
Szafranski M, Poland
Tait Robert, Canada
Tanner William E, Canada
Tarling Raymond, Canada
Tatajczak R, Poland
Taubman Harold, Australia, 460 Sqn
Taylor B
Taylor Dennis
Taylor EA
Taylor George F, Australia
Taylor John E
Tebbit DF, 41 Sqn
Thomas AG
Thomas J, Canada
Thompson Douglas L, Canada, 106 Sqn
Thompson John J
Thompson JMV
Tiplady George W

Tollemache Anthony Henry, 800 Sqn, GC
Toper John J, 'Jack', 166 Sqn, MBE
Tosh James, 'Jock', 466 Sqn
Towers-Perkins William, UK*, 238 Sqn, First
    Secretary GPC
Townsend Ken N
Trask JK, Australia, 231 Sqn
Treagust John R
Tremblay Leonard, Canada
Truhlar Francisek, 'Frankie', Czechoslovakia, 311/312
    Sqns
Tugwell KS
Tully L
Turnbull Richard L, Canada, 952 Sqn
Turner Guy, UK*, 32 Sqn
Varty J
Verran James, New Zealand, DFC†
Vince Douglas L
Vincent E, Canada
Vivian R
Voges Thomas E
Wainwright Les, Canada, 425 Sqn, DFC
Wakley A Edward, 16 Sqn
Walker Charles, Australia
Walshe Timothy C, 220 Sqn
Warburton Kenneth C
Ward Colin GA
Ward HC
Warman William C
Warren Paul S, USA, 35 Sqn RCAF
Warwick CR
Watkins Charles
Watkins F
Watkins H, 149 Sqn
Waterson JT
Weber Paul John, Canada
Webster Frank
Weeks Peter C, 607 Sqn, First, Treasurer GPC
Wells Patrick HV, SA*, 249 Sqn
Welsh John, 428 Sqn
Weston John
Whale Frederick V
Whalley Bernard G
Wham R
White J
White N
Whitehorn R Frederick, 78 Sqn
Wild MWE
Wilkes C

Wilkins Les R, 76 Sqn
Wilkinson George, Canada, 419 Sqn
Williams Henry
Williams SR
Williams T, 50 Sqn
Williams TW, 141 Sqn
Willie V, Canada
Wilson George A, 'Curly', Canada, 427 Sqn
Wilson H
Wilton Michael, 4 Sqn
Wishart John J 'Jack', Australia
Wood IA, Australia
Woodward Harold W
Woodwark PAS
Woolf Arthur S, 'Red'
Wooley George E
Woollard FG, 41 Sqn
Worn Richard L
Wright CM
Wright Donald V, Canada
Wright James Ernest Frederick, 'Jimmy', OBE, DFC
Wright Robert C, 85 Sqn

Perhaps to avoid nationalism, no record of the country of origin of individual members was kept by the Guinea Pig Club and unless otherwise stated the members are assumed to be from the UK. The Canadian names are based on those included in *As*

For the Canadians (2000) by Rita Donovan and are a reasonably complete record. Additional information came from *McIndoe's Army* (2001) by Edward Bishop. Barry Cardno tirelessly searched all the *Guinea Pig* magazines for information on other nationalities, complicated by GPs emigrating after the war, particularly to Australia, New Zealand and South Africa. Entries such as 'In Aust 1947' etc are based on items in the GP magazine about where particular GPs happened to be living at the time. His research together with that of Sergeant Chris Turner of RAF Shawbury and Bob Marchant uncovered the names of several GPs not recorded on the honours board in the Canadian Wing. They are as follows:

Allen Claude
Avery Harold F, Canada
Doe Robert Francis Thomas, UK*, 234, 238 Sqs, DSO, DFC[†]
Edwards James Keith O'Neill, 'Jimmy', DFC, comedian
Hay JF
McLennan Kenneth C, Canada
Marchcourt René, France
Nield Norman
Pickard Walter
Prusski Creslay, Poland
Shaughnessy Gerard, Canada

Army maxillofacial units 1939–45

Dieppe
RJV Battle; P Wren (dental)

Boulogne
CL Heanley; GT Hankey (dental)

MFU No 1 (Middle East Forces; based at various times in Alexandria, Tripoli, Sicily and Italy)
R Champion (1940–43)
RS Murley (1941–44)
RJV Battle (1943–45)
RPG Sandon (1944–45)
EJ Dalling (1940–45) (dental)
BV Janes (1943–45)
JF Lockwood (1945)

Ad hoc Unit (Italy)
A Smith-Walker (1944–45)
Hribajevsky (1944–45) (dental)
R Grewcock (1944–45)

MFU No 2 (Middle East Forces; based in Cairo)
MC Oldfield (1940–43)
MH Shaw (1943–45)
WR Roberts (1940–45) (dental)
RS Pook (1940–45)

MFU No 3 (Far East, India, Burma)
CL Heanley (1942–45)
JH Hovell (1942–45) (dental)

MFU No 4 (North Africa, Italy)
PW Clarkson (1942–45)
R Lawrie (1943–45)

W Grossman
TH Wilson (1942–45; died on active service) (dental)
J Hancock

MFU No 5 (Normandy and Germany)
GM FitzGibbon (1944–45)
T Gibson (1944–45)
NH Holland (1944–45) (dental)

MFU No 6 (France and Belgium)
W Hynes (1944–45)
W Cowell (1944–45)
WB Hales (1944–45) (dental)

Indian MFU No 1
FW Pickard (Canada; 1943–45)
T Gibson (1945–46)
N Thompson (1945–46) (dental)

Indian MFU No 2
E Peet (1943–45)

Lone Ranger (India)
HE Blake (1942–43)

Data from: PW Clarkson & FA Walker (1955). 'Gun-shot wounds of the face and jaws', in NL Rowe & HC Killey (eds), *Fractures of the Facial Skeleton*, E&S Livingstone Ltd, Edinburgh and London, pp. 493–585; RJV Battle (1978), 'Plastic surgery in the two world wars and in the years between', *Journal of the Royal Society of Medicine* 71, pp. 844–48.

GLOSSARY

acromio-thoracic pedicle: flap raised from the shoulder and chest

ala: lateral wall of the nose

antrum: cavity or chamber

autogenous bone: bone grafted from the same individual

bony callus: deposit formed between broken bones

cancellous bone: the tissue that makes up the interior of bones

cell-mediated immunity: immune response involving cells such as T-cells (lymphocytes)

columella: central column of nose

costal cartilage: cartilage attached to the ribs

ectropion/eversion: outwardly turned

edentulous: without teeth

debridement: removal of dead, damaged or infected tissue

dermatome: a surgical instrument to produce thin slices of skin

epithelium: tissue lining the cavities and surfaces of the body

gangrene: death of tissue following injury or infection

gutta percha: an inelastic latex produced from the sap of trees

haemorrhage: loss of blood, bleeding

helix: the prominent rim of the outer ear or auricula

heterograft (xenograft): tissue transplanted between different species

homograft (allograft): tissue transplanted between same species

humoral immunity: immune response involving antibodies

hyoscine: an antispasmodic used to treat nausea and motion sickness

iliac crest: the curved upper border of the pelvis

inner or medial canthus: point where the upper and lower eyelids meet

keloid scar: scar with an excessive growth of fibrous tissue

Kingsley splint: splint used to apply traction or support to the upper jaw

lachrymal sac: sac from which the tears drain via a duct into the nose

leucocytes: white blood cells

lupus: an autoimmune disease where the body's immune system attacks normal tissue

lymphocyte: white blood cell; part of the immune system

lymphoedema: localised fluid retention and tissue swelling

malar prominence: prominence formed by cheekbone

mandible: lower jaw

mandibular symphysis: midline of the mandible

masseter muscle: muscle from zygomatic arch to the angle of the mandible

maxilla: upper jaw

mesenchymal cells: undifferentiated connective tissue cells

metacarpo-phalangeal joint: joint between the bones of the hand and fingers

mucous membrane: epithelial coverings lining cavities such as the nose and mouth

nasal septum: structure dividing nasal airway into two halves

necrosis: death of cells and tissues

orthognathic surgery: corrective surgery of the jaws

osteoblasts: mononucleate cells responsible for bone formation

osteoclasts: multinucleate cells responsible for bone resorption

pedicle flap: flap attached to the donor site to provide blood supply

periosteum: tissue covering the outer surface of bones

perpendicular plate of ethmoid: part of the nasal septum

phagocytic action: the ingestion and destruction of bacteria, cells or foreign particles

philtrum: vertical groove in middle of upper lip

premaxilla: part of the maxilla which bears the incisor teeth

prognathic: prominence of the upper or lower jaws

prosthesis: artificial device replacing lost tissue

proteoglycans: protein-polysaccharide molecules prominent in cartilage

rhinoplasty: operation for correcting the form or function of the nose

sepsis: whole body inflammation caused by infection

septicaemia: presence of pathogenic organisms in the blood leading to sepsis

serum: blood minus cells and clotting factors

sulcus: furrow or fissure

suture/interrupted suture: stitch to close wound

temporal muscle: muscle from side of skull to the mandible

temporomandibular joint: jaw joint or articulation

tibial graft: bone from the tibia or shin bone

Thiersch graft: split-skin graft with the thickness of tissue paper

vulcanite: a rubber hardened with sulphur

Wolfe graft: a full-thickness skin graft without any subcutaneous fat

Notes

Chapter 1

1 J Heslop (1998). 'The Murray Clarke Oration: A brief history of burn treatment and the contribution of four New Zealand pioneers of plastic surgery', in *Australian and New Zealand Journal of Surgery* 68, 746–51. Meikle MC (2006). 'The evolution of plastic and maxillofacial surgery in the twentieth century: The Dunedin connection', *The Surgeon* 4, pp. 325–34.

2 AH McLintock (1949). *The History of Otago: The origins and growth of a Wakefield class settlement.* Otago Centennial Historical Publications, Dunedin.

3 E Olssen (1984). *A History of Otago.* John McIndoe Ltd, Dunedin.

4 AH Reed (1956). *The Story of Early Dunedin.* AH & AW Reed, Wellington.

5 AH McLintock (1966). 'Cargill, William (1784–1860), Otago coloniser', in *An Encyclopaedia of New Zealand.* vol 1, ed. AH McLintock. RE Owen, Government Printer, Wellington).

6 AH McLintock (1958). *Crown Colony Government in New Zealand.* RE Owen, Government Printer, Wellington; P Bloomfield (1961). *Edward Gibbon Wakefield: Builder of the British Commonwealth.* Longmans, Green & Co, London.

7 KC McDonald (1965). *City of Dunedin: A century of civic enterprise.* Dunedin City Corporation. Coulls Somerville Wilkie Ltd, Dunedin.

8 DW Carmalt Jones (1945). *Annals of the University of Otago Medical School 1875-1939.* AH & AW Reed, Wellington and Dunedin.

9 GE Thompson (1919). *A History of the University of Otago (1869-1919).* J Wilkie & Co, Dunedin.

10 GL Pearce (1976). *The Scots of New Zealand.* William Collins Ltd, Auckland.

11 WP Morrell (1969). *The University of Otago: A centennial history.* University of Otago Press, Dunedin.

12 Dorothy Page (2008). *Anatomy of a Medical School: A history of medicine at the University of Otago 1875-2000.* Otago University Press, Dunedin.

13 SFW Holloway (1966). 'The Apothecaries' Act 1815: A reinterpretation. Part I: The origins of the Act', *Medical History* 10, 107–29; J Menzies Campbell (1958). *From a Trade to a Profession: Byways in dental history.* Limited edition of 350 copies published privately by the author; ND Richards (1968). 'Dentistry in England in the 1840s: The first indications of a movement towards professionalization', *Medical History* 12, 137–52; MGH Bishop & S Gelbier (2002). 'Ethics: How the Apothecaries' Act of 1815 shaped the dental profession. Part 1: The apothecaries and the emergence of the dental profession', *British Dental Journal* 193, 627–31.

14 TWH Brooking (1980). *A History of Dentistry in New Zealand.* New Zealand Dental Association, John McIndoe Ltd, Dunedin.

15 WJ Gies (1926). *Dental Education in the United States and Canada: A report to the Carnegie Foundation for the Advancement of Teaching.* Carnegie Foundation for the Advancement of Teaching, New York.

Chapter 2

1 BJ Fraser (1966). 'Gillies, John (1802–1871), Otago Resident Magistrate', in *An Encyclopaedia of New Zealand.* vol I, ed. AH McLintock. RE Owen, Government Printer, Wellington.

2 Jane Thomson (ed.) (1998). 'John Gillies 1802–1871'. *Southern People: A dictionary of Otago Southland biography.* Longacre Press in association with Dunedin City Council.

3 JW Stack (1936). *More Maoriland Adventures.* AH & AW Reed, Dunedin, pp. 102–08.

4 'Arrival of the *Slains Castle* (from the *Otago Witness*, November 13, 1852)'. Accessed at freepages. genealogy.rootsweb.ancestry.com/~nzbound/ slainscastle.htm

5 AH McLintock (1958). *Crown Colony Government in New Zealand.* RE Owen, Government Printer, Wellington.

6 BJ Fraser (1966). 'Gillies, Thomas Bannatyne (1828–1889)', in *An Encyclopaedia of New Zealand.*

vol I, ed. AH McLintock. RE Owen, Government Printer, Wellington.

7   Lois Galer (1995). 'Transit House', in *Houses of Dunedin: An illustrated collection of the city's historic homes.* Hyndman Publishing, Dunedin. pp. 60–02.

8   Jane Thomson (ed.) (1998). 'Robert Craig Gillies, 1835–1886'. *Southern People: A dictionary of Otago Southland biography.* Longacre Press in association with the Dunedin City Council.

9   HD Gillies. 'Sir Harold Gillies KBE, FRCS, 1895–1900', in *The Wanganui Collegian* 1954, pp. 33–34.

10 B Hamilton & D Hamilton (2003). *Never a Footstep Back: A history of the Wanganui Collegiate School 1854–2003.* Whanganui College Board of Trustees, Whanganui, p. 115.

11 P Pierce (1990). 'Hugh Trumble, 1867–1938'. *Australian Dictionary of Biography.* vol 12, Melbourne University Press, Melbourne, p. 268.

12 E Grayland (1967). 'Sir Harold Gillies: Maker of new faces'. *Famous New Zealanders.* Whitcombe & Tombs, Christchurch, pp. 37–46.

13 Reginald Pound (1964). *Gillies: Surgeon Extraordinary.* Michael Joseph, London.

14 England Golf Internationals: Complete Player Records. www.archive.englishgolfunion.org.uk

15 D Sugrue (1997). 'A memorable interview: None of his business', *British Medical Journal* 314: 0.08 (11 January).

16 WP Morrell (1969). *The University of Otago: A centennial history.* University of Otago Press, Dunedin.

17 E Ives (2000). *The First Civic University: Birmingham 1880–1980: An introductory history.* Birmingham University Press, Birmingham.

18 RA Cohen (1958). *The History of the Birmingham Dental Hospital and Dental School, 1858–1958.* Board of Governors of the United Birmingham Hospitals.

19 Speech given by Ronald Cohen to the Dental Students' Society at the celebration of their jubilee in November 1945. www.dentistry.bham.ac.uk

20 RH Brown (2007). *Pickerill: Pioneer in plastic surgery, dental education, and dental research.* Otago University Press, Dunedin; Obituary: HP Pickerill CBE, MD, ChM, MDS, FRACS. *British Medical Journal* 2 (25 August 1956). p. 483.

21 Dental Surgery. Regulations of the General Medical Council. University of Birmingham. Degrees in Dentistry – namely Bachelor and Master of Dental Surgery (BDS and MDS). *British Medical Journal* (25 August 25 1900). pp. 525–26.

22 'A message from the late Dr HP Pickerill' (1956), *New Zealand Dental Journal* 52, pp. 193–94.

23 RF Stockwell (1970). 'Owen Vivian Davies', *New Zealand Dental Journal* 66, pp. 364–68.

24 TWH Brooking (1980). *A History of Dentistry in New Zealand.* New Zealand Dental Association, John McIndoe Ltd, Dunedin.

25 HP Pickerill (1912). 'Double resection of the mandible'. *Dental Cosmos* 54, pp. 114–19; HP Pickerill & ST Champtaloup (1914). 'An investigation into the causes of immunity to dental disease in the Maori of the Urewera', *New Zealand Dental Journal* 9, pp. 169–82; HP Pickerill (1915). 'The etiology of dental caries', *British Dental Journal* 36, pp. 361–85; HP Pickerill (1915). 'Cleft palate', *Dental Cosmos* 57, pp. 1304–05.

26 HP Pickerill (1912). *The Prevention of Dental Caries and Oral Sepsis.* Baillière, Tindall and Cox. Covent Garden, London.

27 HP Pickerill (1912). *Stomatology in General Practice.* Oxford Medical Publications, London.

Chapter 3

1   W Stanley Macbean Knight (1914–20). *The History of the Great European War: Its causes and effects.* vol I. Caxton Publishing Company, Surrey Street, London: www.bbc.co.uk/history/world wars/wwone/

2   John Keegan (1976). *The Face of Battle.* Jonathan Cape, London.

3   RT Foley & H McCartney (2006). *The Somme: An eyewitness history.* Folio Society, London.

4   JS Davis (1926). 'The art and science of plastic surgery', *Annals of Surgery* 84, pp. 203–10.

5   AA Bowlby (1915). 'The Bradshaw lecture on wounds in war', *British Journal of Surgery* 3, pp. 451–74. Sir Anthony Alfred Bowlby (1855–1929) Bart, KCB, KCMG, KCVO was Surgeon-in-Ordinary to King George V and consulting surgeon to the BEF in France during the First World War.

6   Frank Richards (1933). *Old Soldiers Never Die.* Faber & Faber Ltd, London. Frank 'Big Dick' Richards' classic account of the war is arguably the most famous of all the memoirs written by a common soldier. A reservist when war broke out, in 1914 he joined the 2nd Battalion Royal Welch Fusiliers, and served throughout every major battle of the war as

a private. He was awarded both the Distinguished Conduct Medal (DCM) and the Military Medal (MM) for distinguished conduct in the field. The DCM was the second highest award for gallantry in action (after the Victoria Cross) for all army ranks below commissioned officers, and the MM was the equivalent of the Military Cross.

7   Sir A Bowlby & C Wallace (1917). 'The development of British surgery at the front', *British Medical Journal* (2 June), pp. 705–21.

8   Anon ('A Royal Field Leech') (1917). *The Tale of a Casualty Clearing Station*. William Blackwood & Sons, Edinburgh and London. Originally published in monthly instalments in *Blackwood's Magazine*; the author has not been identified.

9   *Diary of a Nursing Sister on the Western Front, 1914–1915*. William Blackwood & Sons, Edinburgh and London. Published anonymously in 1915, but since attributed to Katherine Luard (1872–1962). A member of the Army Nursing Service Reserve, Luard was mobilised on the outbreak of war; this account details the early days of confusion and her life as a nursing sister on an ambulance train. (Accessible online as a Project Gutenberg ebook courtesy of The Internet Archive/Canadian Libraries.)

10 WH Dolamore (1916). 'The treatment in Germany of gunshot injuries of the face and jaws', *British Dental Journal* 37 (war supplement), pp. 105–84.

11 Sir Harold Gillies & D Ralph Millard Jr (1957). *The Principles and Art of Plastic Surgery*, 2 vols. Little, Brown & Co, Boston; Reginald Pound (1964). *Gillies: Surgeon Extraordinary*. Michael Joseph Ltd, London.

12 A Lindemann (1915). 'Zur Deckung grösserer Defekte der Weichteile bei Kieferschuss-verletzungen', in C Bruhn (ed.), *Die gegenwärtigen Behandlungswege der Kieferschussverletzungen: Ergebnisse aus dem Düsseldorfer Lazarette für Kieferveletzte. (Kgl. Reservelazarett)*, Heft 1. Verlag von JF Bergmann, Wiesbaden, pp. 13–29. (I am grateful to Dirk Bister for translating relevant sections for notes 12 and 13.)

13 A Lindemann (1916). 'Über die Beseitigung der traumatischen Defekte der Gesichtsknochen: Ein Beitrag zur fieren Osteoplastik', in C Bruhn (ed.), *Die gegenwärtigen Behandlungswege der Kieferschussverletzungen: Ergebnisse aus dem Düsseldorfer Lazarette für Kieferveletzte. (Kgl.*

Reservelazarett), Heft IV–VI, Verlag von JF Bergmann, Wiesbaden (1916–1917), pp. 243–328.

14 WH Dollamore (1917). 'The treatment of injuries of the face and jaws at Düsseldorf', *British Dental Journal* 38 (war supplement) pp. 1–37. An abridged translation of C Bruhn (ed.) (1916–17), *Die gegenwärtigen Behandlungswege der Kieferschussverletzungen*, Heft IV–VI, Verlag von JF Bergmann, Wiesbaden, pp. 243–455.

15 RH Ivy (1971). 'The mysterious AC Valadier', *Plastic and Reconstructive Surgery* 47, pp. 365–70.

16 McAuley JE (1974). 'Charles Valadier: A forgotten pioneer in the treatment of jaw injuries', *Proceedings of the Royal Society of Medicine* 67, pp. 785–89; JE McAuley (1990). 'Valadier revisited', *Dental History* 19, pp. 16–21.

17 WP Cruse (1987). 'Auguste Charles Valadier: A pioneer in maxillofacial surgery', *Military Medicine* 152, pp. 337–41.

18 'Particulars of Civil Surgeons desirous of service with the Royal Army Medical Corps. Valadier describes himself as an oral surgeon.' (Copy of document in Valadier's Service and Career File, RADC/1914/1918/39 1914–1918, Army Medical Services Museum Archives, Keogh Barracks, Aldershot, England.)

19 In the *New York Times* dated 11 January 1891, under Columbia College, the honour men for 1889–90 are listed: Sophomore Class, Charles A Valadier achieved honours in Greek, Latin, English Literature, Rhetorical Composition and German. On 9 June 1892 the *New York Times* reported that Charles A Valadier was a member of the 138th graduating class of Columbia College with an AB (Bachelor of Arts). He achieved honours in Latin, Ethics, Botany, Experimental Psychology and History of Philosophy and received one of the 18 university fellowships awarded that year.

20 LJ Godden (1971). *History of the Royal Army Dental Corps*. Royal Army Dental Corps, Aldershot; VH Ward & MJ Newell (1997). *Ex Dentibus Ensis: A history of the Army Dental Service*. RADC Historical Museum.

21 M Rauer (ed. S Marble). *Yanks in the King's Forces: American Physicians serving with the British Expeditionary Force in World War I*. Office of Medical History, Office of the Surgeon General, United States Army. www.history.amedd.army.mil/booksdocs/wwi/AmericanArmyMCOfficersBEF.pdf

22 Ian Hay (1953). *One Hundred Years of Army Nursing: The story of the British Army nursing services from the time of Florence Nightingale to the present day.* Cassell, London.

23 Lieut-Colonel Guy N Stephen RAMC (1919). 'Notes on the history of Boulogne as a military medical base', *Royal United Services Institution Journal* 63, pp. 39–48, 271–87; 64, pp. 393–409.

24 The Official War Diary of Maud McCarthy (1859–1949), Matron-in-Chief, BEF in France and Flanders, is held at the National Archives under the references WO95/3988, 3989, 3990 and 3991. (Accessible on the Internet under scarletfinders.co.uk) The following entries refer directly to Major Valadier by name:
12 April 1916: Letter from A/Matron 13 Stationary, giving particulars for Major Valadier's special ward for jaw cases. Mrs. Johnston put in charge, operating theatre attached; all the latest appliances for these special cases have been supplied.
12 September 1916: Official correspondence from DDMS, Boulogne – Major Valadier now satisfied with the number of nursing staff provided for his wards and considered them quite efficient.
1 March 1917: Major Valadier: Miss Hordley, A/Principal Matron, Boulogne, wrote that Major Valadier was very ill with pneumonia and was being nursed at 7 Stationary Hospital.
19 October 1917: From there they [a group of visiting dignitaries] went to 83 General Hospital, where they were shown Major Valadier's wonderful jaw wards and the therapeutic department of Major Curtis Webb. (With acknowledgements and gratitude to Sue Light, who transcribed the Official War Diary of Maud McCarthy for information about Valadier, and went to the trouble of visiting the National Archives to clarify the name change of No 13 Stationary to 83rd General Hospital in May 1917.)

25 DJ Smithson (2001). 'The Royal Army Dental Corps Museum archive (ca 1917–1920)', *Journal of Audiovisual Media in Medicine* 24, pp. 184–88. The Army Medical Services Museum at Aldershot has a collection of stereographic glass slides and stereographic cards taken by Mr Fullerton, chief clerk to Valadier, illustrating a variety of maxillofacial injuries, which were used as teaching material for dental personnel during the Second World War.

26 P Martinier & G Lemerle (1917). *Injuries of the Face and Jaw and their Repair and the Treatment of Fractured Jaws.* Translated by H Lawson Whale. Baillière, Tindall and Cox, London.

27 AC Valadier (1916). 'A few suggestions for the treatment of fractured jaws', *British Journal of Surgery* 4, pp. 64–73.

28 AC Valadier & H Lawson Whale (1917). 'A report on oral and plastic surgery and on prosthetic appliances', *British Journal of Surgery* 5, pp. 151–71; AC Valadier & H Lawson Whale (1917). 'A note on oral surgery', *British Medical Journal* 2, pp. 5–6.

29 H Lawson Whale (1919). *Injuries to the Head and Neck.* Baillière, Tindall & Cox, London; Paul Hoeber, New York. The book consists of 322 pages and 130 illustrations, many of them reproduced courtesy of Major Valadier. As he points out in the introduction, the volume is in no sense a textbook, but a systematised attempt to make useful generalisations from cases he had treated during the war – mainly involving the neck, nose and face – from emergency treatment at a CCS to reconstruction at a base hospital.

30 A Codivilla (1905). 'On the means of lengthening, in the lower limbs, the muscles and tissues which are shortened through deformity', *Journal of Bone and Joint Surgery* Am s2-2, pp. 353–69.

31 Letter from Philip Thorpe, a former patient of Major Sir Charles Valadier, to Mr JE McAuley, dated 29 May 1965; it includes his impressions of Valadier and the treatment he received for a wound to his face. (This and several other letters from Thorpe to McAuley dated 1965/66 are in Valadier's Service and Career File, RADC/1914/1918/39 1914–1918, Army Medical Services Museum Archives, Keogh Barracks, Aldershot, England.)

32 Letter from Field-Marshal Sir John French, Commander-in Chief of the BEF, dated 8 October 1915, requesting the War Office grant Mr Auguste Charles Valadier the honorary rank of major while serving with His Majesty's Army in France. (Copy in Valadier's Service and Career File, RADC/1914/1918/39 1914–1918.

33 Letter from General Sir Douglas Haig, Commander-in-Chief of the BEF from December 1915, dated 30 April 1916, in support of a decoration for Valadier. (Copy Valadier's Service and Career File, RADC/1914/1918/39 1914–1918.

34 On 4 February 1899 Auguste Charles Valadier married Marion Stowe in Manhattan, New York

(source: Family Search International Genealogical Index). The following two items relating to Valadier's abandonment of his wife and young son appeared in the *New York Times*: 'Dentist accused by wife' (24 August 1903) and 'Erlanger denies charges' (12 July 1904): '… the charges were preferred by Dr Auguste Charles Valadier, who spent more than three months in the jail after he had been arrested on the complaint of his wife, who sued for separation.'

35 During 1916 a number of hospitals and universities in the US supplied volunteer medical staff for service with the BEF. The original six units assigned for duty and the BEF hospitals they took over were as follows: US Army Base Hospital No 2 (No 1 General) at Etretat. Parent institution: Presbyterian Hospital, New York, Director Dr George Brewer (active June 1917–January 1919); US Army Base Hospital No 4 (No 9 General) at Rouen. Parent institution: Lakeside Hospital, Cleveland, Director Dr George Crile (May 1917–March 1919); US Army Base Hospital No 5 (No 11 General) at Camiers, then (No 13 General) at Boulogne. Parent institution: Harvard University, Director Dr Harvey Cushing (June 1917–January 1919); US Army Base Hospital No 10 (No 16 General) at Le Treport. Parent institution: Pennsylvania Hospital, Philadelphia, Director Dr RH Harte (June 1917–February 1919); US Army Base Hospital No 12 (No 18 General) at Dannes-Camiers. Parent institution: Northwestern University Medical School, Chicago, Director Dr FA Beasley (June 1917–March 1919). US Army Base Hospital No 21 (No 12 General) at Rouen. Parent institution: Washington University, St Louis, Director Dr Fred T Murphy (May 1917–January 1919). (With acknowledgements to William Chapin (1926). *The Lost Legion: The story of the fifteen hundred American doctors who served with the BEF in the Great War*. Published privately, Springfield, Massachusetts; George Crile (1947). *An Autobiography*. JB Lippincott, Philadelphia; Harvey Cushing (1936). *From a Surgeon's Journal 1915-1918*. Little, Brown, Boston.)

36 SR Aziz (2001). 'Harvard dental school and the fight for "the ideals of democracy"', *Journal of Oral and Maxillofacial Surgery* 59, pp. 428–33.

37 H Martin Deranian (2007). *Miracle Man of the Western Front*. Chandler House Press, Worcester, Massachusetts. An excellent and comprehensive account of Kazanjian's life and work. Copiously illustrated, it is particularly informative about his surgery during the First World War.

38 Floyd Gibbons (1918). *And They Thought We Wouldn't Fight*. George H Doran Co., New York. Floyd Gibbons, a foreign correspondent for the *Chicago Tribune*, was en route to cover the war in Europe on the RMS *Laconia* when it was torpedoed on the night of 25 February 1917. After six hours in open boats most of the passengers and crew were rescued by HMS *Laburnum*. That night Gibbons cabled a 4000-word article 'The sinking of the Laconia', which was syndicated in metropolitan dailies across the US. The story caused a sensation; it was read from the floor of both houses of Congress and played a role in changing American anti-isolationist feeling; war was declared against Germany five weeks later. At the Battle of Belleau Wood in June 1918 Gibbons was shot in the face, losing an eye while attempting to rescue an American soldier, and was awarded the Croix de Guerre.

39 Gordon Bell (1968). *Surgeon's Saga*. AH & AW Reed, Wellington.

40 VH Kazanjian (1916). 'Immediate treatment of gunshot fractures of the jaws', *British Dental Journal* 37 (war supplement), pp. 297–336; VH Kasanjian (1917). 'The department of oral surgery of the Harvard Surgical Unit', *British Medical Journal* 2, pp. 3–5; VH Kazanjian (1918). 'Splints combined with sutures through the bone for the immobilisation of extensive fractures of the lower jaw', *Proceedings of the Royal Society of Medicine* 11 (Odontology Section), pp. 67–86.

41 VH Kazanjian & H Burrows (1917). 'The treatment of haemorrhage caused by gunshot wounds of the face and jaws', *British Journal of Surgery* 5, pp. 126–50; VH Kazanjian & H Burrows (1918). 'The treatment of gunshot wounds of the face accompanied by extensive destruction of the lower lip and mandible', *British Journal of Surgery* 6, pp. 74–85.

42 HD Gillies (1920). *Plastic Surgery of the Face: Based on selected cases of war injuries of the face including burns*. Published by the Joint Committee of Henry Frowde and Hodder & Stoughton, Oxford University Press, London. Reprinted (1986), Classics of Surgery Library, Gryphon Editions Ltd, Birmingham, Alabama.

Chapter 4

1 Anne Pitcher (1996). *The Cambridge Military Hospital Aldershot: An illustrated history.* Holmes & Sons, 10 High St, Andover, Hampshire. Prince George, 2nd Duke of Cambridge, was the only son of Prince Adolphus, 1st Duke and seventh son of King George III, and since he had no legitimate heirs, on his death in 1904 the title lapsed. It was restored in 2011 (the Fifth creation) when, hours before his wedding to Catherine Middleton on 29 April 2011, Prince William of Wales was created Duke of Cambridge, Earl of Strathearn and Baron Carrickfergus.

2 'Blackie' (Sister Catherine Black) (1939). *King's Nurse, Beggar's Nurse.* Hurst & Blackett, London. Catherine Black (1883–?) MBE, ARRC (Associate Royal Red Cross) was on the nursing staff of the London Hospital and on the outbreak of war joined the QAIMNS and was sent to the Cambridge Military Hospital, Aldershot. In the autumn of 1916 she was transferred to No 7 General Hospital in St Omer, where she treated officers with shell-shock. She later moved to a CCS in Poperhinge, No 41 Stationary Hospital in Sailly-Laurette and No 5 General Hospital in Rouen. She was the personal nurse to King George V from 1928 until his death from cardiorespiratory failure in 1936. (With many thanks to Sue Light, who kindly provided copies of the relevant pages from her copy of Catherine Black's autobiography recalling her experiences at Aldershot.)

3 Sir Harold Gillies, D Ralph Millard Jr (1957). *The Principles and Art of Plastic Surgery.* 2 vols. Little, Brown & Co, Boston; Reginald Pound (1964). *Gillies: Surgeon Extraordinary.* Michael Joseph Ltd, London.

4 As Robert Graves explained in *Goodbye to All That* (p. 75), permission to spell Welch with a *c* was granted by a special Army Council Instruction of 1919, which went on to say, 'Welch referred us somehow to the archaic North Wales of Henry Tudor and Owen Glendower and Lord Herbert of Cherbury, the founder of the regiment; it dissociated us from the modern North Wales of chapels, Liberalism, the dairy and drapery business, slate mines, and the tourist trade.'

5 Ian Whitehead (1996). 'Not a doctor's work? The role of the British regimental medical officer in the field', in Hugh Cecil and Peter H Liddle (eds) *Facing Armageddon: The First World War experienced.* Leo Cooper, London, pp. 466–74.

6 Peter Lovegrove (1951). *Not Least in the Crusade: A short history of the Royal Army Medical Corps.* Gale & Polden, Aldershot (p. 47); Keith Simpson (1996). 'Dr James Dunn and shell shock', in Hugh Cecil and Peter Liddle (eds) *Facing Armageddon: The First World War experienced.* Leo Cooper, London. pp. 502–20.

7 Chapin WAR (1926). *The Lost Legion: The story of the fifteen hundred American doctors who served with the BEF in the Great War.* Published privately, Springfield, Massachusetts. William Andrew Robertson Chapin (1890–1969), MC, MD from Massachusetts, was attached to the 6th Battalion, The Queen's Own Royal West Kent Regiment, for the last 14 months of the war. Of the 1427 American doctors loaned to the British in 1918, over 1200 saw service at the Front, 30 were captured, 18 killed, 250 wounded and 163 were decorated for bravery; Nick Bosanquet (1996). 'Health systems in khaki: The British and American medical experience' in *Facing Armageddon,* in Hugh Cecil and Peter Liddle (eds) *Facing Armageddon: The First World War experienced.* Leo Cooper, London, pp. 451–65.

8 Viscount Gladstone (1918). *William GC Gladstone: A memoir.* Nisbet & Co, London. William Glynne Charles Gladstone (1885–1915) was a grandson of the Liberal Prime Minister William Ewart Gladstone, and the last of four generations of Gladstones to serve in the House of Commons as MP for Kilmarnock Burghs. At the beginning of the First World War he enlisted as a second lieutenant in the Royal Welch Fusiliers and was fatally shot through the head by a German sniper at Poperhinge on 13 April 1915, aged 29.

9 Siegfried Sassoon (1930). *Memoirs of an Infantry Officer.* Faber & Faber Ltd, London. The page numbers quoted in the text come from a paperback edition by Simon Publications, Safety Harbour, Florida.

10 Jean Moorcroft Wilson (1998). *Siegfried Sassoon: The making of a war poet: A biography (1886–1918).* Gerald Duckworth & Co Ltd, London.

11 Frank Richards (1933). *Old Soldiers Never Die.* Faber & Faber Ltd, London.

12 Captain JC Dunn (1987). *The War the Infantry Knew 1914–1919: A chronicle of service in France and Belgium with the Second Battalion, His Majesty's*

Twenty-Third Foot, The Royal Welch Fusiliers: Founded on personal records, recollections and reflections, assembled, edited and partly written by one of their medical officers. Jane's Publishing Co Ltd, London. The book was first published in the United Kingdom by PS King Ltd in 1938 in a private edition of 500 copies. James Churchill Dunn (1871–1955) had a New Zealand connection. His father Richard emigrated to New Zealand from Lanarkshire in the 1860s, married an Irish girl, and Dunn was born on a farm at Churchill in the Waikato on 14.2.1871. A few months later both his parents were killed by a Maori raiding party, but Dunn survived and was discovered by a neighbouring farmer and sent back to Scotland, where he was raised by two spinster aunts. (With acknowledgements to the Introduction by Keith Simpson in the 1987 edition of *The War the Infantry Knew*.)

13 RVS Thompson (1995). 'What are the priorities in plastic surgery?' Kay–Kilner Prize Essay, 1994. *British Journal of Plastic Surgery* 48, pp. 410–18.

14 Joseph Hone (1939). *The Life of Henry Tonks*. William Heinemann Ltd, London; L Morris (2004). www.oxforddnb.com/view/article/36535. *Oxford Dictionary of National Biography*, Oxford University Press, Oxford.

15 JP Bennett (1968). 'Henry Tonks and his contemporaries'. *British Journal of Plastic Surgery* 39, pp. 1–34.

16 J Freeman (1985). 'Professor Tonks: War artist', *Burlington Magazine* 127, pp. 284–91, 293.

17 David Boyd Haycock (2009). *A Crisis of Brilliance: Five young British artists and the Great War*. Old Street Publishing, London.

18 Diane 'Dickie' Orpen. 'Henry Tonks'. Personal memoir in the Antony Wallace Archive, British Association of Plastic, Reconstructive and Aesthetic Surgeons, Royal College of Surgeons of England. Date unknown.

19 E Chambers (2009). 'Fragmented identities: Reading subjectivity in Henry Tonks' surgical portraits'. *Art History* 32, pp. 578–607; S Biernoff (2010). 'Flesh poems: Henry Tonks and the art of surgery'. *Visual Culture in Britain* 11, pp. 25–47; S Helmers (2010). 'Iconic images of wounded soldiers by Henry Tonks'. *Journal of War and Cultural Studies* 3, pp. 181–99.

20 HP Pickerill (1953). The Queen's Hospital, Sidcup. *British Journal of Plastic Surgery* 6, pp. 247–49.

21 S Callister (2007). '"Broken gargoyles": The photographic representation of severely wounded New Zealand soldiers'. *Social History of Medicine* 20, pp. 111–30; S Callister (2007). *The Face of War: New Zealand's Great War photography*. Auckland University Press, Auckland.

22 Ward Muir (1917). *Observations of an Orderly: Some glimpses of life and work in an English war hospital.* Simpkin, Marshall, Hamilton, Kent & Co, London (accessible on the Internet); Ward Muir (1918). *The Happy Hospital*. Simpkin, Marshall, Hamilton, Kent & Co, London. Lance-Corporal Ward Muir (1878–1927) RAMC(T), a writer, journalist and photographer, was editor of the *Gazette of the 3rd London General Hospital*, a monthly magazine started in October 1915 by the CO of the hospital, Lt-Col HE Bruce Porter.

23 FD Wood (1917). 'Masks for facial wounds', *The Lancet* (23 June), pp. 949–51.

24 K Feo (2007). 'Invisibility: memory, masks and masculinities in the Great War', *Journal of Design History* 20, pp. 17–27. According to the Gillies Archives at Queen Mary's Hospital, Sidcup, Anna Coleman Ladd's American Red Cross Studio in Paris produced 220 masks, but other secondary sources claim she produced just 97.

25 John Glubb (1978). *Into Battle: A soldier's diary of the Great War*. Book Club Associates, London.

26 W Warwick James & BW Fickling (1940). *Injuries of the Jaws and Face: With special reference to war casualties.* John Bale & Staples Ltd, London. Produced at the beginning of the war for the benefit of dental surgeons and others involved in the treatment of facial injuries.

27 M Weinberg (1916). 'Bacteriological and experimental researches on gas gangrene', *Proceedings of the Royal Society of Medicine* 9, pp. 119–44. Professor Weinberg was head of the bacteriology laboratories at the Pasteur Institute; GL Keynes (1981). *The Gates of Memory*. Oxford University Press, Oxford.

28 George Crile (1947). *An Autobiography*. 2 vols. JB Lippincott Co, Philadelphia. Edited by his wife, Grace Crile, and published posthumously.

29 J Lister (1867). 'On a new method of treating compound fractures, abscess, etc, with observations on the conditions of suppuration', *The Lancet* 1, pp. 326–29, 357–59, 387–89, 507–09; 295–96; J Lister (1867). 'On the antiseptic principle in the practice of surgery', *The Lancet* 2, pp. 353–56, 668–69.

30 J Lorraine Smith, AM Drennan, T Bettie & W Campbell (1915). 'Antiseptic action of hypochlorous

acid and its application to wound treatment', *British Medical Journal* (24 July), pp. 129–36.

31 HD Dakin (1915). 'On the use of certain antiseptic substances in the treatment of infected wounds', *British Medical Journal* 2 (28 August), pp. 318–20. The work described in this article was carried out in laboratories at Compiègne supported by the Rockefeller Institute attached to Hospital 21 of the French Army. It was here that the French surgeon and 1912 Nobel Laureate Alexis Carrel with the English chemist Henry Dakin developed the Carrel–Dakin method for cleansing infected wounds.

32 TS Helling & E Daon (1998). 'In Flanders fields: The Great War, Antoine Depage, and the resurgence of debridement', *Annals of Surgery* 228, pp. 173–81; EF Hirsch (2008). 'The treatment of infected wounds, Alexis Carrel's contribution to the care of wounded soldiers during World War I', *Journal of Trauma* 64, S209–10.

33 Sir AA Bowlby (1918). 'An address on primary suture of wounds at the front in France', *British Medical Journal* (13 March), pp. 333–37.

34 HMW Gray (1915). 'Treatment of gunshot wounds by excision and primary suture', *British Medical Journal* (28 August), p. 317; HMW Gray (1918). 'Primary suture of war wounds', *British Medical Journal* (20 April), p. 467. Letter in response to Sir Anthony Bowlby's article in the March 13 *BMJ*, naming the surgeons who had laid the foundations of excision and primary suture in 1914 and 1915 whom Bowlby had failed to acknowledge. Sir Henry Gray was a pioneer of *aseptic* as opposed to *antiseptic* surgery.

35 C de Costa & F Miller (2007). 'Sarah Bernhardt's "Doctor God": Jean-Samuel Pozzi (1846–1918)', *Australian and New Zealand Journal of Obstetrics and Gynaecology* 47, pp. 352–56.

36 A Fleming (1915). 'On the bacteriology of septic wounds', *The Lancet* (18 September), pp. 638–43; Sir AE Wright (1917). 'Conditions which govern the growth of the bacillus "gas gangrene" in artificial culture media, in the blood fluids *in vitro* and in the dead and living organism', *The Lancet* (6 January), pp. 1–9; Sir AE Wright & A Fleming (1918). 'Acidaemia in gas gangrene and on the conditions which favour the growth of its infective agent in the blood fluids', *The Lancet* (9 February), pp. 204–10: A Fleming (1919). 'The action of chemical and physiological antiseptics in a septic wound', *British Journal of Surgery* 7, pp. 99–129. Hunterian Lecture delivered at the Royal College of Surgeons of England, 12 February 1919.

37 Sir AE Wright, A Fleming & L Colebrook (1918). 'The conditions under which the sterilisation of wounds by physiological agency can be obtained', *The Lancet* (15 June), pp. 831–38.

38 Before the Boer War, Wright had been responsible for developing an anti-typhoid vaccine, but fewer than 12,000 men (about 4 percent) had been inoculated – during the three years of the war the army had nearly 58,000 cases of typhoid with about 9000 deaths. During the First World War the majority of British troops were voluntarily immunised with typhoid-specific vaccine and TAB (also protective against paratyphoid A and B) that saved thousands of lives. Compulsory immunisation had been rejected by the government as the result of a vociferous campaign by those opposed to vaccination on the grounds that it was a gross interference with personal liberty. For further discussion see: A Hardy (2000). 'Straight back to barbarism: Antityphoid inoculation and the Great War, 1914', *Bulletin of the History of Medicine* 74, pp. 265–90.

39 GM FitzGibbon (1968). 'The commandments of Gillies'. Gillies Memorial Lecture 1967. *British Journal of Plastic Surgery* 21, pp. 226–39.

40 HD Gillies & LAB King (1917). 'Mechanical supports in plastic surgery', *The Lancet* (17 March), pp. 412–14.

41 HD Gillies (1917). 'Some cases of facial deformity treated in the Department of Plastic Surgery at the Cambridge Hospital, Aldershot', *St Bartholomew's Hospital Journal* 79–83. The article was reprinted the same year in the *Journal of Laryngology, Rhinology and Otology* 32, pp. 274–83.

Chapter 5

1 'The Queen's Hospital, Frognal, Sidcup (1917)', *The Lancet* 190 (3 November), pp. 687–89.

2 'The Queen's Hospital Sidcup'. This small, soft-covered brochure of 19 pages traces the origins and history of the hospital up until its closure in 1929, together with the names of the officers who worked there. The committee that approached Sir Charles Kenderdine for advice which led to the foundation of the hospital was composed of Lady Rodney, Lady Gough, the Earl of Clarendon and

Sir William Arbuthnot Lane. (The copy of the brochure consulted by the author is in the Hocken Collections, Uare Taoka o Hakena, University of Otago. Pickerill papers, reference number MS-3094/021).

3   A Keogh (1916). 'Surgical organization in war', *British Journal of Surgery* 4, pp. 1–8.

4   Reginald Pound (1964). *Gillies: Surgeon Extraordinary*. Michael Joseph Limited, London, p. 42.

5   HP Pickerill (1953). 'The Queen's Hospital, Sidcup', *British Journal of Plastic Surgery* 6, pp. 247–49.

6   G Seccombe Hett (1917). 'The use of the turbinals and the septum in the repair of injuries and defects in the wall of the nasal cavity', *The Lancet* (15 December), pp. 892–97; G Seccombe Hett (1919). 'Methods of repair of wounds of the nose and nasal accessory sinuses', *Proceedings of the Royal Society of Medicine* 12 (Laryngology Section), pp. 136–47; W Kelsey Fry, GS Hett (1918). 'Case of total loss of hard palate and exposure of the antral cavities in the mouth', *PRSM* 11, pp. 90–94.

7   J Eastcourt Hughes (1972). *Henry Simpson Newland: A Biography*. Published by the South Australian Fellows of the Royal Australasian College of Surgeons; N Hicks & E Leopold (1988). 'Newland, Sir Henry Simpson (1873–1969)', *Australian Dictionary of Biography*. vol 11, Melbourne University Press, pp. 8–9.

8   HD Gillies (1920). *Plastic Surgery of the Face: Based on selected cases of war injuries of the face including burns*. Published by the Joint Committee of Henry Frowde and Hodder & Stoughton at the Oxford University Press, London. Reprinted (1986) by the Classics of Surgery Library, Gryphon Editions Ltd, Birmingham, Alabama. Accessible online at Internet Archive.

9   VP Blair (1920). *Surgery and Diseases of the Mouth and Jaws: A practical treatise on the surgery and diseases of the mouth and allied structures*. 3rd edn. CV Mosby Co, St Louis. The third edition was updated to include data from the First World War concerning gunshot wounds of the face and jaws.

10 RH Ivy (1962). *A Link with the Past*. Williams & Wilkins Co, Baltimore.

11 John Staige Davis (1919). *Plastic Surgery: Its principles and practice*. P Blakiston's Son & Co, Philadelphia. Accessible online at Internet Archive.

12 JS Davis (1926). 'The art and science of plastic surgery', *Annals of Plastic Surgery* 84, pp. 203–10.

13 W Kelsey Fry (1917). 'On the treatment of gunshot wounds of the maxilla and mandible', *The Lancet* 2 (8 December), pp. 852–65; W Kelsey Fry (1919). 'Prosthetic treatment of old injuries of the maxilla', *Proceedings of the Royal Society of Medicine* 12 (Odontology Section), pp. 73–94; W Kelsey Fry, G Seccombe Hett (1918). 'Case of total loss of hard palate and exposure of the antral cavities in the mouth'. *PRSM* 11 (Laryngology Section), pp. 90–94.

14 JL Aymard (1917). 'Nasal reconstruction. With a note on Nature's plastic surgery', *The Lancet* 2 (15 December), pp. 888–92.

15 HD Gillies (1920). 'The tubed pedicle in plastic surgery', *The Lancet* 2 (7 August), p. 320; Reprinted (1923) in the *Journal of Laryngology and Otology* 38, p. 503.

16 VP Filatov (1917). 'Plastika na kruglom stebl', *Vestnik Oftalmologii* 34, pp. 149–58. Reprinted (1959). 'Plastic procedure using a round pedicle'. Translated from the Russian by M Labunka, MT Gnudi and JP Webster. *Surgical Clinics of North America* 39, pp. 277–87.

17 H Ganzer (1917). 'Die Bildung von langgestielten Stranglappen bei Gesichtsplastik', *Berliner Klinische Wochenschrift* 54, pp. 1095–96.

18 JF Esser (1917). 'Studies in plastic surgery of face. I. Use of skin from the neck to replace face defects. II. Plastic operations about the mouth. III. The epidermic inlay', *Annals of Surgery* 65, pp. 297–331.

19 HD Gillies (1918). 'Discussion on plastic operation of the eyelids', *Transactions of the Ophthalmological Society of the UK* 38, pp. 1–18, 70–100, 348–54.

20 ME Ring (2001). 'How a dentist's name became a synonym for a life-saving device: The story of Dr Charles Stent', *Journal of the History of Dentistry* 49, pp. 77–80.

21 *Suśruta Samhitā* (2004). Illustrated in 3 vols. Translated into English with explanatory notes by Professor KR Srikantha Murthy. Chaukhamba Orientalia, Varanasi.

22 G Tagliocozzi (1597). *De Curtorum Chirurgia per Insitionem*. Gasparum Bindorum, Venice.

23 JP Bennett (1983). 'Aspects of the history of plastic surgery since the 16th century', *Journal of the Royal Society of Medicine* 76, pp. 152–56.

24 Daryl Lindsay (1965). *The Leafy Tree: My Family*. FW Chester Pty Ltd, Melbourne, Victoria.

25 T Gibson & PB Medawar (1943). 'The fate of skin homografts in man', *Journal of Anatomy* 77, pp. 299–310.

26 PB Medawar (1944). 'The behaviour and fate of skin autografts and skin homografts in rabbits', *Journal of Anatomy* 78, pp. 176–99.

27 PB Medawar (1945). 'A second study of the behaviour and fate of skin homografts in rabbits', *Journal of Anatomy* 79, pp. 157–76.

28 RE Billingham, L Brent & PB Medawar (1956). 'The antigenic stimulus in transplantation immunity', *Nature* 178, pp. 514–19.

29 HD Gillies & HK Kristensen (1951). 'Ox cartilage in plastic surgery', *British Journal of Plastic Surgery* 4, pp. 63–73.

30 MBL Craigmyle (1955). 'Studies of cartilage autografts and homografts in the rabbit', *British Journal of Plastic Surgery* 8, pp. 93–100.

31 MBL Craigmyle (1958). 'Regional lymph node changes induced by cartilage homo- and heterografts in the rabbit', *Journal of Anatomy* 92, pp. 74–83.

32 L Peer (1954). 'Cartilage grafting', *British Journal of Plastic Surgery* 7, pp. 250–62.

33 T Gibson & WB Davis (1953). 'The fate of preserved bovine cartilage implants in man', *British Journal of Plastic Surgery* 6, pp. 4–25.

34 T Gibson & WB Davis (1955). 'Some further observations on the use of preserved animal cartilage', *British Journal of Plastic Surgery* 8, pp. 85–92.

35 R Mowlem (1941). 'Bone and cartilage transplants: their use and behaviour', *British Journal of Surgery* 29, pp. 182–93.

36 RJV Battle (1964). 'Thomas Pomfret Kilner, CBE, DM, FRCS', *British Journal of Plastic Surgery* 17, pp. 330–34.

37 HA Condon & E Gilchrist (1986). 'Stanley Rowbotham: Twentieth century pioneer anaesthetist', *Anaesthesia* 41, pp. 46–52.

38 AN Bamji (2006). 'Sir Harold Gillies: Surgical pioneer', *Trauma* 8, pp. 143–56.

Chapter 6

1 HTB Drew (1923). *The War Effort in New Zealand*, vol IV, HTB Brew (ed.), Whitcombe & Tombs Ltd, Auckland, pp. xi–xxii.

2 TA Hunter (1923). 'New Zealand Dental Corps', in HTB Brew (ed.) *The War Effort in New Zealand*, vol IV, Whitcombe & Tombs Ltd, Auckland, pp. 138–48.

3 HP Pickerill (1917). 'New Zealand Expeditionary Force, Jaw Department', *New Zealand Dental Journal* 13, pp. 35–38.

4 Lieut-Col Myers CMG, NZMC (1923). 'New Zealand Hospitals in the United Kingdom', in HTB Brew (ed.) *The War Effort in New Zealand*, vol IV, Whitcombe & Tombs Ltd, Auckland, pp. 115–26.

5 RH Brown (2007). *Pickerill: Pioneer in plastic surgery, dental education, and dental research*. University of Otago Press, Dunedin.

6 HP Pickerill (1912). 'Double resection of the mandible', *Dental Cosmos* 54, pp. 114–19.

7 HP Pickerill (1915). 'Cleft palate', *Dental Cosmos* 57, pp. 1304–05.

8 HP Pickerill (1916). 'Treatment of fractured mandible accompanying gunshot wounds', *New Zealand Dental Journal* 12, pp. 75–80.

9 FH Albee (1915). *Bone Graft Surgery*. WB Saunders Ltd, Philadelphia.

10 FH Albee (1943). *A Surgeon's Fight to Rebuild Men: An autobiography*. EP Dutton & Co, New York, p. 64.

11 MC Meikle (2007). 'On the transplantation, regeneration and induction of bone: The path to bone morphogenetic proteins and other skeletal growth factors', *The Surgeon* 5, pp. 232–43.

12 Sir Frank Bowerbank (1958). *A Doctor's Story*. Wingfield Press, Wellington.

13 Lieut-Col AD Carbery CBE, NZMC (1924). *The New Zealand Medical Service in the Great War 1914–1918: Based on official documents*. Whitcombe & Tombs Ltd, Auckland, p. 488. Reprinted (2002) by Naval & Military Press, Uckfield, East Sussex.

14 HP Pickerill (1918). 'Intra-oral skin grafting: The establishment of the buccal sulcus', *Proceedings of the Royal Society of Medicine* 12, p. 17.

15 HP Pickerill (1918). 'Methods of control of fragments in gunshot wounds of the jaws', *New Zealand Dental Journal* 14, pp. 109–18.

16 HP Pickerill (1919). 'Orthodontics in war surgery', *New Zealand Dental Journal* 14, pp. 140–41.

17 HP Pickerill (1919). 'Cases illustrative of plastic surgery of the face', *New Zealand Dental Journal* 14, pp. 184–85. Before and after photographs of six cases under the care of Major HP Pickerill at Sidcup. No accompanying text.

18 HP Pickerill (1924). *Facial Surgery*. E & S Livingstone, Edinburgh.

19 FH Albee (1943). *A Surgeon's Fight to Rebuild Men: An autobiography*. EP Dutton & Co, New York, p. 129.

20 HP Pickerill & JR White (1922). 'The tube skin-flap in plastic surgery', *British Journal of Surgery* 9, pp. 321–33.

21 Lois Galer (1981). 'Castlemore holds its king to ransom', in *More Houses and Homes*. Allied Press Ltd, Dunedin, pp. 18–19.

22 Coroner's report into the death of Angus McPhee Marshall, 1 April 1927. Archives New Zealand, Wellington (J 46 1927/926). Kindly provided by Dr Basil R Hutchinson.

23 Dr Marion Whyte (later Cameron): Interview with Dr Basil R Hutchinson, 12 August 1969, in Dunedin. (Basil Hutchinson, personal communication.)

24 AD Macalister (1987). 'The Queen's Hospital, Sidcup: The foundation of British Oral Surgery'. Menzies Campbell Lecture, Royal College of Surgeons of England. (Unpublished manuscript, Hocken Collections, Uare Taoka o Hakena, University of Otago, MS-3094/014.)

25 AN Bamji (1993). 'The Macalister archive: Records from the Queen's Hospital, Sidcup, 1917–1921', *Journal of Audiovisual Media in Medicine* 16, pp. 76–84.

Chapter 7

1 John Hector 'Jock' McIndoe, Archibald McIndoe's nephew (personal communication). During the Second World War, JH McIndoe (b. 1924) joined the Royal New Zealand Air Force and, after pilot training at RNZAF Taieri near Dunedin and then in Canada, flew Hawker Typhoons on ground-attack missions across Europe with 198 Squadron RAF. He attended several Guinea Pig functions while staying with his uncle on leave, and after the war followed his father into managing the family printing and publishing business.

2 Arrival of the *Alpine*. *Otago Witness* arrivals 1859. www.genealogy.rootsweb.ancestry.com

3 James McIndoe (1899). 'Reminiscence: Voyage of the *Alpine*', *Otago Witness*, 28 September 1899, p. 59.

4 AH Reed (1956). *The Story of Early Dunedin*. AH & AW Reed, Wellington.

5 KID Maslen (2007). 'McIndoe, John 1858–1916', *Dictionary of New Zealand Biography*. www.dnzb.govt.nz

6 DW Carmalt Jones (1945). *Annals of the University of Otago Medical School 1875–1939*. AH & AW Reed, Wellington and Dunedin.

7 CE Hercus (1966). 'McIndoe, Sir Archibald Hector CBE (1900–1960)', *An Encyclopaedia of New Zealand*. vol 2 (ed. AH McLintock). RE Owen, Government Printer, Wellington.

8 Sir Arthur Porritt's speech made at a meeting of the college council, 14 April 1960, following the death of McIndoe can be found in the college journal: 'In memoriam: Sir Archibald Hector McIndoe, CBE, MSc, MS, FRCS, FACS 1900–1960', *Annals of the Royal College of Surgeons of England* 26, pp. 332–35.

9 Hugh McLeave (1961). *McIndoe: Plastic Surgeon*. Frederick Muller Ltd, London.

10 Leonard Moseley (1962). *Faces from the Fire: The biography of Sir Archibald McIndoe*. The Quality Book Club, 121 Charing Cross Road, London WC2.

11 Sir Archibald Hector McIndoe (1900–1960). *Lives of the Fellows of the Royal College of Surgeons of England 1952–1964*. E&S Livingstone, Edinburgh and London 1970, pp. 266–68.

12 John Mowlem (1934). *Moulham – a Dorset Place and Surname – Mowlem*. Printed privately for the author by E Dwelley, Greenside, Kenilworth Road, UK. Dorothy Mowlem (personal communication).

13 Hamish Keith (2007). *The Big Picture: A history of New Zealand art from 1642*. Godwit, Random House, Auckland.

14 KA Trembath (1969). *Ad Augusta: A centennial history of Auckland Grammar School 1869–1969*. Wilson & Horton Ltd, Auckland, for the Auckland Grammar School Old Boys' Association.

15 Auckland Grammar School Archives. Paul Paton, curator (personal communication).

16 Obituary, Rainsford Mowlem MB NZ, FRCS (1986). *The Lancet* 1 (15 March), pp. 629–30. Other obituaries appeared in *The Times* 18 February 1986; *Daily Telegraph* 18 February 1986; *British Medical Journal* 1986, 292, p. 774 with portrait; *British Journal of Plastic Surgery* 1987, 40, pp. 102–03 with portrait; New Zealand *Medical Journal* 1986, 99, p. 252.

17 RLG Dawson (1988). 'The history, antecedents and progress of the Mount Vernon Centre for Plastic Surgery and Jaw Injuries, Northwood, Middlesex 1939–1983', *British Journal of Plastic Surgery* 41, pp. 83–91.

18 Sir Harold Gillies & D Ralph Millard Jr (1957). *The Principles and Art of Plastic Surgery*. 2 vols. Little, Brown & Co, Boston; Reginald Pound (1964). *Gillies: Surgeon Extraordinary*. Michael Joseph, London.

19 Benjamin K Rank (1987). *Heads and Hands: An era of plastic surgery*. Gower Medical Publications Ltd, London.

20 'Book review: *Plastic Surgery of the Face*', *The Lancet* 196, Issue 5056, (24 July 1920), p. 194.

21 CW Chapman (1987). 'Two World Wars and the years between', in *The History of the British Association of Plastic Surgery: The first 40 years*. Published by the British Association of Plastic Surgery.

22 TP Kilner (1947). 'Cases and case records illustrating orthopaedic and plastic surgical teamwork', *Proceedings of the Royal Society of Medicine* 40, pp. 892–95.

23 'Visits to clinics. Mr Norman Tanner's gastroenterological unit, St James' Hospital, London', *British Journal of Surgery* (1964) 51, pp. 141–46.

24 Robert H Ivy (1962). *A Link with the Past*. Williams & Wilkins Co, Baltimore.

25 JF Fraser & CS Hultman (2010). 'America's fertile frontier: How America surpassed Britain in the development and growth of plastic surgery during the interwar years of 1920–1940', *Annals of Plastic Surgery* 64, pp. 610–13.

26 PJ Sykes & AN Bamji (2010). 'Plastic surgery during the interwar years and the development of the specialty in Britain', *Annals of Plastic Surgery* 65, pp. 374–77.

27 Abraham Flexner (1910). *Medical Education in the United States and Canada: A report to the Carnegie Foundation for the Advancement of Teaching*. Bulletin 4, New York. In 1908 the Council on Medical Education (CME) of the American Medical Association asked the Carnegie Foundation to survey American medical education. Abraham Flexner was chosen to conduct the survey. At the time there were 155 medical schools in North America (14 in Chicago alone), many of them 'propriety', ie, owned by one or more doctors, unaffiliated with a college or university. The aim of the CME was the elimination of medical schools that failed to meet their standards. Flexner regarded the Johns Hopkins School of Medicine as the ideal model for American medical schools and recommended: (1) Two years of college or university study as the minimum entry requirement. (2) The length of medical education should be four years. (3) Proprietary medical schools should either close or be incorporated into existing universities. All these recommendations were adopted and by 1935 there were only 66 medical schools operating in the US. One consequence of the report was that medical education became much more expensive, putting it beyond the reach of all but upper- and middle-class white males: African Americans, women and students of limited financial means could not usually afford six to eight years of university education. (The report is accessible at www.carnegiefoundation.org/sites/Flexner_Report)

28 P Randell, JG McCarthy & RC Wray (1996). 'History of the American Association of Plastic Surgeons', *Plastic and Reconstructive Surgery* 97, pp. 1254–92.

29 Alexis de Tocqueville (1848). *Democracy in America*. Translated by Henry Reeve. Pratt, Woodford & Co, New York. (Accessible at www.gutenberg.org/ebooks/815)

30 Brian Kingcome (1999). *A Willingness to Die: Life and memories from Fighter Command and beyond*. Tempus Publishing Ltd, Stroud, Gloucestershire. Reprinted (2008) by The History Press, Stroud, Gloucestershire. One of the most interesting memoirs by a fighter pilot, edited by Peter Ford and published posthumously.

31 Kenneth J Valentine (1983). 'The founding of Saint Andrew's Hospital, Dollis Hill'. A six-page history published by the Willesden Local History Society. www.willesden-local-history.co.uk/books.htm

Chapter 8

1 *Report to the Army Council of the Army Advisory Standing Committee on Maxillo-Facial Injuries*. The War Office, June 1935. Printed and published by His Majesty's Stationery Office, 1939.

2 Dr Ian Kelsey Fry (personal communication).

3 EJ Dennison (1963). *A Cottage Hospital Grows Up: The story of the Queen Victoria Hospital East Grinstead*. Anthony Blond Ltd, London.

4 JP Bennett (1988). 'A history of the Queen Victoria Hospital, East Grinstead', *British Journal of Plastic Surgery* 41, pp. 422–40.

5 Geert Hofstede (2001). *Culture's Consequences: Comparing values, behaviors, institutions and organizations across nation*, 2nd edn. Sage Publications, Thousand Oaks, California. The data on which the power distance index (PDI) is based were collected by IBM in the company's international employee attitude survey programme, conducted in two survey rounds between 1967 and

1973 from 72 countries. For a discussion of the influence of the PDI on airline pilot behaviour, read the chapter on 'The ethnic theory of plane crashes' in Malcolm Gladwell's entertaining book entitled *Outliers: The story of success* (2008). Little, Brown & Co, New York.

6   RM Davies (1977). 'Relationships: Archibald McIndoe, his times, society, and hospital'. McIndoe Lecture 1976. *Annals of the Royal College of Surgeons of England* 59, pp. 359–67.

7   Hugh McLeave (1961). *McIndoe: Plastic Surgeon.* Frederick Muller Ltd, London.

8   Patrick Bishop (2003). *Fighter Boys: Saving Britain 1940.* HarperCollins Ltd, London.

9   Lord Moran (1945). *The Anatomy of Courage.* Constable, London. pp 36–37.

10   AH McIndoe (1983). 'Total reconstruction of the burned face. The Bradshaw Lecture 1958. The Late Sir Archibald Hector McIndoe, CBE, MS, FRC', *British Journal of Plastic Surgery* 36, pp. 410–20. Sir Archibald McIndoe died in 1960 and this lecture, which had been delivered at the Royal College of Surgeons of England in 1958, was never published. In view of the importance of both the subject and its author, the college council granted permission for it to be published posthumously.

11   DM Jackson (1964). 'Burns: McIndoe's contribution and subsequent advances', *Annals of the Royal College of Surgeons of England* 61, pp. 335–40.

12   EC Davidson (1925). 'Tannic acid in the treatment of burns', *Surgery, Gynecology and Obstetrics* 41, pp. 202–21.

13   'The use of tannic acid in the local treatment of burn wounds: Intriguing old and new perspectives', *Wounds* 13, pp. 144–58 (2001). www.medscape.com.

14   AH McIndoe (1940). 'Discussion at a joint meeting on the treatment of burns. Sections of Surgery and of Therapeutics and Pharmacology, Royal Society of Medicine, 6 November 1940. Meeting chaired by JB Hunter and Sir William Wilcox', *The Lancet* 2 (16 November), pp. 621–22.

15   R Mowlem (1941). 'The treatment of burns', *Proceedings of the Royal Society of Medicine* 34, pp. 221–24.

16   TP Kilner (1934). 'The Thiersch graft: Its preparation and uses', *Post-graduate Medical Journal* 10, pp. 176–81; BK Rank (1940). 'Use of the Thiersch skin graft', *British Medical Journal* 1(4142), pp. 46–49.

17   Thiersch or split-skin graft. In 1872 Léopold Ollier devised a method of skin grafting which was later modified by Karl Thiersch and sometimes called the Ollier-Thiersch graft, though the term Thiersch graft is now commonly used. A thin graft consisting of the surface epithelial layers. When cut, it should have the appearance of thin tissue paper and should leave a donor surface with only tiny punctuate haemorrhages on which epithelial healing should be complete in seven days. The graft is applied to the raw surface of the wound and maintained in place by firm pressure applied by either a crêpe bandage or elastoplast strapping.

18   Emily Mayhew (2004). *The Reconstruction of Warriors: Archibald McIndoe, the Royal Air Force and the Guinea Pig Club.* Greenhill Books, London.

19   AH McIndoe. Foreword to Colin Hodgkinson (1957). *Best Foot Forward: The autobiography of Colin Hodgkinson.* WW Norton & Co, New York.

20   Colin Hodgkinson (1957). *Best Foot Forward: The autobiography of Colin Hodgkinson.* WW Norton & Co, New York.

21   AH McIndoe quoted in Leonard Mosley (1962). *Faces from the Fire.* The Quality Book Club, London, p. 94.

22   Peter Williams & Ted Harrison (1979). *McIndoe's Army: The injured airmen who faced the world.* Pelham Books, London.

23   In 1930 Mrs Gordon Clemetson, writing as 'Aunt Agatha', started the Peanut Club in the children's section of the *Kent and Sussex Courier.* Mrs Clemetson promised a bag of peanuts to anyone giving 12 new pennies to raise money for the Kent and Sussex Hospital in Tunbridge Wells. The idea was to collect small sums of money from a large number of people and it was remarkably successful. Financial help was extended to the Queen Victoria Hospital, East Grinstead in 1936, and the club continued to provide amenities for the hospital outside the NHS for many years.

24   Rita Donovan (2000). *As for the Canadians: The remarkable story of the RCAF's 'Guinea Pigs' of World War II.* Buschel Books, Ottawa.

25   KW Fry, PR Shepherd, AC McLeod & GJ Parfitt (1942). *The Dental Treatment of Maxillo-Facial Injuries.* Blackwell Scientific Publications Ltd, Oxford.

26   Bf 109 or Me 109? Some confusion exists regarding the correct prefix for the Messerschmitt 109 (as well

as the Messerschmitt 110) and both are found in the English literature. Wilhelm Messerschmitt was the chief designer of the Bayerische Flugzeugwerke AG (BFW; Bavarian Aircraft Works) where the 109 was first developed, hence the prefix Bf. In July 1938 Messerschmitt was appointed chairman and managing director of BFW and the company renamed Messerschmitt AG; aircraft developed by the company after that date (such as the jet engined Me 262) received the Me prefix. However, the official *Reichsluftfahrtministerium* (German Air Ministry) designation for the aircraft remained the Bf 109 throughout the war and is used in this book.

27 Edward Bishop (2001). *McIndoe's Army: The story of the Guinea Pig Club and its indomitable members.* Grub Street, London. A rewritten version of *The Guinea Pig Club* (1963) published for the 60th anniversary of the club's foundation.

Chapter 9

1 *The Battle of Britain, August–October 1940: An Air Ministry account of the great days from 8th August–31st October 1940.* Issued by the Ministry of Information on behalf of the Air Ministry, first published 1941, His Majesty's Stationery Office, London; *The Battle of Britain.* Air Ministry Pamphlet 156: Issued by the Department of the Air Member for Training, August 1943. (Both can be accessed online at ww2airfronts.org/Theatres/eto/hmso.)

2 Edward Bishop (2001). *McIndoe's Army: The story of the Guinea Pig Club and its indomitable members.* Grub Street, London. A rewritten version of *The Guinea Pig Club* (1963) published for the 60th anniversary of the club's foundation; Peter Williams & Ted Harrison (1979). *McIndoe's Army: The injured airmen who faced the world.* Pelham Books, London. Based on the Thames Television documentary *The Guinea Pig Club,* screened in 1979.

3 Group-Captain AJL Scott (1920). *Sixty Squadron RAF: A history of the squadron from its formation.* William Heinemann, London. George H Doran Co, New York. (Accessible online.)

4 Vincent Orange (2004). 'Smith-Barry, Robert Raymond (1886–1949), Air Force Officer', *Oxford Dictionary of National Biography.* Oxford University Press. Orange was educated at Eton College and Trinity College, Cambridge. He was awarded the AFC in 1918 and the Order of Leopold of Belgium.

5 William Simpson (1955). *I Burned My Fingers.* Putnam, London.

6 Tom Gleave (1988). 'Tribute to Blackie'. *Guinea Pig* magazine.

7 RM Davies (1977). McIndoe Lecture 1976. 'Relationships: Archibald McIndoe, his times, society, and hospital'. *Annals of the Royal College of Surgeons of England* 59, pp. 359–67.

8 RAF Casualty (1941). *I Had a Row with a German.* Macmillan & Co Ltd, London. 'RAF Casualty' was the nom de plume of Squadron Leader Tom Gleave.

9 Anon (1941). *Fighter Pilot: A personal record of the campaign in France September 8th 1939 to June 13th 1940.* BT Batsford Ltd, London. The personal memoir of Pilot Officer Paul HM Richey (1916–1989) DFC & Bar. One of the classic books of the war, *Fighter Pilot* sold 75,000 copies as soon as they could be produced and has been republished several times, most recently in 2001 by Cassell & Co. Before he was wounded on 19 May, Richey had claimed 10 victories. After a long period of rehabilitation, he returned to active duty in 1941 and ended the war as a wing commander.

10 Cuthbert Orde (1942). *Pilots of Fighter Command: Sixty-four Portraits.* GG Harrap & Co, London. During the Battle of Britain, artist Cuthbert Julian Orde (1888–1968) was commissioned by the Air Ministry to draw the heroes of RAF Fighter Command. He visited almost every operational station in the country and produced 160 drawings. A selection, *Some of the Few: Portraits by Cuthbert Orde* by Reid JPM (1960), was published by MacDonald Publishing, London.

11 Richard Hillary (1942). *The Last Enemy.* Macmillan & Co Ltd, London.

12 Lovat Dickson (1950). *Richard Hillary.* Macmillan & Co Ltd, London. Horatio Henry Lovat Dickson (1902–1987) was general editor and a director of Macmillan who commissioned *The Last Enemy.* Hillary and Dickson became friends and the book includes material from Hillary's letters and diaries describing the psychological struggle that eventually led to his tragic death.

13 Richard Hillary (1942). *Falling Through Space.* Reynal & Hitchcock, New York. The American edition of *The Last Enemy.*

14 Foreword by DMW in a commemorative edition of *The Last Enemy* published in 2003 on 20 April, Richard Hillary's birthday, 60 years after his death,

by Pippin Publishing Corporation, Don Mills, Ontario, Canada. 'DMW' was Denise Maxwell-Woosnam, Peter Pease's fiancée.

15 Arthur Koestler (1945). *The Yogi and the Commissar and other Essays*. Macmillan Press, New York; Eric Linklater (1947). *The Art of Adventure*. Macmillan & Co, London; Sebastian Faulks (1996). *The Fatal Englishman: Three short lives*. Hutchinson Books Limited, London.

16 David Ross (2000). *Richard Hillary: The definitive biography of a Battle of Britain fighter pilot and author of* The Last Enemy. Grub Street, London.

17 William Simpson (1943). *One of Our Pilots Is Safe*. Hamish Hamilton, London; William Simpson (1944). *The Way of Recovery*. Hamish Hamilton, London; William Simpson (1955). *I Burned My Fingers*. Putnam, London.

18 Geoffrey Page (1981). *Tale of a Guinea Pig*. Pelham Books, London. Reissued in 1999 as *Shot Down in Flames*.

19 TP Kilner (1934). 'The Thiersch graft: Its preparation and uses', *British Medical Journal* (25 May), pp. 846–89.

20 S Cade (1944). 'War surgery in the Royal Air Force', *British Journal of Surgery* 32, pp. 12–24.

21 Brian Cull & Roland Symons (2003). *One-Armed Mac: The story of Squadron Leader James MacLachlan DSO, DFC and 2 Bars, Czech War Cross based upon his diaries and letters*. Grub Street, London.

22 Richard Pape (1953). *Boldness Be My Friend*. Paul Elek Ltd, London.

23 Colin Hodgkinson (1957). *Best Foot Forward: The autobiography of Colin Hodgkinson*. Odhams Press Ltd, London. WW Norton & Co, New York.

24 Sir William Rothenstein (1942). *Men of the RAF*. Oxford University Press, London. At the beginning of the Second World War, Sir William Rothenstein (1872–1945) offered his services as a war artist making portrait drawings of airmen at RAF bases in England. *Men of the RAF* contains 40 portraits together with an account of life in the service.

25 Vítek Formánek (1998). *The Stories of Brave Guinea Pigs*. J&HK Publishing, Hailsham, East Sussex.

26 Jo Capka (1958). *Red Sky at Night: The story of Jo Capka DFM as told to Kendall McDonald*. Anthony Blond Ltd, London.

27 Alois Siska (2008). *Flying for Freedom: The flying, survival and captivity experiences of a Czech pilot in the Second World War*. Translated by his daughter, Dagmar Johnson-Siska. Pen and Sword Books, Barnsley, Yorkshire.

28 John Harding (1988). *The Dancin' Navigator*. Asterisk Communications, Guelph, Ontario.

29 Rita Donovan (2000). *As for the Canadians: The remarkable story of the RCAF's 'Guinea Pigs' of World War II*. Buschek Books, Ottawa. The title *As for the Canadians* comes from the Guinea Pig Anthem.

Chapter 10

1 RLG Dawson (1988). 'The history, antecedents and progress of the Mount Vernon Centre for Plastic Surgery and Jaw Injuries, Northwood, Middlesex 1939–1983', *British Journal of Plastic Surgery* 41, pp. 83–91. Dawson was appointed to Hill End as a senior registrar in 1949 and much of which we know about Mowlem and the unit comes from his pen.

2 Lord Moran (1966). *Winston Churchill: The struggle for survival 1940–1965*. Taken from the diaries of Lord Moran, Heron Books, London. Charles McMoran Wilson MC, 1st Baron Moran of Manton (1882–1977), was Sir Winston Churchill's personal physician from 1940 until Churchill's death in 1965. In the book (p. 518) Moran gives an account of Mowlem's attendance on Churchill, who had badly burned his hand by exploding a box of matches with his cigar:

At that moment Mowlem, the plastic surgeon who had been looking after his hand while he was at Chequers, came into the room. Winston had already related how Mowlem had told him: 'The recuperative powers shown by your hand are those of a much younger man.' That is the kind of patter that Winston likes. It showed on Mowlem's part, a good working knowledge of psychology. I had not met him before, but I knew without asking that the PM liked him and had confidence in his skill, so that he did not suggest that Dunhill should see him again; in the field of surgery Winston can usually spot a master craftsman. His answers to Winston's questions were clear and decisive. There were no doubts in his mind; his manner was full of easy assurances.

When we left the room Mowlem recalled the first time he saw the PM at Chequers; how he sat on the bed for nearly an hour while Winston talked about Omdurman. It took me about a year to reach that stage with Winston. I left Mowlem and returned to the PM.

The Omdurman incident is described by Churchill in *My Early Life: A roving commission*, (1930), Thornton Butterworth Ltd, London. Reprinted (2007) by the Folio Society, London. Lieutenant RF Molyneux, a subaltern in the Blues, who like Churchill had been attached to the 21st Lancers at the Battle of Omdurman (2 September 1898), had been seriously wounded by a sword cut on his right wrist. On the way back to England, a nurse and Churchill were both prevailed upon by Molyneux's doctor, a great raw-boned Irishman, into providing skin grafts to cover the wound. Churchill's was the size of a shilling, cut from the inside of his forearm. Churchill later claimed, 'It remains there to this day and did him lasting good in many ways. I for my part keep the scar as a souvenir.' (In the Folio Society edition, the incident is described on pp. 196–97.)

3   BK Rank (1987). *Heads and Hands: An era of plastic surgery*. Gower Medical Publications Ltd, London; BK Rank (1987). 'The contribution of Rainsford Mowlem (1903–1986) to the development of plastic surgery', *Australia and New Zealand Journal of Surgery* 57, p. 127.

4   R Mowlem (1941). 'Discussion on chemotherapy and wound infection', *Proceedings of the Royal Society of Medicine* 34 (Section of Therapeutics and Pharmacology), pp. 340–42; JM Barron et al. (1953). 'Organisation and work of plastic units', in Sir Zachary Cope (ed.) *History of the Second World War: Surgery*, Her Majesty's Stationery Office, London, pp. 325–40. Colebrook was another protégé of Sir Almroth Wright and, like Fleming, had worked as an RAMC captain on wound infection in Wright's laboratory at No 13 General Hospital, Boulogne-sur-Mer.

5   *Report to the Army Council of the Army Advisory Standing Committee on Maxillo-Facial Injuries*. The War Office, June 1935. His Majesty's Stationery Office, 1939.

6   AH McIndoe (1941). 'Diagnosis and treatment of injuries of the middle third of the face', *British Dental Journal* 71, pp. 235–45.

7   AC McLeod & PR Shepherd (1941). 'Cap splints', *British Dental Journal* 71, pp. 267–77.

8   JL Dudley Buxton, GJ Parfitt & AB MacGregor (1941). 'Arch-wires for the immobilisation of fractures of the mandible', *British Dental Journal* 71, pp. 285–97.

9   R Mowlem (1941). 'A review of fixation methods from the standpoint of the plastic surgeon', *British Dental Journal* 71, pp. 323–31.

10 HD Gillies (1941). 'The replacement and control of maxillo-facial fractures', *British Dental Journal* 71, pp. 351–59.

11 Roger Anderson (1934). 'Fractures of the radius and ulna. A new anatomical method of treatment', *Journal of Bone and Joint Surgery* 16A, pp. 379–93.

12 R Mowlem, AB MacGregor, JL Dudley Buxton & JN Barron (1941). 'External pin fixation for fractures of the mandible', *The Lancet* 238 (4 October), pp. 391–93.

13 R Mowlem (1942). 'Experiences with various methods of skeletal fixation in fractures of the jaws', *Proceedings of the Royal Society of Medicine* 35 (Odontology Section), pp. 415–26.

14 AB MacGregor (1941). 'Sepsis in relation to fractures of the mandible', *British Dental Journal* 71, pp. 246–48.

15 W Warwick James & BW Fickling (1940). *Injuries of the Jaws and Face: With special reference to war casualties*. John Bale & Staples Ltd, London.

16 R Mowlem (1941). 'Bone and cartilage transplants: Their use and behaviour', *British Journal of Surgery* 29, pp. 182–93.

17 W Macewen (1881). 'Observations concerning transplantation of bone, illustrated by a case of interhuman osseous transplantation, whereby two-thirds of the shaft of a humerus was restored', *Proceedings of the Royal Society, London* 32, pp. 232–47.

18 W Macewen (1912). *The Growth of Bone: Observations on osteogenesis: An experimental enquiry into the development and reproduction of diaphyseal bone*. James Maclehose & Sons, Glasgow.

19 FH Albee (1915). *Bone Graft Surgery*. WB Saunders Ltd, Philadelphia.

20 EW Hey Groves (1917). 'Methods and results of transplantation of bone in the repair of defects caused by injury or disease', *British Journal of Surgery* 5, pp. 185–242.

21 A Lindemann (1916). 'Über die Beseitigung der traumatischen Defekte der Gesichtsknochen. Ein Beitrag zur fieren Osteoplastik'. Heft IV–VI, *Die gegenwärtigen Behandlungswege der Kieferschussverletzungen: Ergebnisse aus dem Düsseldorfer Lazarette für Kieferveletzte. (Kgl.*

Reservelazarett) (ed. C Bruhn). Verlag von JF Bergmann, Wiesbaden, pp. 243–328.

22 Sir Harold Gillies & D Ralph Millard Jr (1957). *The Principles and Art of Plastic Surgery*. 2 vols. Little, Brown & Co, Boston.

23 Sir Arthur Keith (1919). 'The introduction of certain orthopaedic methods to British surgery', *Menders of the Maimed: The anatomical & physiological principles underlying the treatment of injuries to muscles, nerves, bones & joints*. Henry Froude, Hodder & Stoughton, London, pp. 155–69.

24 Sir William Arbuthnot Lane carried out his first open operation on a fracture on 8 January 1894, when the broken ends of a non-united tibial fracture in a 34-year-old man were exposed and two screws inserted across the oblique line of the fracture to keep the fragments in place. He was not the first, however, to use direct methods to secure exact reapposition of the bone ends. Lister had wired the fragments of a broken patella together in 1877, and Albin Lambotte in Antwerp had wired oblique fractures of the tibia in the late 1880s, but apparently discontinued the practice. Carl Hansmann (1852–1917) of Hamburg is usually credited with being the first to use plates and screws for fracture fixation in 1886, but Lane made open reduction and internal fixation for the treatment of fractures a reliable and – in the face of conservative opinion – an acceptable procedure. It was not until 1968 that Hans-Georg Luhr in Göttingen proposed that plates and screws could be used in maxillofacial surgery for fracture and osteotomy fixation. Nevertheless, the method did not become widely used until the mid-1980s.

25 W Arbuthnot Lane (1905). *The Operative Treatment of Fractures*. The Medical Publishing Company Ltd, London; W Arbuthnot Lane (1907). 'Clinical remarks on the operative treatment of fractures', *British Medical Journal* (4 May), pp. 1037–48; W Arbuthnot Lane (1909). 'The operative treatment of fractures', *Annals of Surgery* 50, pp. 1106–13.

26 TB Layton (1956). *Sir William Arbuthnot Lane, Bt.* E&S Livingstone Ltd, Edinburgh. Chapter XII, 'Fractures', pp. 73–78.

27 WE Gallie & DE Robertson (1918). 'The transplantation of bone', *Journal of the American Medical Association* 70, pp. 1134–40.

28 CW Waldron & EF Risdon (1919). 'Mandibular bone-grafts', *Proceedings of the Royal Society of Medicine* 12 (Surgery Section), pp. 11–21. Presented at a discussion on bone grafting held on 22 January 1919 at the Royal Society of Medicine, London. The first English-language report of the use of bone from the iliac crest to reconstruct the mandible, although Albee in his autobiography *A Surgeon's Fight to Rebuild Men* (1943) mentions in passing that he restored the contour of the mandible of a French poilu with a U-shaped graft from the pelvic bone (p. 137) during his four-month stay in France in 1916.

29 WE Gallie (1919). 'Discussion on bone-grafting', *Proceedings of the Royal Society of Medicine* 12 (Surgery Section), pp. 22–23. William Gallie MD, FRCS was a Captain in the Canadian Army Medical Corps at the time and was later appointed Professor of Surgery at the University of Toronto.

30 G Chubb (1920). 'Bone-grafting of the fractured mandible with an account of sixty cases', *The Lancet* (3 July), pp. 9–14; G Chubb (1921). 'A further series of forty cases of bone-grafted mandibles', *The Lancet* (26 March), pp. 640–41.

31 R Mowlem (1944). 'Cancellous chip bone-grafts. Report on 75 cases', *The Lancet* 2 (9 December), pp. 746–48.

32 R Mowlem (1963). 'Bone grafting'. The Gillies Memorial Lecture, *British Journal of Plastic Surgery* 16, pp. 293–304.

33 MC Meikle (2007). 'On the transplantation, regeneration and induction of bone: The path to bone morphogenetic proteins and other skeletal growth factors', *The Surgeon* 5, pp. 232–43.

34 A Fleming (1929). 'On the antibacterial action of cultures of penicillin with special reference to their use in the isolation of *B. influenzae*', *British Journal of Experimental Pathology* 10, pp. 226–36.

35 E Chain, HW Florey, AD Gardner, NG Heatley, MA Jennings, J Orr-Ewing & AG Sanders (1940). 'Penicillin as a therapeutic agent', *The Lancet* 236 (24 August), pp. 226–28.

36 EP Abraham, E Chain, CM Fletcher, AD Gardiner, NG Heatley, MA Jennings & HW Florey (1941). 'Further observations on penicillin', *The Lancet* 238 (16 August), pp. 177–89.

37 P Neushul (1993). 'Science, government and the mass production of penicillin', *Journal of the History of Medicine and Allied Sciences* 48, pp. 371–95.

38 C Fletcher (1984). 'First clinical use of penicillin', *British Medical Journal* 289 (22–29 December), pp. 1721–23. Charles Fletcher MD, FRCP was Professor of Clinical Epidemiology at the University of London. In 1941 he was a Nuffield Research

Fellow at Oxford and the man who gave the first injection of penicillin to a patient. This occurred on 12 February 1941 at the Radcliffe Infirmary, Oxford.

39 Eric Lax (2004). *The Mould in Dr Florey's Coat: The remarkable true story of the penicillin miracle.* Little, Brown, London. The title comes from members of Florey's team having secreted spores of *Penicillium notatum* into their clothing, so that in the event of a German invasion and they had to flee the country, they would still have samples on which to continue their research.

40 RHH Lovell (2004). 'Wilson, Charles McMoran, first Baron Moran (1882–1977), physician and writer', in *Oxford Dictionary of National Biography*, Oxford University Press.

41 WH Schmidt & AJ Moyer (1944). 'Penicillin. I. Methods of assay', *Journal of Bacteriology* 47, pp. 199–208; AJ Moyer & RN Coghill (1946). 'Penicillin. VIII. Production of penicillin in surface cultures', *Journal of Bacteriology* 51, pp. 57–78; AJ Moyer & RN Coghill (1946). 'Penicillin. IX. The laboratory scale production of penicillin in submerged cultures by *Penicillium notatum* Westling (NRRL 832)', *Journal of Bacteriology* 51, pp. 79–93.

42 JN Barron, RV Christie, DB Fraser, LP Garrod, OT Mansfield, HV Morgan, R Mowlem, IM Robertson, AC Roxburgh & IA Roxburgh (1944). 'An investigation of the therapeutic properties of penicillin. A report to the Medical Research Council', *British Medical Journal* (15 April), pp. 513–30.

43 R Mowlem (1944). 'Surgery and penicillin in mandibular infection', *British Medical Journal* (15 April), pp. 517–19; R Mowlem (1945). 'Osteomyelitis of the jaws', *Proceedings of the Royal Society of Medicine* 38 (Odontology Section), pp. 452–55.

44 JN Barron & OT Mansfield (1944). 'The local application of penicillin in soft-tissue lesions', *British Medical Journal* (15 April), pp. 521–23.

45 Diana Orpen. 'Henry Tonks'. Personal memoir in the Antony Wallace Archive, British Association of Plastic, Reconstructive and Aesthetic Surgeons, Royal College of Surgeons of England (undated manuscript).

Chapter 11

1 Sir Harold Gillies & D Ralph Millard Jr (1957). *The Principles and Art of Plastic Surgery*, vol 2. Little, Brown & Co, Boston; Reginald Pound (1964). *Gillies: Surgeon Extraordinary.* Michael Joseph Ltd, London.

2 JC Mustardé (1987). 'The way it was', *European Journal of Plastic Surgery* 10, pp. 93–98. John Mustardé was a consultant ophthalmologist who retrained as a plastic surgeon after the war, with Gillies at Rooksdown and Kilner at Oxford. The paper is an amusing account of how Mustardé survived the contrasting personalities and cultures of the two centres.

3 William L Shirer (1959). *The Rise and Fall of the Third Reich: A history of Nazi Germany.* Simon & Schuster, New York.

4 J Rickard (19 February 2008). *Operation Aerial: The evacuation from Northwestern France, 15–25 June 1940.* (http://www.historyofwar.org/articles/operation_aerial.html)

5 Colin Smith (2009). *England's Last War Against France: Fighting Vichy, 1940–1942.* Weidenfeld & Nicolson, London.

6 Patrick Bishop (2003). *Fighter Boys: Saving Britain 1940.* HarperCollins, London.

7 John A Gillies (1912–1993) MBE QSO, the eldest son of Sir Harold Gillies, was educated at Winchester College and Gonville and Caius College, Cambridge, where he read law. He qualified as a chartered accountant in London and learned to fly with 604 (County of Middlesex) Squadron, RAuxAF. On the evening of 23 May 1940 during a fighter sweep with 92 Squadron Gillies was shot down over Dunkirk. Captured by the Germans, he became a POW in Stalag Luft III and part of the prisoners' organisation that led to the 'Great Escape'. In January 1949 Gillies and his wife Eileen emigrated to Invercargill, New Zealand, where he joined fellow POW Bob Stark as a partner in the accounting firm of Webb Stark & Co. He died in Wanaka, Central Otago. (With thanks to JA Gillies' daughter Jane Waller, Michael Fenton and Max Lambert.)

8 Winston Churchill, speaking in the House of Commons, 18 June 1940:

What General Weygand called the Battle of France is over. I expect that the Battle of Britain is about to begin. Upon this battle depends the survival of Christian civilisation. Upon it depends our own British life and the long continuity of our institutions and our Empire. The whole fury and might of the enemy must very soon be turned on us. Hitler knows that he will have to break us in this island or lose the war. If we can stand up to him, all Europe may be free and the life of the world may move forward into broad, sunlit uplands. But if we fail, then the whole world, including the United States, including all that we have known and cared for, will sink into the abyss of a new Dark Age, made more sinister, and perhaps more protracted, by the lights of perverted science. Let us therefore brace ourselves to our duties, and so bear ourselves that, if the British Empire and its Commonwealth last for a thousand years, men will still say, 'This was their finest hour.'

9   Michael JF Bowyer (1990). *The Battle of Britain: 50 years on.* Patrick Stephens Ltd, Wellingborough, Northamptonshire; Stephen Bungay (2000). *The Most Dangerous Enemy: An illustrated history of the Battle of Britain.* Aurum Press, London; Horst Boog (2000). 'The Luftwaffe's assault', in Paul Addison & Jeremy A Crang (eds). *The Burning Blue: A new history of the Battle of Britain.* Pimlico, Random House, London, pp. 39–54; James Holland (2010). *The Battle of Britain: Five months that changed history May–October 1940.* Bantam Press, London.

10   DB Levine (2008). 'The Hospital for the Ruptured and Crippled renamed the Hospital for Special Surgery 1940: The war years 1941–1945', *Hospital for Special Surgery Journal* 5, pp. 1–8. When the Hospital for the Ruptured and Crippled first opened its doors on 1 May 1863, the name of the hospital was not unusual, since it described the type of patients it treated. Hospitals founded during the nineteenth century were often known by a disease, a condition, or affiliation with a religious or ethnic group.

11   HD Gillies (1941). 'The replacement and control of maxillo-facial fractures', *British Dental Journal* 71, pp. 351–59.

12   JM Converse & FW Waknitz (1942). 'External skeletal fixation in fractures of the mandibular angle', *Journal of Bone and Joint Surgery* 24A, pp. 143–60. This article describes the first case in which the method of external pin fixation developed by Roger Anderson for long bones was used to immobilise a fracture of the mandible. The patient was a 21-year-old British soldier and the operation took place on 8 January 1941 at Rooksdown House, Park Prewett Hospital, Basingstoke, England. Frederick Waknitz (1906–2006) received his MD from the University of Kansas in 1933. During

the war he served in the European and Pacific Theatres until 1946, retiring with the rank of lieutenant colonel. After the war he settled in Seattle, Washington, where he practised orthopaedic surgery.

13   MA Rushton & FA Walker (1942). 'Mandibular fractures treated by pin fixation: Twenty-one cases', *American Journal of Orthodontics and Oral Surgery* 28, B307–15; Reprinted as: MA Rushton & FA Walker (1943). 'Mandibular fractures treated by pin fixation', *British Dental Journal* 74, pp. 4–11; TH Clouston & FA Walker (1943). 'The Clouston-Walker splint for pin fixation', *British Dental Journal* 74, pp. 147–52.

14   S Cade (1944). 'War surgery in the Royal Air Force', *British Journal of Surgery* 32, pp. 12–24.

15   PW Clarkson & FA Walker (1955). 'Gun-shot wounds of the face and jaws', in NL Rowe & HC Killey, *Fractures of the Facial Skeleton*. E&S Livingstone Ltd, Edinburgh and London.

16   Brian Kingcome (1999). *A Willingness to Die: Life & memories from Fighter Command and beyond.* Tempus Publishing Ltd, Stroud, Gloucestershire. Reprinted (2008) by The History Press, Stroud, Gloucestershire.

17   Bob Doe (1999). *Fighter Pilot: The story of one of the few.* CCB Associates, Selsdon, Surrey.

18   Helen Doe, personal communication.

19   Numbers of enemy aircraft shot down during the Battle of Britain by individual pilots tend to vary, but these figures are taken from Appendix 2: High-scoring RAF fighter pilots 1 July–31 October 1940 in Michael JF Bowyer (1990). *The Battle of Britain: 50 years on.* Patrick Stephens Ltd, Wellingborough, Northamptonshire, pp. 226–29.

20   Thomas Hardy. *The Dynasts: An epic drama of the war with Napoleon.* (Accessible on the Internet.)

21   RJV Battle (1953). 'War history of plastic surgery in the army', in Sir Zachary Cope (ed.) *History of the Second World War: Surgery.* Her Majesty's Stationery Office, London, pp. 341–59; CW Chapman (1987). 'Two world wars and the years between', *The History of the British Association of Plastic Surgery: The first 40 years.* British Association of Plastic Surgery, pp. 1–11; VH Ward & MJ Newell (1997). *Ex Dentibus Ensis: A history of the Army Dental Service.* Royal Army Dental Corps, Historical Museum.

22   JHW Clarkson, JJ Kirkpatrick & RS Lawrie (2008). 'Prevention by organization: The story of No 4 maxillofacial surgical unit in North Africa and

Italy during the Second World War', *Plastic and Reconstructive Surgery* 121, pp. 657–68.

23 PW Clarkson & RS Lawrie (1946). 'The management and surgical resurfacing of serious burns', *British Journal of Surgery* 33, pp. 311–23.

24 PW Clarkson, THH Wilson & RS Lawrie (1946). 'Treatment of jaw and face casualties in the British Army', *Annals of Surgery* 123, pp. 190–208.

25 Gillies HD & Harrison SH (1950). 'Operative correction by osteotomy of recessed malar maxillary compound in a case of oxycephaly', *British Journal of Plastic Surgery* 2, pp. 123–27; Sir Harold Gillies & D Ralph Millard Jr (1957). *The Principles and Art of Plastic Surgery*, vol II. Little, Brown & Co, Boston, pp. 551–53.

26 Murray C Meikle (2002). *Craniofacial Development, Growth and Evolution*. Bateson Publishing, Bressingham, Norfolk.

27 Le Fort Classification. René Le Fort (1869–1951) was a French Army surgeon from Lille. In 1901 he published *Etude expérimentale sur les fractures de la machoire supérieure* based on experimental injuries he had made to the face of cadavers with a blunt instrument. From these he concluded that fractures of the midface occurred along lines of weakness in the facial skeleton and could be grouped into three main categories: Le Fort I: a horizontal fracture above the teeth and palate; also known as a Guerin fracture. Le Fort II: pyramidal in shape extending from the maxilla below the zygomatic buttress to the orbital rim. Le Fort III: a high transverse fracture involving the zygomatic bones and extending across the orbit to the nasal and frontal processes of the maxilla. The Le Fort classification was subsequently used as a guide for designing osteotomies to correct abnormalities of the midface skeleton.

28 P Tessier (1967). 'Osteotomies totals de la face. Syndrome de Crouzon, syndrome d'Apert: oxycephalies, scaphocephalies, turricaphalies', *Annales de Chirurgie Plastique* 12, pp. 273–86; P Tessier (1971). 'The definitive plastic surgical treatment of the severe facial deformities of craniofacial dysostosis: Crouzon's and Apert's diseases', *Plastic and Reconstructive Surgery* 48, pp. 419–42.

29 H Gillies & NL Rowe (1954). 'L'osteotomie du maxillaire superieur enviségée essentiellement dans les cas de bec-de-lièvre totale'. [Osteotomy of the maxilla with special reference to total harelip], *Revue Stomatologie* 55, pp. 545–52.

30 SH Harrison (1951). 'Treacher Collins syndrome', *British Journal of Plastic Surgery* 3, pp. 282–90.

31 HL Obwegeser (2007). 'Orthognathic surgery and a tale of how three procedures came to be: a letter to the next generation of surgeons', *Clinics in Plastic Surgery* 34, pp. 331–55.

32 R Trauner & H Obwegeser (1957). 'The surgical correction of mandibular prognathism and retrognathia with consideration of genioplasty. I. Surgical procedures to correct mandibular prognathism and reshaping of the chin', *Oral Surgery, Oral Medicine, Oral Pathology* 10, pp. 677–89; H Obwegeser (1963). 'The indications for surgical correction of mandibular deformity by the sagittal splitting technique', *British Journal of Oral Surgery* 1, pp. 157–71; H Obwegeser (1969). 'Surgical correction of small or retrodisplaced maxillae', *Journal of Plastic and Reconstructive Surgery* 44, pp. 351–65.

Chapter 12

1 RH Brown (2007). *Pickerill: Pioneer in plastic surgery, dental education and dental research*. Otago University Press, Dunedin.

2 Lord Arthur Porritt (1978). 'As I remember: Sir Archibald McIndoe, CBE, FRCS', *Annals of Plastic Surgery* 2, pp. 174–75.

3 Richard Battle, rev. HCG Matthew (2004). 'McIndoe, Sir Archibald Hector (1900–1960)', *Oxford Dictionary of National Biography*, Oxford University Press.

4 CW Chapman (1987). 'Two world wars and the years between', *The History of the British Association of Plastic Surgery: The first 40 years*. British Association of Plastic Surgery, pp. 1–11.

5 Reginald Pound (1964). *Gillies: Surgeon Extraordinary*. Michael Joseph Ltd, London.

6 Richard Battle (2004). 'Gillies, Sir Harold Delf (1882–1960)', *Oxford Dictionary of National Biography*, Oxford University Press.

7 Eugene Grayland (1967). 'Sir Harold Gillies', *Famous New Zealanders*. Whitcombe & Tombs Ltd, Christchurch, pp. 37–46.

8 BK Rank (1987). 'The contribution of Rainsford Mowlem (1903-1986) to the development of plastic surgery', *ANZ Journal of Surgery* 57, p. 127.

9 'Obituary: Rainsford Mowlem MB, FRCS', *The Lancet* (15 March 1986), pp. 629–30.

10 Ross J Paterson (1948). 'Plastic surgery in the training of a surgeon', *British Journal of Plastic*

Surgery 1, pp. 4–8. Sir James Paterson Ross (1895–1980), Bart, KCVO, later became president of the Royal College of Surgeons of England, 1957–60.

11 James Percy Moss (1934–2010), late Emeritus Professor of Orthodontics, University College and Middlesex School of Dentistry (personal communication).

12 RLG Dawson (1986). 'Obituary: Rainsford Mowlem MB, FRCS', *British Journal of Plastic Surgery* 40, pp. 102–03.

13 Benjamin K Rank (1987). *Heads and Hands: An era of plastic surgery*. Gower Medical Publications Ltd, London.

14 Mowlem Land Trust: Registered Charity Number: 1049323. Assent dated 11 May 1990. Objects: Open spaces, footways and roadways for the benefit of the inhabitants of the Town of Swanage gifted by the will of the late Arthur Rainsford Mowlem FRCS together with the benefit of covenants attaching to the land. The income in 2010 was £300,000.

15 Sister Catherine ('Blackie') Black (1939). *King's Nurse, Beggar's Nurse*. Hurst & Blackett, London.

16 The television programmes include the six-part series *A Perfect Hero*, starring Nigel Havers as Pilot-Officer Hugh Fleming and James Fox as the famous plastic surgeon Angus Meikle. First broadcast in 1991, it is a fictional account of the experiences of Richard Hillary, after being shot down and badly burned in September 1940 during the Battle of Britain. It was adapted from the novel by Christopher Matthew, first published in 1980 as *The Long-Haired Boy* (Hamish Hamilton Ltd), and reissued as a paperback in 1991 as *A Perfect Hero* (Mandarin Publishing) to accompany the TV series.

Select bibliography

Addison P & JA Crang (eds) (2000). *The Burning Blue: A new history of the Battle of Britain*. Pimlico, London.

Albee FH (1915). *Bone Graft Surgery*. WB Saunders Ltd, Philadelphia.

— (1943). *A Surgeon's Fight to Rebuild Men: An Autobiography*. EP Dutton & Co, New York.

Anon ('A Royal Field Leech') (1917). *The Tale of a Casualty Clearing Station*. William Blackwood and Sons, Edinburgh and London. The author has not been identified.

Arbuthnot Lane W (1905). *The Operative Treatment of Fractures*. Medical Publishing Co Ltd, London.

Bell G (1968). *Surgeon's Saga*. AH & AW Reed, Wellington.

Bishop E (2001). *McIndoe's Army: The story of the Guinea Pig Club and its indomitable members*. Grub Street, London. A rewritten version of *The Guinea Pig Club* (1963) published for the 60th anniversary of the club's foundation.

Bishop P (2003). *Fighter Boys: Saving Britain 1940*. HarperCollins, London.

Black C (1939). *King's Nurse, Beggar's Nurse*. Hurst & Blackett, London.

Blair VP (1920). *Surgery and Diseases of the Mouth and Jaws: A practical treatise on the surgery and diseases of the mouth and allied structures*. 3rd edn. CV Mosby Co, St Louis.

Bowerbank FT (1958). *A Doctor's Story*. Wingfield Press, Wellington.

Bowyer MJF (1990). *The Battle of Britain: 50 years on*. Patrick Stephens Ltd, Wellingborough, Northamptonshire.

Brooking TWH (1980). *A History of Dentistry in New Zealand*. NZ Dental Association. John McIndoe Ltd, Dunedin.

Brown RH (2007). *Pickerill: Pioneer in plastic surgery, dental education and dental research*. Otago University Press, Dunedin.

Bungay S (2000). *The Most Dangerous Enemy: An illustrated history of the Battle of Britain*. Aurum Press, London.

Callister S (2007). *The Face of War: New Zealand's Great War photography*. Auckland University Press, Auckland.

Capka J (1958). *Red Sky at Night: The story of Jo Capka DFM as told to Kendall McDonald*. Anthony Blond, London.

Carbery AD (1924). *The New Zealand Medical Service in the Great War 1914–1918: Based on official documents*. Whitcombe & Tombs Ltd, Auckland. Reprinted (2002) by the Naval & Military Press, Uckfield, East Sussex.

Carmalt Jones DW (1945). *Annals of the University of Otago Medical School 1875–1939*. AH & AW Reed, Wellington and Dunedin.

Cecil H & PH Liddle (1996). *Facing Armageddon: The First World War experienced*. Leo Cooper, London.

Chapin WAR (1926). *The Lost Legion: The story of the fifteen hundred American doctors who served with the BEF in the Great War*. Published privately, Springfield, Massachusetts.

Churchill WS (1930). *My Early Life: A roving commission*. Thornton Butterworth, London.

Crile GW (1947). *An Autobiography*. 2 vols. JB Lippincott Co, Philadelphia.

Cull B, Symons R (2003). *One-Armed Mac: The story of Squadron Leader James MacLachlan*. Grub Street, London.

Cushing HW (1936). *From a Surgeon's Journal 1915–1918*. Little, Brown and Co , Boston, Massachusetts.

Dennison EJ (1963). *A Cottage Hospital Grows Up: The story of the Queen Victoria Hospital East Grinstead*. Anthony Blond Ltd, London.

Deranian HM (2007). *Miracle Man of the Western Front*. Chandler House Press, Worcester, Massachusetts.

Dickson L (1950). *Richard Hillary*. Macmillan, London.

Doe RFT (1999). *Fighter Pilot: The story of one of the few*. CCB Associates, Selsdon, England.

Donovan R (2000). *As for the Canadians: The remarkable story of the RCAF's 'Guinea Pigs' of World War II*. Buschel Books, Ottawa.

Drew HTB (1923). *The War Effort in New Zealand*, vol IV (ed. HTB Brew). Whitcombe & Tombs Ltd, Auckland.

Dunn JC (1987). *The War the Infantry Knew 1914–1919*. Jane's Publishing, London.

Eastcourt Hughes J (1972). *Henry Simpson Newland: A Biography*. South Australian Fellows of the Royal Australasian College of Surgeons.

Faulks S (1996). *The Fatal Englishman: Three short lives*. Hutchinson Books, London.

Foley RT & H McCartney (2006). *The Somme: An eyewitness history*. Folio Society, London.

Formánek V (1998). *The Stories of Brave Guinea Pigs*. J&HK Publishing, Hailsham, East Sussex.

Fry WK, PR Shepherd, AC McLeod & GJ Parfitt (1942). *The Dental Treatment of Maxillo-Facial Injuries*. Blackwell Scientific Publications, Oxford.

L Galer (1981). *More Houses and Homes*. Allied Press, Dunedin.

— (1995). *Houses of Dunedin: An illustrated collection of the city's historic homes*. Hyndman, Dunedin.

Gibbons F (1918). *And They Thought We Wouldn't Fight*. George H Doran Co, New York.

Gillies HD (1920). *Plastic Surgery of the Face: Based on selected cases of war injuries of the face including burns*. Henry Frowde and Hodder & Stoughton, London.

Gillies HD & RD Millard Jr (1957). *The Principles and Art of Plastic Surgery*. 2 vols. Little, Brown & Co, Boston.

Gladstone, Viscount (1918). *William GC Gladstone: A Memoir*. Nisbet and Co Ltd, London.

Gleave TP (1941). *I Had a Row with a German*. Macmillan, London. Originally authored by 'RAF Casualty'.

Glubb JB (1978). *Into Battle: A soldier's diary of the Great War*. Book Club Associates, London.

Godden LJ (1971). *History of the Royal Army Dental Corps*. Royal Army Dental Corps, Aldershot.

Graves RR (1929). *Good-bye to All That*. Jonathan Cape, London.

Grayland E (1967). *Famous New Zealanders*. Whitcombe & Tombs Ltd, Christchurch.

Hamilton B & D Hamilton (2003). *Never a Footstep Back: A History of the Wanganui Collegiate School 1854–2003*. Whanganui College Board of Trustees, Whanganui.

Harding J (1988). *The Dancin' Navigator*. Asterisk Communications, Guelph, Ontario.

Hay I (1953). *One Hundred Years of Army Nursing*. Cassell & Co, London.

Haycock DB (2009). *A Crisis of Brilliance: Five young British artists and the Great War*. Old Street Publishing, London.

Hillary RH (1942). *The Last Enemy*. Macmillan, London. First published in America in 1942 as *Falling Through Space*. Reynal & Hitchcock, New York.

Hodgkinson C (1957). *Best Foot Forward: The autobiography of Colin Hodgkinson*. WW Norton & Co, New York.

Hofstede G (2001). *Culture's Consequences: Comparing values, behaviors, institutions and organizations across nations*, 2nd edn. Sage Publications, Thousand Oaks, California.

Holland J (2010). *The Battle of Britain: Five months that changed history May–October 1940*. Bantam Press, London.

Hone J (1939). *The Life of Henry Tonks*. William Heinemann, London.

Ives E (2000). *The First Civic University: Birmingham 1880–1980: An introductory history*. Birmingham University Press, Birmingham.

Ivy RH (1962). *A Link with the Past*. Williams & Wilkins Co, Baltimore.

Keegan J (1976). *The Face of Battle*. Jonathan Cape, London.

Keith A (1919). *Menders of the Maimed*. Henry Froude, Hodder & Stoughton, London.

Keith H (2007). *The Big Picture: A history of New Zealand art from 1642*. Godwit, Auckland.

Kennington E (1942). *Drawing the RAF: A book of portraits*. Oxford University Press, London.

Kingcome CBF (1999). *A Willingness to Die: Life & memories from Fighter Command and beyond*. Tempus Publishing Ltd, Stroud, Gloucestershire.

Koestler A (1945). *The Yogi and the Commissar and Other Essays*. Macmillan, New York.

Lawson Whale H (1919). *Injuries to the Head and Neck*. Baillière, Tindall & Cox, London; Paul Hoeber, New York.

Lax E (2004). *The Mould in Dr Florey's Coat: The remarkable true story of the penicillin miracle*. Little Brown, London.

Layton TB (1956). *Sir William Arbuthnot Lane, Bt.* E&S Livingstone Ltd, Edinburgh.

Lindsay D (1965). *The Leafy Tree: My Family*. FW Chester Pty Ltd, Melbourne, Victoria.

Linklater E (1947). *The Art of Adventure*. Macmillan, London.

Lovegrove P (1951). *Not Least in the Crusade: A short history of the Royal Army Medical Corps*. Gale & Polden, Aldershot.

Luard K (1915). *Diary of a Nursing Sister on the Western Front, 1914–1915.* William Blackwood & Sons, Edinburgh and London. Published anonymously but since attributed to Katherine Luard.

Macbean Knight WS (1914–1920). *The History of the Great European War: Its causes and effects.* vol I. Caxton Publishing, London.

Macewen W (1912). *The Growth of Bone.* James Maclehose & Sons, Glasgow.

McDonald KC (1965). *City of Dunedin: A century of civic enterprise.* Dunedin City Corporation, Dunedin.

McLeave H (1961). *McIndoe: Plastic Surgeon.* Frederick Muller Ltd, London.

McLintock AH (1949). *The History of Otago: The origins and growth of a Wakefield class settlement.* Otago Centennial Historical Publications, Dunedin.

McLintock AH (1958). *Crown Colony Government in New Zealand.* RE Owen, Government Printer, Wellington.

Martinier P & G Lemerle (1917). *Injuries of the Face and Jaw and Their Repair and the Treatment of Fractured Jaws.* Translated by H Lawson Whale. Baillière, Tindall and Cox, London.

Matthew C (1980). *The Long-Haired Boy.* Hamish Hamilton, London. Reprinted in 1991 as *A Perfect Hero.* Mandarin Paperbacks, London.

Mayhew E (2004). *The Reconstruction of Warriors: Archibald McIndoe, the Royal Air Force and the Guinea Pig Club.* Greenhill Books, London.

Meikle MC (2002). *Craniofacial Development, Growth and Evolution.* Bateson Publishing, Bressingham, Norfolk, England.

Moran, Lord (1945). *The Anatomy of Courage.* Constable, London.

— (1966). *Winston Churchill: The struggle for survival 1940–1965.* Heron Books, London.

Morrell WP (1969). *The University of Otago: A centennial history.* University of Otago Press, Dunedin.

Moseley L (1962). *Faces from the Fire: The biography of Sir Archibald McIndoe.* Quality Book Club, London.

Muir W (1917). *Observations of an Orderly: Some glimpses of life and work in an English war hospital.* Simpkin, Marshall, Hamilton, Kent & Co Ltd, London.

— (1918). *The Happy Hospital.* Simpkin, Marshall, Hamilton, Kent & Co Ltd, London.

Olssen E (1984). *A History of Otago.* John McIndoe Ltd, Dunedin.

Orde C (1942). *Pilots of Fighter Command: Sixty-four portraits.* GG Harrap & Co, London.

Page AG (1981). *Tale of a Guinea Pig.* Pelham Books, London. Grub Street. Reissued in 1999 as *Shot Down in Flames.*

Page D (2008). *Anatomy of a Medical School: A history of medicine at the University of Otago 1875–2000.* Otago University Press, Dunedin.

Pape R (1953). *Boldness Be My Friend.* Paul Elek Ltd, London.

Pearce GL (1976). *The Scots of New Zealand.* William Collins Ltd, Auckland.

Pickerill HP (1912). *The Prevention of Dental Caries and Oral Sepsis.* Baillière, Tindall & Cox, Covent Garden, London.

Pickerill HP (1912). *Stomatology in General Practice.* Oxford Medical Publications, London.

— (1924). *Facial Surgery.* E&S Livingstone, Edinburgh.

Pitcher A (1996). *The Cambridge Military Hospital Aldershot: An illustrated history.* Holmes & Sons, Andover, Hampshire.

Pound R (1964). *Gillies: Surgeon Extraordinary.* Michael Joseph, London.

Rank BK (1987). *Heads and Hands: An era of plastic surgery.* Gower Medical Publications Ltd, London.

Reed AH (1956). *The Story of Early Dunedin.* AH & AW Reed, Wellington.

Richards F (1933). *Old Soldiers Never Die.* Faber & Faber Ltd, London.

Richey PHM (1941). *Fighter Pilot: A personal record of the campaign in France September 8th 1939 to June 13th 1940.* BT Batsford Ltd, London. Originally authored by 'Anon'.

Ross D (2000). *Richard Hillary: The definitive biography of a Battle of Britain fighter pilot and author of* The Last Enemy. Grub Street, London.

Rothenstein W (1942). *Men of the RAF.* Oxford University Press, London.

Rowe NL & HC Killey (1955). *Fractures of the facial skeleton.* E&S Livingstone Ltd, Edinburgh and London.

Sassoon S (1930). *Memoirs of an Infantry Officer.* Faber & Faber Ltd, London.

Scott AJL (1920). *Sixty Squadron RAF: A history of the squadron from its formation.* William Heinemann, London. George H Doran Co, New York.

Shirer WL (1959). *The Rise and Fall of the Third Reich: A history of Nazi Germany*. Simon & Schuster, New York.

Simpson W (1943). *One of Our Pilots Is Safe*. Hamish Hamilton, London.

— (1944). *The Way of Recovery*. Hamish Hamilton, London.

— (1955). *I Burned My Fingers*. Putnam, London.

Siska A (2008). *Flying for Freedom: The flying, survival and captivity experiences of a Czech pilot in the Second World War*. Pen and Sword Books, Barnsley, Yorkshire.

Smith C (2009). *England's Last War Against France: Fighting Vichy, 1940–1942*. Weidenfeld & Nicolson, London.

Stack JW (1936). *More Maoriland Adventures*. (ed. AH Reed), AH & AW Reed, Dunedin.

Staige Davis J (1919). *Plastic Surgery: Its principles and practice*. P Blakiston's Son & Co, Philadelphia.

Tagliocozzi G (1597). *De Curtorum Chirurgia per Insitionem*. Gasparum Bindorum, Venice.

Thompson GE (1919). *A History of the University of Otago (1869–1919)*. J Wilkie & Co, Dunedin.

Trembath KA (1969). *Ad Augusta: A centennial history of Auckland Grammar School 1869–1969*. Wilson and Horton Ltd, Auckland, for the Auckland Grammar School Old Boys' Association.

Ward VH, Newell MJ (1997). *Ex Dentibus Ensis: A history of the Army Dental Service*. RADC Historical Museum, Aldershot.

Warwick James W, Fickling BW (1940). *Injuries of the Jaws and Face: With special reference to war casualties*. John Bale & Staples Ltd, London.

Williams P, Harrison T (1979). *McIndoe's Army: The injured airmen who faced the world*. Pelham Books, Bedford Square, London.

Wilson JM (1998). *Siegfried Sassoon: The making of a war poet: A biography (1886–1918)*. Gerald Duckworth & Co Ltd, London.

INDEX

Page numbers in **bold** refer to illustrations.